# High Dose Rate Brachytherapy:
# A Textbook

**Edited by**

**Subir Nag, M.D.**
*Chief of Brachytherapy*
*Arthur G. James Cancer Hospital and*
*Research Institute*
*Ohio State University*
*Columbus, Ohio*

**Library of Congress Cataloging-in-Publication Data**

High dose rate brachytherapy : a textbook / edited by Subir Nag.
     p.    cm.
     Includes bibliographical references and index.
     ISBN 0-87993-588-X
     1. Radioisotope brachytherapy.   2. Cancer—Radiotherapy.   I. Nag.
Subir.
     [DNLM:   1. Neoplasms—radiotherapy.   2. Brachytherapy—methods.
3. Radiotherapy Dosage.   QZ 269 H6375 1994]
RC271.R27H53   1994
616.99′406424—dc20
DNLM/DLC
for Library of Congress                                      94-5083
                                                         CIP

Copyright 1994
Futura Publishing Company, Inc.

*Published by*
Futura Publishing Company, Inc.
135 Bedford Road
Armonk, New York 10504

LC#:94-5083
ISBN #: 0-87993-588-X

Printed in the United States of America.

This book is printed on acid-free paper.

nwst
IAFF7844

# Contributors

**André Abitbol, M.D.**
*Department of Radiation Oncology, Baptist Hospital of Miami, Miami, Florida*

**Lowell L. Anderson, Ph.D.**
*Department of Medical Physics, Memorial Sloan-Kettering Cancer Center, New York, New York*

**David J. Brenner, Ph.D.**
*Center for Radiologic Research, Columbia University, New York, New York*

**Debra M. Brown, R.N., B.S.N., O.C.N.**
*Department of Radiation Oncology, William Beaumont Hospital, Royal Oak, Michigan*

**Daniel H. Clarke, M.D.**
*Director of Brachytherapy, Northern Virginia Cancer Center, Alexandria, Virginia*

**Roger G. Dale, Ph.D.**
*Department of Medical Physics, Charing Cross Hospital, Furham Palace Road, London, England*

**Larry DeWerd, Ph.D.**
*Director of Radiation Calibration Laboratory, University of Wisconsin, Madison, Wisconsin*

**David Donath, M.D.**
*Division of Radiation Oncology, McGill University, Montreal, Canada*

**Anatoly Dritschilo, M.D.**
*Department of Radiation Medicine, Georgetown University Medical Center, Washington, D.C.*

**Gregory Edmunson, R.T.**
*Department of Radiation Oncology, William Beaumont Hospital, Royal Oak, Michigan*

**Gary Ezzell, M.S.**
*Gershenson Radiation Oncology Center, Harper Hospital, Detroit, Michigan*

**Albino Flores, M.D.**
*Clinical Professor, Department of Surgery, University of British Columbia, and Department of Radiation Oncology, British Columbia Cancer Agency, Vancouver, British Columbia, Canada*

**James Fontanesi, M.D.**
*Radiation Oncology Department, Harper Hospital, Detroit, Michigan*

**John F. Fowler, Ph.D.**
*Division of Radiation Oncology, University of Wisconsin, Madison, Wisconsin*

**Delia Garcia, M.D.**
*Director of Radiation Oncology, Missouri Baptist Medical Center, St. Louis, Missouri*

**Glenn Glasgow, Ph.D.**
*Professor, Division of Medical Physics, Loyola Hines Department of Radiotherapy, Stritch School of Medicine, Maywood, Illinois*

**Cherylann Gregory, R.N., B.S.N., O.C.N.**
*Nurse Manager, Department of Radiation Oncology, William Beaumont Hospital, Royal Oak, Michigan*

**Louis Harrison, M.D.**
*Chief of Brachytherapy Service, Department of Radiation Oncology, Memorial Sloan-Kettering Cancer Center, New York, New York*

**Basil S. Hilaris, M.D., F.A.C.R.**
*Chairman, Department of Radiation Medicine, New York Medical College, Valhalla, New York*

**Pavel Houdek, Ph.D.**
*Department of Radiation Oncology, University of Miami School of Medicine, Sylvester Comprehensive Cancer Center, Miami, Florida*

**H. Jacobs, M.D.**
*Saarbrucker Winterbergkliniken, Klinik für Strahlentherapic und Radioonkologic, Saarbrucken, Germany*

**Janet Jancs, R.N.**
*Nursing Supervisor, Department of Radiation Oncology, New York Hospital Medical Center of Queens, Flushing, New York*

**Inger-Karine K. Kolkman-Deurloo, M.Sc.**
*Departments of Clinical Physics and Radiation Oncology, Dr. Daniel den Hoed Cancer Center, Rotterdam, The Netherlands*

**György Kovács, M.D.**
*Professor and Deputy Chairman, Clinic for Radiation Therapy, Christian Albrechts University of Kiel, Kiel, Germany*

**Robert R. Kuske, M.D.**
*Department of Radiation Oncology, Ochsner Clinic, New Orleans, Louisiana*

**Peter C. Levendag, M.D., Ph.D.**
*Professor and Chairman, Department of Radiation Oncology, Dr. Daniel den Hoed Cancer Center, Rotterdam, The Netherlands*

**Alan A. Lewin, M.D.**
*Department of Radiation Oncology, Baptist Hospital of Miami, Miami, Florida*

**Peter Lukas, M.D.**
*Professor and Chairman, Clinic for Radiotherapy, University of Innsbruck, Innsbruck, Austria*

**Hans N. Macha, M.D.**
*Lungenklinik Hemer, Hemer, Germany*

**Alvaro A. Martinez, M.D., F.A.C.R.**
*Chairman, Department of Radiation Onclogy, William Beaumont Hospital, Royal Oak, Michigan*

**Timothy P. Mate, M.D.**
*Radiation Oncologist, Swedish Hospital Medical Center, Seattle, Washington*

**Minesh P. Mehta, M.D.**
*Assistant Professor of Human Oncology, University of Wisconsin Hospitals, Madison, Wisconsin*

**Fritz Mundinger, M.D.**
*Department of Neurosurgery, St. Joseph Krakenhaus, Freiberg, Germany*

**Subir Nag, M.D.**
*Chief of Brachytherapy, Division of Radiation Oncology, Arthur G. James Cancer Hospital, Ohio State University, Columbus, Ohio*

**Dattatreyudu Nori, M.D., F.A.C.R.**
*Chairman, Department of Radiation Oncology, New York Hospital Medical Center of Queens, Flushing, New York*

**Arthur Olch, Ph.D.**
*Department of Radiation Oncology, Kaiser Permanente Medical Center, Los Angeles, California*

**Colin Orton, Ph.D.**
*Director of Medical Physics, Gershenson Radiation Oncology Center, Harper Hospital, Detroit, Michigan*

**Lincoln Pao, M.D.**
*Department of Radiation Oncology, New York Hospital Medical Center of Queens, Flushing, New York*

**Theodore Phillips, M.D.**
*Professor and Chairman, Department of Radiation Oncology, University of California, San Francisco, California*

**Arthur T. Porter, M.D.**
*Professor and Chairman, Wayne State University School of Medicine, Detroit, Michigan*

**David Rogers, M.D.**
*Department of Radiation Oncology, New York Hospital Medical Center of Queens, Flushing, New York*

**Chris G. Rowland, M.D.**
*Department of Radiotherapy, Royal Devon and Exeter Hospital, Exeter, England*

**Frederick B. Ruymann, M.D.**
*Section Chief, Division of Hematology and Oncology, Children's Hospital, Columbus, Ohio*

**James G. Schwade, M.D.**
*Professor and Chairman, Department of Radiation Oncology, Sylvester Comprehensive Cancer Center, University of Miami School of Medicine, Miami, Florida*

**Burton L. Speiser, M.D.**
*Chairman, Department of Radiation Oncology, St. Joseph's Hospital, Phoenix, Arizona*

**Judith A. Stitt, M.D.**
*Clinical Director and Associate Professor, Department of Human Oncology, University of Wisconsin, Madison, Wisconsin*

**Bruce R. Thomadsen, Ph.D.**
*Departments of Human Oncology and Medical Physics, University of Wisconsin, Madison, Wisconsin*

**David S. Thomas, M.D.**
*Director, Scranton Regional Cancer Center, Clarks Summit, Pennsylvania*

**Rob van der Laarse, Ph.D.**
*Nucletron Research, B.V., Veenendaal, The Netherlands*

**Bhadrassain Vikram, M.D.**
*Chairman and Professor, Department of Radiation Oncology, Albert Einstein College of Medicine, Bronx, New York*

**Frank Vicini, M.D.**
*Education Director, Department of Radiation Oncology, William Beaumont Hospital, Royal Oak, Michigan*

**A.G. Visser**
*Departments of Clinical Physics and Radiation Oncology, Dr. Daniel den Hoed Cancer Center, Rotterdam, The Netherlands*

**Jeffrey Williamson, Ph.D.**
*Mallinckrodt Institute of Radiology, Washington University School of Medicine, St. Louis, Missouri*

**Wei-bo Yin, M.D.**
*Professor, Radiation Oncology, Cancer Hospital, Chinese Academy of Medical Sciences, Beijing, People's Republic of China*

**Lucia Zamorano, M.D.**
*Department of Neurosurgery, Wayne State University, Detroit, Michigan*

# Foreword

Brachytherapy, also known as curietherapy or endocurietherapy, was one of the first uses of radiation therapy shortly after the discovery of radium. Until the 1930s, the low energy of external beam devices limited much successful radiotherapy to the use of radium.

Techniques were developed to insert sources into almost any part of the body—either externally or during surgery—and remove them through the use of retraction sutures. As the equipment for delivering x-rays of energies higher than 130 to 200 kilovolts emerged in the late 1930s, and in particular in the 1950s and 1960s, the use of brachytherapy declined. It became evident, however, that local control rates in many sites were not as high as desirable, and that higher local control rates would certainly impact on survival.

On the basis of these findings, a rebirth of the use of brachytherapy evolved. This was due to many factors, including the availability of new isotopes, better instrumentation for source introduction and retention, and computerized treatment planning and dose calculations.

Finally, the introduction of afterloading in the late 1960s and the introduction of remote afterloading in the early 1980s has made brachytherapy safer and much more available and effective than in the past. It is an extremely important part of the armamentarium of the radiation oncologist.

Delivery of radiation over a short time period, that is, less than 1 week, has major advantages in that it does not allow significant tumor-cell proliferation, which could occur with protraction of treatment over 5 to 7 weeks as is common with external-beam irradiation. It has been calculated that at least 60 centigray or more per day increased dose is required for each day of prolongation of the overall treatment. Most high dose rate (HDR) brachytherapy schedules significantly shorten the overall time of treatment.

The use of interstitial or intracavity techniques in brachytherapy places the highest concentration of the radiation source directly within the tumor. Because of the inverse square law, the dose of radiation drops rapidly as an inverse function of the square of the distance from the source. Thus, with proper geometric placement of the sources, the tumor will receive far higher doses than the surrounding normal tissues. These advantages can be further augmented by varying the strength of the sources or by varying the dwell time of remote afterloading sources in order to shape the dose distribution to fit the geometric borders of the tumor.

A major reason for the progress of brachytherapy and its future potentials is the development of new sources. Prior to the onset of the atomic age, the only available sources were radium and its daughter products, particularly radon. The former has an extremely long half-life and is very expensive and quite bulky when encapsulated for safety. The latter, radon, has very high energy and a very short half-life, leading to very high dose rates over short periods that are not biologically advantageous and posing very serious hazards for medical personnel.

The isotopes that are produced in a reactor or, in some cases, through cyclotron neutron bombardment, have characteristics far superior to that of radium. First, most of the isotopes do not emit a gas, that is, radon, which was a major hazard because of leakage from radium sources or needles. Second, most of these isotopes selected have the desired energy of the gamma or nuclear x-rays and a half-life that is compatible with repeat reutilization or permanent implantation.

A very wide range of isotopes has been studied and utilized in the clinic, but a limited number have found permanent use, particularly for remote afterloading. Only $^{60}$Co, $^{192}$Ir and $^{137}$Cs are of high enough specific activity and have long enough half-lives to be used in remote afterloading.

Over the past 25 years, the available instrumentation for brachytherapy has improved markedly. Initially, sources were available only as needles or tubes that had to be inserted directly into the tissues. The first major advance was the development of a technique by Ulrich Henschke in which plastic catheters were drawn behind stainless steel needles through the tissue. These catheters could then be afterloaded with iridium wires or seeds or with a remote afterloaded iridium source. The combination of guide needles, flexible catheters, and buttons was developed at Oxford University in England by Frank Ellis and at Memorial-Sloan Kettering Cancer Center in New York by Henschke. This technique made it possible to do large implants either intraoperatively or percutaneously with much greater ease and with much less radiation exposure to the oncologist than was previously the case for radium sources.

Gynecologic insertions, which have been one of the major uses of brachytherapy throughout its history, were performed with hot-loaded applicators in which the radium tubes were inserted. There were three primary techniques—the Stockholm technique, the Paris technique, and the Manchester technique. Each involved the use of a uterine tube or tandem and a method of applying sources to the surface of the cervix. In the Manchester system, it was in the form of two ovoids shaped to mimic the confirmation of the isodose curves from a radium tube. In the Paris technique, it was a pair of wine-cork-shaped devices separated with a spring, and in the Stockholm technique, it was in a box-shaped device sized for the cervix. All of these techniques required insertion of the loaded radium in the operating room by the surgeon and high exposures to personnel.

The pioneering work of Henschke, followed by the work of many others in Europe and the United States, led to an evolution of afterloaded applicators for gynecologic treatment. All of these applicators were designed to replace the intrauterine tandem and culpostats. They were devices that protruded through the vaginal pack and could be loaded with radioactive sources after the patient reached the hospital room. They provided the stage on which HDR brachytherapy evolved.

Other important instruments for brachytherapy include multiple catheter designs that can be inserted into the bronchi, the esophagus, the biliary ducts, the nasopharynx, and other sites to deliver high doses to limited volumes. More recently, remote afterloading molds have seen extensive intraoperative use. Essentially, any part of the body can be treated by using either percutaneous or intraoperative techniques.

Templates are a newer innovation that allow the insertion of multiple needles in a parallel fashion to cover a volume of tumor. They have been particularly useful in the pelvis because of the availability of perineal insertion. Such templates are highly effective in the treatment of advanced carcinoma of the cervix and of carcinoma of the prostrate, rectum, and anus.

Over the past 10 years, there has been a major increase in the interest in brachytherapy, based primarily on the development of automated remote afterloading devices. These devices allow the insertion of the radioactive sources from a storage safe that is remote from but attached to the patient by various tube arrangements. There are a number of advantages to remote afterloading: (1) There is no radiation exposure to patient-care personnel or visitors; (2) Radiation source selection and positioning is highly variable and, in some cases, infinitely variable; (3) Radiation sources are confined to the closed environment of the safe and delivery tubes. Source losses are eliminated, and the delivery of much more optimized dose distributions is possible.

Remote afterloading devices are classified into four types. They include low dose rate (LDR) between 40 and 100 centigray per hour at the assigned tumor dose point. Intermediate dose rates can deliver anything between 100 centigray per hour to as high as 400 or 600 centigray per hour. High dose rate remote afterloaders generally deliver 100 centigray per minute and allow treatments within minutes rather than hours. In an interesting application, an HDR machine has been designed to pulse for 10 to 15 minutes each hour and mimic LDR with a 1 Ci $^{192}$Ir source. It is known as pulsed dose rate (PDR).

Iridium afterloaders are available in two forms. The HDR iridium afterloading system, which is offered by at least two companies in the United States, is widely sold. It employs a small-size iridium source, generally 1 cm or less in length, which will fit in the standard catheters and other applicators of almost any type. This source of 10 Ci can be used for all applications in the HDR mode. The other form is the PDR machine.

High dose rate brachytherapy has proven to be as effective as LDR brachytherapy in the treatment of carcinoma of the cervix. Its usefulness with interstitial techniques as compared to LDR is as yet unproven since the optimum dose per treatment and total dose have not yet been determined. High dose rate brachytherapy, obviously, has an advantage in endobronchial and esophageal applications because of the markedly reduced application time required. So far the data suggest that in these two sites HDR is as effective and, with the clinically used doses to date, induces similar complications.

There are certain biological advantages of LDR that may be lost with HDR unless the physical distribution is superior. In spite of this unproven assumption, HDR brachytherapy has seen an explosion in sites of application and in equipment installed. There are a number of reasons that this has occurred. Radiation safety has become an increasing problem, and regulators annually con strict what can be done with direct-loaded sources. Source accountability and source loss are continuing problems. Without remote afterloading, it is hard to justify the radiation exposure that occurs to nursing personnel and to the radiation oncology personnel loading the applicators. Afterloaded LDR and PDR solve these problems but still require lengthy hospitalization, with patients often bedridden. This leads to increased hospital costs, patient inconvenience, and a definite incidence of serious pulmonary embolism.

High dose rate brachytherapy solves these problems since it is an outpatient procedure for many sites. In others the implant catheters can be placed in an operating room, and the patient is treated daily after discharge. It remains to be seen if HDR will completely replace all other forms of brachytherapy. If clinically equivalent fractionation schemes that equal LDR in tumor control and complications can be found, HDR may well do so.

Unfortunately, the number of persons trained in and practicing brachytherapy has been shrinking so that many radiation oncologists are unwilling to undertake any brachytherapy, or at least anything beyond simple gynecologic intracavity placements. The specialty needs to address this problem through the establishment of fellowships that provide positions for an additional year of training in brachytherapy, with significant experience in HDR brachytherapy.

Against this background this is a very important book. It provides the necessary physics and biology background to apply HDR. Safety and quality assurance issues are well covered, as are specific techniques. Individual chapters cover all of the sites in which there is HDR experience. Indeed, these include essentially all of the sites now treated by brachytherapy, except the eye. Special topics include the nursing care of these patients and the rapidly developing intraoperative techniques. The authors are experienced with techniques for the sites about which they write. They tell you "how to do it" with practical examples. Anyone starting an HDR service or expanding to new sites will find this book an excellent source.

**Theodore L. Phillips, M.D.**

*Professor and Chair*
*Department of Radiation Oncology*
*University of California*
*San Francisco, California*

# Preface

Radiation therapy has a long history as a treatment for most forms of cancer, and the continuing struggle to control this disease gives constant impetus to efforts to refine the various available treatment modalities. Growing experience with high dose rate (HDR) brachytherapy has demonstrated that it can provide advantages in radiation protection, length of treatment time, and treatment optimization on an out-patient basis. As result of these advantages, use of this methodology has also grown. Presently, many different HDR techniques are being employed in centers around the world, and consensus is lacking regarding indications and approach. Although this diverse clinical experience is sometimes reported at some brachytherapy meetings, there is no common source of information about this treatment modality. This text has been written to try to meet the need for a comprehensive textbook on HDR brachytherapy in the hope that drawing together a detailed review from a number of centers and numerous practitioners might contribute to a more general understanding of the utility of HDR brachytherapy and help in the development of guidelines for its safe and efficacious use.

*HDR Brachytherapy: A Textbook* is intended to serve as a reference text for radiation oncologists and residents, physicists, dosimetrists, technologists, and other physicians interested in this form of radiation therapy. The text includes sections on the basic physics and radiobiology of HDR brachytherapy, clinical methods and experience (organized to include the full range of body sites), and investigational applications and potential future uses of this methodology. Our purpose has been to provide a comprehensive and detailed overview of HDR brachytherapy that would be of practical benefit to a broad range of clinicians, medical technologists, and scientists. Each chapter has been multiauthored to give a broad view of the approaches to and use of this methodology, and each chapter also includes a detailed description of the specific methodology, with the intention of providing the reader a step-by-step explanation of the procedure used. The coauthors have both contributed their specific expertise and critically reviewed the entire chapter that includes their contribution. We hope that this approach has produced a comprehensive, detailed, and balanced discussion of the subject.

With any technology, time and use lead to changes and refinements. We expect that the same will be true of HDR brachytherapy; those inevitable changes are certain to make necessary new descriptions of the advances achieved with the methodology outlined in this text. Thus, we hope that this book will be only the beginning of attempts to provide a specific, broad-based understanding of HDR brachytherapy and that this understanding will enable us to use this exciting modality more effectively.

Subir Nag, M.D.

# Acknowledgments

I would like to thank the many authors who contributed chapters to this text. No one knows better than they what a daunting task it is to draw together and correlate the contributions of multiple authors. Their hard work and continued cooperation throughout the process of assembling this text are greatly appreciated. I also want to thank my colleagues at The Ohio State University Medical Center, Drs. Reinhard Gahbauer and Demetrious Spigos, for their encouragement and support for this project. Thanks are also due to the staff at Futura Publishing Co., Steven Korn, Louise Farkas, and Helen Powers, whose understanding, patience, and ability to adapt to last-minute changes and missed deadlines made timely publication possible. In the same light, thanks are due to David Carpenter for his assistance in editing this text and coordinating the details of publication at Ohio State. Finally, I want to thank my wife, Sima, and daughters, Sunita and Sumona, for their understanding during this process that required many long hours away from them.

S.N.

# Contents

Contributors                                                        iii
Foreword                                                            vii
Preface                                                             xi

**Part I.   Introduction, Physics, and Radiobiology**

Chapter 1: Evolution and General Principles of High Dose Rate
           Brachytherapy
           *Basil S. Hilaris*                                       3

Chapter 2: Radiobiology
           *Colin G. Orton, David J. Brenner, Roger G. Dale, and*
           *John F. Fowler*                                         11

Chapter 3: Design and Implementation of a Program for High Dose
           Rate Brachytherapy
           *Pavel V. Houdek, Glenn P. Glasgow, James G. Schwade, and*
           *André A. Abitbol*                                       27

Chapter 4: High Dose Rate Remote Afterloading Equipment
           *Glenn P. Glasgow and Lowell L. Anderson*               41

Chapter 5: Calibration Principles and Techniques
           *Larry A. DeWerd, Gary A. Ezzell, and Jeffrey F. Williamson*   59

Chapter 6: Treatment Planning and Optimization
           *Bruce R. Thomadsen, Pavel V. Houdek, Rob van der Laarse,*
           *Gregory Edmunson, Inger-Karine K. Kolkman-Deurloo,*
           *and A.G. Visser*                                        79

Chapter 7: Quality Assurance for High Dose Rate Brachytherapy
           *Jeffrey F. Williamson, Gary A. Ezzell, Arthur Olch, and*
           *Bruce R. Thomadsen*                                     147

**Part II:   Clinical Body Sites**

Chapter 8: High Dose Rate Brachytherapy in the Treatment of Malig-
           nant Gliomas
           *Delia M. Garcia, Lucia Zamorano, and Fritz Mundinger*   215

Chapter 9: High Dose Rate Brachytherapy for Cancer of the Head and Neck
*Peter C. Levendag, Bhadrassain Vikram, Albino D. Flores, and and Wei-bo Yin*          237

Chapter 10: High Dose Rate Brachytherapy for Carcinoma of the Esophagus
*Albino D. Flores, Chris G. Rowland, and Wei-bo Yin*          275

Chapter 11: High Dose Rate Brachytherapy for Lung Cancer
*Minesh P. Mehta, Burton L. Speiser, and Hans N. Macha*          295

Chapter 12: High Dose Rate Brachytherapy for Breast Cancer
*Daniel H. Clarke, Frank Vicini, H. Jacobs, Chris G. Rowland, and Robert R. Kuske*          321

Chapter 13: Remote Afterloading High Dose Rate Brachytherapy for Carcinoma of the Bile Duct
*Dattatreyudu Nori, Subir Nag, David Rogers, and Bhadrassain Vikram*          331

Chapter 14: Interstitial High Dose Rate Irradiation for Hepatic Tumors
*David S. Thomas and Anatoly Dritschilo*          339

Chapter 15: The Role of High Dose Rate Brachytherapy in Rectal Cancer
*Dattatreyudu Nori and Lincoln Pao*          347

Chapter 16: High Dose Rate Brachytherapy of the Prostate
*Timothy P. Mate, György Kovács, and Alvaro A. Martinez*          355

Chapter 17: High Dose Rate Brachytherapy for Carcinoma of the Cervix
*André A. Abitbol, Judith A. Stitt, James G. Schwade, and Alan A. Lewin*          373

Chapter 18: The Role of High Dose Rate Brachytherapy in Carcinoma of the Endometrium
*Dattatreyudu Nori, Judith A. Stitt, and Lincoln Pao*          385

Chapter 19: The Role of High Dose Rate Brachytherapy in the Management of Adult Soft Tissue Sarcomas
*Subir Nag, Arthur T. Porter, and David Donath*          393

Chapter 20: High Dose Rate Remote Brachytherapy in the Treatment of Pediatric Tumors
*Subir Nag, Frederick B. Ruymann, and James Fontanesi*          399

**Part III:    Special Topics**

Chapter 21: High Dose Rate Brachytherapy Nursing
*Debra M. Brown, Janet Janes, and Cherylann Gregory*          411

Chapter 22: Intraoperative High Dose Rate Remote Brachytherapy
*Subir Nag, Peter Lukas, David S. Thomas, and
Louis Harrison*                                                427

Chapter 23: The Future of High Dose Rate Brachytherapy
*Subir Nag, Alvaro A. Martinez, Arthur T. Porter, and
Basil S. Hilaris*                                              447

Index                                                          455

# Part I

# Introduction, Physics, and Radiobiology

# Chapter 1

# Evolution and General Principles of High Dose Rate Brachytherapy

*Basil S. Hilaris*

## Introduction

In the early 1950s, professional concern regarding the harmful effects of radiation caused a serious decline in the use of brachytherapy. Although the techniques using radium and radon were well established for almost 50 years and the clinical results were excellent, their application was complicated and time consuming. It involved a radiation hazard to hospital personnel and necessitated general anesthesia during the insertion of the preloaded applicators and/or sources, followed by a hospital stay in an isolation room.

The development of afterloading of radioactive sources and the introduction of artificial radionuclides received considerable attention in the literature and contributed to a renaissance of brachytherapy. The principal advantage of manual afterloading of radioactive sources was improvement of the treatment procedure, which could be done with more care and deliberation and with a significant reduction of radiation exposure to staff. The principle of afterloading was very simple: unloaded tubes or applicators were inserted in the tumor, and these were subsequently loaded (thus the term "afterloading") with radioactive sources.[1-3]

Initially, afterloading was used either operatively or postoperatively. In operative afterloading, the radioactive sources were inserted in the operating room after unloaded needles had been placed inside the tumor. This technique, used mainly for permanent implantation, reduced exposure in the operating room but did not eliminate radiation exposure in other hospital areas. In postoperative afterloading, the insertion of radioactive sources was done in the patient's hospital room hours or days after the implantation of empty needles or tubes. This technique, adopted for temporary implantation and intracavitary applications, eliminated all radiation exposure in the operating room, recovery room, radiology department, and hallways and elevators of the hospital[4,5]; however, the problem of radiation exposure to the nursing and resident staff and anyone else who entered the patient's room still remained.

From: Nag, S. (ed.): *High Dose Rate Brachytherapy: A Textbook*, Futura Publishing Company, Inc., Armonk, NY, © 1994.

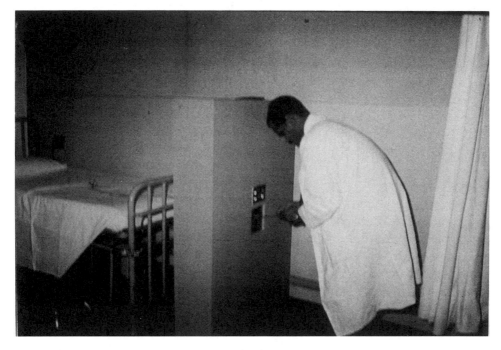

**Fig. 1.** Manual remote after loading of iridium-192.

## Development of Remote Afterloading

Remote afterloading of radioactive sources was a logical extension of the manual afterloading concept for the purpose of completely eliminating staff radiation exposure. Figure 1 shows the early attempts by our group at Memorial Hospital in New York to handle radioactive iridium-192 sources by manual remote afterloading. Specially designed iridium sources of up to 50 mg radium equivalent were placed in a container located inside a lead screen at the foot of the patient's bed. The sources were moved manually to and from the applicator in the patient through plastic tubes. The operator stood behind the lead screen during the loading and/or the removal of sources. With this apparatus, the duration of the treatment lasted a few hours instead of the conventional 2 to 3 days.

## High Dose Rate Remote Afterloading

High dose rate (HDR) remote afterloading was favored by the Memorial Hospital group from the beginning, starting in 1961. Small cobalt sources of high activity moving back and forth to simulate sources of different longer active lengths were used. It was concluded in the first paper on this subject that ". . . on the basis of our limited experience with such short treatment times in the last three years, we feel that they may be used with impunity if the total

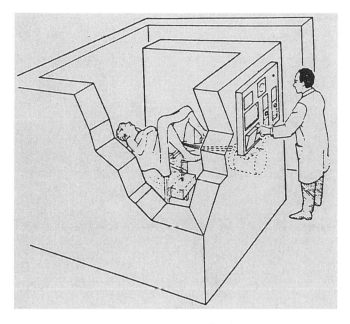

**Fig. 2.** HDR remote afterloader.

dose is divided into more fractions."[6] In a subsequent paper, it was stated that ". . . moving source remote afterloaders can be used with all gamma emitting radioisotopes, but cesium-137 appears most suitable, except in the case of short treatment times, for which cobalt-60 and iridium-192 are preferable because of their higher specific activity, which, in turn, permits smaller sources and applicators."[7,8]

Figure 2 shows the final version of the HDR remote afterloader installed at Memorial Hospital in 1964.[9] The remotely controlled afterloading device was designed for use principally with cobalt-60 high activity sources and thus constituted a radical departure from traditional brachytherapy methods. No one was exposed to radiation because the radioactive sources were kept in an appropriately designed lead container in a heavily shielded room and were handled from an outside control. Remote afterloading was clearly the best procedure for interstitial and intracavitary brachytherapy in terms of radiation protection.

The HDR remote afterloader developed in 1964 was later commercially marketed by the Atomic Energy of Canada, Ltd., Medical under the name of Brachytron and was installed in several medical centers, including the University of California in San Diego, the University of Southern California in Los Angeles, and the Cancer Institute in Beijing.

The first model at Memorial Hospital in New York was later described as follows: "A nuclear age hot room at New York City's Memorial Hospital is proving valuable in irradiation treatment of tumors in the vagina, nasopharynx and mouth. It is also being used to treat cancers of the cervix and endometrium (the

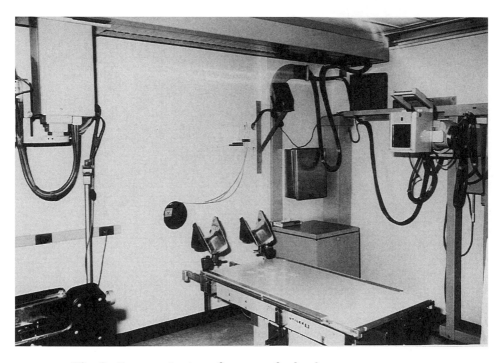

**Fig. 3.** Panoramic view of remote afterloader treatment room.

membrane lining of the uterus). The hot room removes these difficulties (i.e., conventional radium applications are complicated and time consuming, require patient isolation for 2 to 3 days, and involve a radiation hazard to hospital personnel) cuts treatment time from days to minutes, and makes it possible to bombard the tumors with much higher doses of radiation in less time than conventional treatment takes. It consists of a treatment room surrounded by a thick wall (Fig. 3) with a control room on the other side of the wall (Fig. 4). Communication between the treatment room and the control room is by closed circuit TV and a speaker system. A lead safe in the wall holds the radiation sources, tiny stainless steel rods containing radioactive cobalt. The rods are welded to the ends of long cables threaded into flexible plastic tubes, which extend out of the safe into the treatment room. In actual procedure, to irradiate the vagina, for example, a hollow aluminum applicator is inserted into the vagina and three plastic tubes are connected to it. The medical personnel leave the room. From the control room the three sources of radioactive cobalt are advanced electrically out of the safe, through the plastic tubes, and into the applicator. A sensor inserted in the anus of the patient continuously monitors the treatment to avoid over-irradiation and damage to healthy tissue."[10] This HDR remote afterloader remained in use at Memorial Hospital from its installation in 1964 until 1979 when it was replaced by a commercial device (GammaMed; Isotopen-Technik, Germany). The early results of treatment were reported in 1974.[11]

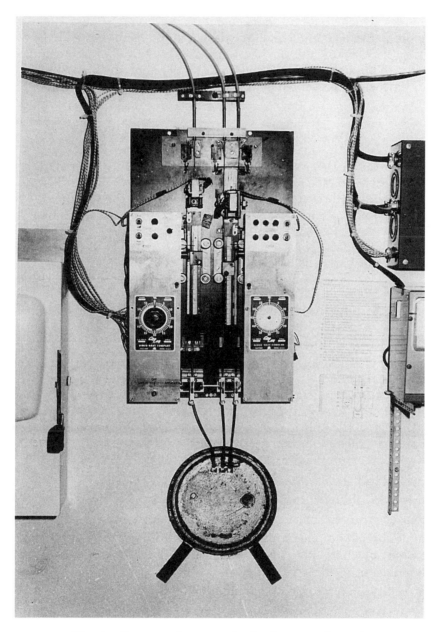

**Fig. 4.** Close-up of remote afterloader control panel.

In England, the TEM Company produced the Cathetron; and in Japan, the Ralston was produced commercially. Both remote afterloaders used high-activity cobalt-60 sources. Reports on the Cathetron were initially published by O'Connell et al.[12] Clinical experience with the Ralston was reported by Wakabayashi.[13] The Cathetron and the Ralston used multiple sources of different strengths, which could be connected to three driving shafts. The use of so many sources greatly complicated the design and increased the chance of human error. In Germany, the Buchler Company produced a remote afterloader that used a high-activity oscillating iridium-192 source. Clinical experience with this device was presented by Rotte.[14]

## Low Dose Rate Remote Afterloading

Low dose rate (LDR) remote afterloaders were initially favored in Sweden, France, and Switzerland. The pioneer work of Walstam[15] in this field resulted in two commercially produced units, the Cervitron and the Curietron (CIS Bio International, Cedex, France). With these devices, the usual treatment time of up to 7 days with the Paris technique were used. The sources were retracted before anyone entered the patient's room. Clinical experience with the Curietron was reported by Chassagne et al.[16]

## Advantages and Disadvantages of High Dose Rate Remote Afterloading

High dose rate afterloading techniques have been in clinical use in Europe, Japan, and the United States for almost three decades. Nevertheless, the clinical experience is limited. Furthermore, continuous quality improvement to monitor radiation exposure and to affirm correct machine operation and proper delivery of the prescribed dose is still lacking. Remote afterloading devices represent a technological advance that offers several important advantages over manual afterloading techniques, including

- improved radiation protection to the staff
- reduced possibility of human error
- increased ease of achieving optimized dose distribution
- elimination of complications associated with prolonged bed confinement, especially in elderly patients
- marked decrease in patient discomfort
- administration of the treatment on an outpatient basis
- avoidance of general anesthesia in selected patients
- and finally, facilitation of scheduling procedures because the radiotherapist and medical physicist do not have to leave the department for long periods of time.

The cost effectiveness of HDR techniques compared with LDR techniques is highly controversial. Although hospitalization is not required, HDR devices tend to be more expensive than the LDR equivalent, and the cost of building a dedicated, heavily shielded room can be considerable.

## Radiobiological Controversies

The convenience of short treatment time for HDR remote afterloading is significantly offset by the need for increased fractionation. In order to achieve clinical results comparable to those with LDR afterloading, most HDR brachytherapy has used doses per fraction in the range of 4 to 9 Gy, with time intervals of about 1 to 2 weeks between fractions. The linear quadratic model has turned out to be a very useful and dependable method of handling both fraction size and overall time.

Traditional LDR of 0.5 to 0.6 Gy per hour caused the same relative biological effects on early and late reacting tissues as conventional external beams of 2 Gy per fraction. The relative effectiveness per Gy was 1.2 for early normal tissue and tumor effects and 1.7 for late normal tissue effects. These relative effectiveness values are greater with higher dose rates, especially with HDR remote afterloading. However, although the relative effectiveness for tumor and early effects rises by 33% to 50% for dose fractions of 6 to 8 Gy, the relative effectiveness for late complications rises by approximately 100%. In HDR remote afterloading, there is a critical radiobiological potential for overdosing with respect to late complications or underdosing with respect to tumor sterilization by significant ratios of 20% to 30% if the usual five large HDR fractions are used. The discrepancy is smaller if larger numbers of smaller fractions are used.

## Physical Dose Distribution

The physical dose distribution is more favorable with HDR insertions of a few minutes than with conventional LDR given over several days, especially in intracavitary applications. Thus, the packing of the rectum and bladder away from the sources is easier to maintain with HDR remote afterloading, and this advantage may offset the radiobiological loss of therapeutic ratio when a few large fractions are used. In addition, because of the short treatment time, there is no patient movement during treatment and no shift of vaginal packing. Dose optimization is significantly easier with HDR in both interstitial and intracavitary brachytherapy.

## Summary

The inherent advantages of remote afterloading techniques, the ready availability of commercially produced HDR devices, and the recent advances in three-dimensional treatment planning provide the means for increased use of brachytherapy on an outpatient basis. Since radiation exposure has been the most serious drawback of brachytherapy and since only remote afterloading can provide complete radiation protection, we expect that all brachytherapy procedures will ultimately be done by remote afterloading with high-activity sources. However, many problems remain to be solved, which makes it important to critically compare HDR programs with the LDR treatments they are replacing. The ultimate test will be controlled clinical trials designed for this comparison. Some trials have already been conducted but with far too few patients to allow for definitive conclusions.

## REFERENCES

1. Henschke UK."Afterloading" applicator for radiation therapy of carcinoma of the uterus. Radiology 74:834, 1960.
2. Henschke UK, Hilaris BS, Mahan GD. Afterloading in interstitial and intracavitary radiation therapy. Am J Roentgenol 90:386-395, 1963.
3. Henschke UK, Hilaris BS, Mahan GD, et al. Afterloading applicator for treatment of cancer of the uterus. N Y State J Med 64:624-628, 1963.
4. Suit HD, Moore EB, Fletcher GH, et al. Modification of Fletcher ovoid system for afterloading, using standard-sized radium tubes (milligram and microgram). Radiology 81:126-131, 1963.
5. Horwitz H, Kereiakes JG, Bahr GK, et al. An afterloading system utilizing cesium 137 for the treatment of carcinoma of the cervix. Am J Roentgenol 91:176-191, 1964.
6. Henschke UK, Hilaris BS, Mahan GD. Remote afterloading for intracavitary radiation therapy. Radiology 83:344-345, 1964.
7. Henschke UK, Hilaris BS, Mahan GD. Remote afterloading for intracavitary radiation therapy. In: Ariel IM, ed. Progress in Clinical Cancer. New York: Grune & Stratton; 1965, 127-136.
8. Henschke UK, Hilaris BS, Mahan GD. Intracavitary radiation therapy of cancer of the uterine cervix by remote afterloading with cycling sources. Am J Roentgenol Radium Ther Nucl Med 96:45-51, 1966.
9. Henschke UK, Hilaris BS, Mahan, GD. Remote afterloading with intracavitary applicators. Radiology 83(2):344-345, 1964.
10. Martin MW. Miracles in Medicine. Middle Village, NY: Jonathan David Publishers, 1974, 39-40.
11. Hilaris BS, Ju H, Lewis JL, et al: Normal and neoplastic tissue effects of high intensity intracavitary irradiation: cancer of the corpus uteri. Radiology 110:459-492, 1974.
12. O'Connell D, Joslin CAF, Howard N, et al. The treatment of uterine carcinoma using the Cathetron: part I: technique. Br J Radiol 40:882-889, 1967.
13. Wakabayashi M. High dose intracavitary radiotherapy using the Ralston: I: treatment of carcinoma of the uterine cervix. Nippon Acta Radiol 31:340-378, 1971.
14. Rotte K. The intracavitary radiation of cervical cancer using an afterloading device with an Ir-192 pinpoint source. In: Simon N, ed. Cancer of the Uterus in Developing Areas. Proceedings of the 4th Encounter of Radiotherapists and Physicists of Brazil. Rio de Janeiro, 1973, 274-282. Sponsor: Mount Sinai School of Medicine, NY.
15. Walstam R. Remotely controlled afterloading apparatus. Acta Radiol (Ther) Suppl 236, Part II, 84, 1965.
16. Chassagne D, Delouche G, Rocoplan JA, et al. Description et premiers essais due Curietron. J Radiol Electrol Med Nucl 50:910-913, 1969.

# Chapter 2

# Radiobiology

*Colin G. Orton, David J. Brenner, Roger G. Dale, and John F. Fowler*

## Introduction

From the standpoint of radiobiology, one of the major rationales for low dose rate (LDR) brachytherapy is to take advantage of the so-called dose-rate effect illustrated in Fig. 1.[1] Other phenomena of potential importance, such as tumor reoxygenation, will be discussed briefly later. As the dose rate is reduced, the curvature of the cell survival curve decreases until it becomes linear (upper dotted line in Fig. 1) with a slope equal to the initial slope of the acute exposure survival curve. This is due to the phenomenon of "repair" of sublethal damage, which occurs at low doses and low dose rates and is represented by the shoulder of the acute exposure (high dose rate (HDR)) cell survival curve (the lowest curve in Fig. 1).

The curves become shallower as the dose rate is reduced because repair takes time, with half-times for repair of the order of 1 hour, and hence repair increases as the irradiation time increases. The limiting value (dotted line) is reached when all available repair has been utilized. In terms of the linear-quadratic (L-Q) model of cell survival (see below), to which Fig. 1 was drawn, this means that only the irreparable component ($\alpha$) of cellular damage remains, and all the reparable damage ($\beta$) has been repaired. Mechanistically, this distinction probably corresponds to damage produced by a single track of radiation ($\alpha$) which is, by definition, dose-rate independent, and damage produced by two independent tracks of radiation ($\beta$) in which damage from the first track can be repaired before it interacts with damage from the second track. But returning to Fig. 1, why is the dose-rate effect so important to LDR brachytherapy since not only does LDR increase the repair of normal tissue cells but also allows increased repair of tumor cells? The reason is shown in Fig. 2: in general, cell survival curves for normal, late responding tissue cells are "curvier" and have more of a shoulder compared with those for tumor cells.[2] Hence, the dose-rate effect is greater for normal cells than for tumor cells. It is this differential in repair at low doses and dose rates that makes fractionation and dose rate so important in teletherapy and brachytherapy, respectively. It is also a major factor to be considered in the radiobiological comparison of HDR

From: Nag, S. (ed.): *High Dose Rate Brachytherapy: A Textbook*, Futura Publishing Company, Inc., Armonk, NY, © 1994.

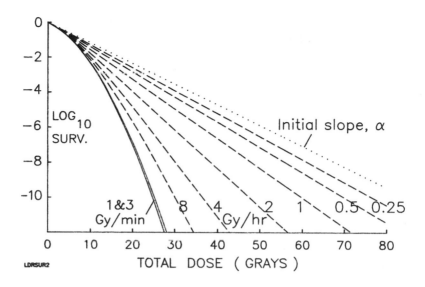

LDRSUR2

**Fig. 1.** As dose rates decrease, cell survival increases because there is more time for repair of sublethal injury to occur. Only the β (dose-squared) component decreases; the α component (initial slope) is not repairable. Assumed values: α/β = 10 Gy, α = 0.28 Gy$^{-1}$, T$_{1/2}$ = 1.5 h (from Stitt JA, et al.[1]).

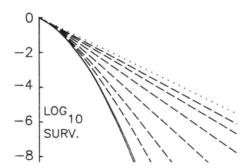

**Fig. 2.** Survival curves (on a log scale) for late-responding normal tissue cells tend to be more curved and have a shallower initial slope compared with tumors. In terms of the L-Q model, this means that for late responding tissues the α/β is lower than for tumors (from Hall EJ[2]).

and LDR brachytherapy. Such comparisons normally involve extensive use of the L-Q model, so this will be discussed first.

## The Linear Quadratic Model

Bioeffect dose in the L-Q model can be represented by the extrapolated response dose (ERD),[3,4] which is sometimes referred to as the biologically effective dose (BED),[5] especially when a time factor is incorporated to account for repopulation. "Extrapolated" means "at the lowest dose rates," so that all the reparable ($\beta$-type) damage has been repaired. The general equation for BED is

$$BED = -(\ln S.F.)/\alpha = NRt \left[ 1 + G \frac{Rt}{(\alpha/\beta)} \right] - kT \qquad (1)$$

where
  S.F. = cell surviving fraction;
  N = number of fractions (either HDR or LDR);
  R = dose rate (in Gy $.h^{-1}$);
  t = time for each fraction (in h);
and
  T = overall time available for repopulation (usually in days).

The other terms in the equation, $\alpha$, $\beta$, G, and k, are all tissue-specific parameters. At the cellular level, G relates to the rate of repair of sublethal damage, $\alpha$ and $\beta$ determine the shape of the cell-survival curve, and k (usually in Gy. $day^{-1}$) refers to the daily dose compensation necessary to combat any concurrent repopulation. Specifically, G is a function of the irradiation time, the dose rate, the cellular repair rate and, if appropriate, the time between fractions; $\alpha$ represents the initial slope of the cell survival curve; and $\beta$ defines its "curviness." The parameter $\alpha/\beta$ is the dose (in Gy) at which the $\alpha$ and $\beta$ components of log cell kill are equal.[3] Finally, k is a function of the doubling time of clonogenic cells ($T_{pot}$) and is given by k = $0.693/\alpha T_{pot}$.[5]

Typical values used for $\alpha/\beta$ are of the order of 1–4 Gy for late-responding normal tissues, and 5–20 Gy for tumors or early responding normal tissues.[5] However, it should be stressed that there is a great deal of variability in these and all other radiobiological parameters discussed here, and that no one parameter value can, a priori, be "correct" for any specific case. Values of k vary from near zero for late reactions, up to 0.6 Gy. $day^{-1}$ for tumors.[6] However, sometimes a biphasic repopulation appears to occur where repopulation is slow initially until a certain time $T_o$, typically 2–4 weeks, after which it accelerates.[7] Hence, for T $\leq T_o$, k is small (or zero) and for T > $T_0$, k is large.

The value of G is highly dependent upon the irradiation conditions, especially with respect to dose rate and time. For example, G = 0 for very long durations (i.e., low dose rates) and G = 1 for very high dose rates, as shown by the following equations for G for a variety of applications.

## Conventional LDR Treatments

For LDR therapy, if only a single fraction is used or when the time between fractions is long compared to the half-time for repair:[4]

$$G = \frac{2}{\mu t} \left[1 - \frac{(1 - e^{-\mu t})}{\mu t}\right] \tag{2}$$

where $\mu$ is the repair-rate constant (in $h^{-1}$), that is, $0.693/\mu$ is the half-time for repair. Typical values used for $\mu$ are $0.46$ $h^{-1}$ for late-reacting normal tissues, corresponding to the half-time for repair of 1.5 $h^8$, and between 0.46 and 1.4 $h^{-1}$ for tumors, corresponding to half-times in the range of 1.5–0.5 h.[9,10]

## Conventional HDR Treatments

For HDR treatments where the duration of each fraction is short and the time between fractions is long compared to the half-time for repair, the value of G is determined from eq. (2) by allowing t to approach zero. Mathematically, the expansion of $e^{-\mu t}$ as a binomial series yields[4]

$$G = 1 \tag{3}$$

This applies to both HDR brachytherapy and HDR fractionated teletherapy.

## Incomplete Repair During and Between Fractions

When the time (x hours) between fractions is not long compared to the repair half-time, *and* the dose rate is low enough to make the time for each fraction not negligible compared to the half-time for repair, then repair both between and during each fraction needs to be taken into account, and the equation for G becomes[9,11-13]

$$G = \frac{2}{\mu t} \left[1 - \frac{(NY - SY^2)}{N\mu t}\right] \tag{4}$$

where

$$Y = 1 - e^{-\mu t}$$

$$S = \frac{NK - K - NK^2 e^{-\mu t} + K^{N+1} e^{-\mu Nt}}{(1 - Ke^{-\mu t})^2}$$

and

$$K = e^{-\mu x}$$

Note that for a single fraction, $S = 0$, and eq. (4) reduces to eq. (2).

### Incomplete Repair Between Fractions: HDR

With HDR treatments, if the time to deliver a fraction is negligible in comparison with the repair half-time, then the above equation for G simplifies to[11]

$$G = \frac{N(1 - K^2) - 2K(1 - K^N)}{N(1 - K)^2} \qquad (5)$$

Note here that, if the time between fractions is long, $K = 0$ and eq. (5) reduces to eq. (3). As before, this equation applies to either HDR brachytherapy or teletherapy.

## Applications of the L-Q Model

### Definitions of HDR and LDR

The major difference between LDR and HDR is that appreciable repair occurs during an LDR exposure, whereas only minimal repair can take place during a short HDR procedure. Indeed, as indicated above, a common definition of HDR therapy is that each HDR treatment is delivered in a time that is short compared to the half-time for repair. Conversely, LDR corresponds to treatment times that are long compared to repair half-times. Unfortunately, however, these definitions leave much to be desired. First, what exactly is meant by the terms "short" and "long"? Second, cellular repair rates have been reported to vary considerably between cell types.[9] A more useful definition might be to relate length of treatment sessions for HDR and LDR to the fraction of the total possible repair that occurs during the irradiation.

But what "fraction" is appropriate? Rationally, this "fraction" ought to be representative of the effect it will have upon clinical outcome. Since a 5–10% change in outcome is probably a realistic estimate of the lower limit of clinical detectability, and since Fowler has estimated that one $\log_{10}$ cell kill can be expected to lead to a difference in local control of about 10–15%,[5,14] it seems reasonable to define dose-rate ranges for HDR and LDR such that they correspond to about one-half of one $\log_{10}$ cell kill. At a typical HDR dose/fraction in the range of 3–10 Gy, about half of the total log cell kill is due to $\alpha$ damage (irreparable) and half to $\beta$ damage (reparable). We know this because $\alpha/\beta$ varies in the range 3 Gy for late-reacting tissues to 10 Gy for tumors, and $\alpha$ damage and $\beta$ damage are equal at the dose $\alpha/\beta$.[3] Hence, if one is eventually aiming for a total $\log_{10}$ cell kill of about 10 from a course of fractionated HDR treatments, the $\beta$-damage will correspond to a $\log_{10}$ cell kill of about 5, so one half of one $\log_{10}$ cell kill will be 10% of this. It is, therefore, reasonable to define a "short" irradiation (i.e., HDR) as a period during which less than 10% of the maximum possible repair capacity of cells occurs, as measured by log cell kill for reparable damage. Conversely, LDR could be defined such that the irradiation time is long enough for at least 90% of this repair to occur. These definitions are demonstrated pictorially by the cell survival curves in Fig. 3: maximal repair is represented by the uppermost curve (infinitely long irradiation time), and minimal repair corresponds to the lower curve (infinitely short irradiation). The difference between these two curves is the "β-type" reparable damage, which represents the maximum repair capacity in terms of log cell survival and is equal to $\beta D^2$. Then the upper shaded area represents LDR, allowing between 90% and 100% of this total repair capacity (log cell kill), that is, within 10% of the infinitely long irradiation time curve, and the lower shaded area corresponds to HDR, or up to 10% more repair than the t = 0 curve.

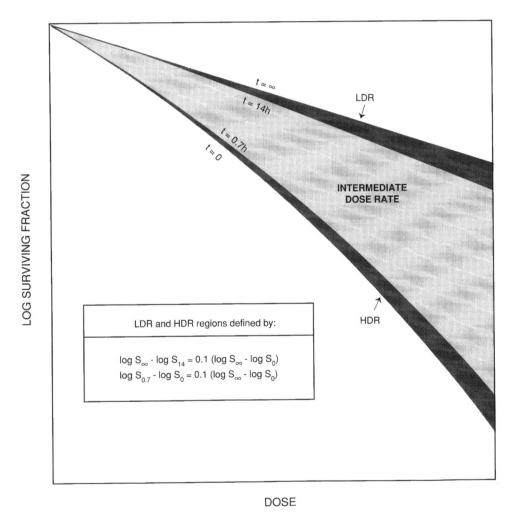

**Fig. 3.** LDR and HDR can be defined in terms of fractional repair: LDR is within 10% of maximum repair, and HDR is within 10% of minimum repair. These correspond to irradiation times of 14 h–∞ for LDR and 0–0.7 h for HDR. Between these limits is the intermediate dose rate.

The limits of these shaded areas can be determined using the L-Q model. If the upper time limit for a treatment to be called HDR is $t_H$, and the lower time limit for LDR is $t_L$, then using eq. (1) without the repopulation parameter (i.e., k = 0) and with N = 1 to calculate cell surviving fractions corresponding to these limits and equating these to 10% of $\beta D^2$, gives G = 0.9 for HDR and G = 0.1 for LDR. Solving eq. (2) for a range of values of $\mu$ between 0.46 h$^{-1}$ and 1.4 h$^{-1}$ yields the following maximum limit for HDR (for $\mu$ = 0.46 h$^{-1}$) and the minimum limit for LDR (for $\mu$ = 1.4 h$^{-1}$) of

$$t_H = 0.7 \text{ h};$$

$$t_L = 14 \text{ h}.$$

Hence, HDR corresponds to treatment times up to a maximum of about 0.7 h, and LDR represents treatments where the time is longer than about 14 h. Note that because solving eq. (2) for t only requires a knowledge of $\mu$, these limits depend solely upon the rates of cellular repair and are independent of $\alpha$, $\beta$, dose, and dose rate. Of course, since repair rates are highly variable, these definitions of HDR and LDR are not hard and fast rules, they are simply guidelines.

Treatments with irradiation times between these limits can be considered as the intermediate (or medium) dose rate.

## HDR Versus LDR

It is clear from Figs. 1 and 3 that a single HDR treatment can produce the same cell kill as an LDR regimen if the dose is reduced accordingly. But in order to truly simulate the cell survival curve of continuous LDR irradiation, HDR treatments must be fractionated so that the same dose leads to identical cell surviving fractions. This is illustrated in Fig. 4, which shows that the survival curve for the HDR regimen falls exactly along that of the continuous LDR irradiation if the equivalent dose/fraction, $d_{eq}$, is used.[15] If the dose/fraction is increased, i.e., fewer fractions are used, then the survival curve falls below that for the continuous irradiation and, conversely, with more fractions at a lower dose/fraction, the HDR curve is above that for LDR.

Conversion from LDR to HDR is not simply a matter of determining the equivalent dose/fraction required to match an LDR survival curve, however, because, as illustrated in Fig. 2, survival curves for tumor and late-reacting normal tissue cells have different shapes. Fortunately, matching the survival curves for both tumor and normal tissue cells can be readily achieved using the L-Q equations for these survival curves. However, the appropriate HDR fractionation depends heavily upon the dose rate of the LDR regime being "matched," the L-Q model parameters assumed, and the physical dose distributions for the LDR and HDR treatments. For example, in one of the earliest papers on this subject, Dale[4] showed that a typical radical course of HDR intracavitary therapy for the treatment of cervical cancer would have to be de-

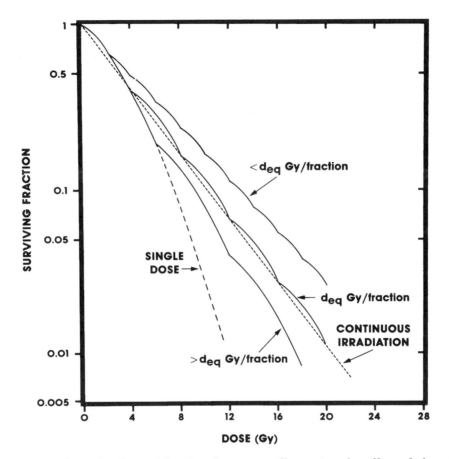

**Fig. 4.** Hypothetical cell surviving fraction curves illustrating the effect of changing the dose per fraction for HDR. At dose per fraction $d_{eq}$ the HDR cell survival curve is equivalent to that of an (unspecified) LDR continuous exposure at all doses (from Orton CG[15]).

livered in about 17 fractions in order to be equivalent to LDR in terms of coincidence of the survival curves for both tumor and late-reacting tissues with the same total dose. For his calculations, he assumed that the LDR dose to Point A was 60 Gy in 72 hours, corresponding to a dose rate to Pt. A of 0.833 Gy h$^{-1}$. This correlates closely to the mean LDR Pt. A dose rate of $(0.85 \pm 0.07)$ Gy h$^{-1}$ determined from a survey of 56 institutions,[16] but is about 50% higher than the dose rate to Pt. A used in the traditional Manchester System and 50% lower than that for the Stockholm System. If the lower (Manchester) LDR dose rate had been assumed for these calculations, more than 17 fractions would have been needed in order to match survival curves. Also, because the total LDR dose would have to be increased above 60 Gy in order to produce the same tumor cell kill as observed at 0.833 Gy h$^{-1}$, the total HDR dose would need to be increased concomitantly. Conversely, to match the higher (Stockholm System) dose rate regime, fewer HDR fractions to a lower total dose would be required.

Although HDR schedules equivalent to LDR can be calculated using the L-Q model, however, it should be realized that, because of the differential sparing of late-reacting tissues at low doses and low dose rates exemplified by the different shapes of the survival curves in Fig. 2, the therapeutic ratio for the lower (Manchester) dose-rate regime (or its matching HDR equivalent) ought to exceed that for the higher (Stockholm) dose rate (or its HDR "match"). Whether or not such a change could be clinically significant is equivocal. Most studies have failed to detect any difference in therapeutic ratio, although a recent report of increased complications with no change in local control or survival for a factor of two increase in LDR dose rate appeared to demonstrate such a difference.[17] However, the overall level of complications in this study was very high (about 70%), and this is in the steep part of the dose-response curve for complications. With more normal complication rates for LDR of less than 20%,[17] we would be in the toe of the dose response curve, and this would make it much less likely that any differences in complication rates would be statistically observable.

In his analysis, Dale[4] assumed that normal tissue and tumor cells repair at the same rate. He later showed,[18] however, that if it is legitimate to assume that tumor cells repair faster than late-reacting normal tissue cells, it might be possible to achieve equivalence with as few as 6–7 fractions, although this would require a reduction in the total dose. In this case, the survival curves would not be coincident, as illustrated in Fig. 5. Several authors have shown that even fewer HDR fractions may be needed if the dose to the critical normal tissues is less than the prescribed "tumor" dose and, furthermore, that the equivalent number of fractions might be even less than this if the ratio of normal tissue dose to tumor dose is lower for HDR than for LDR.[1,19,20] This latter might well be true for treatments for cervical cancer, for example, by improved packing and/or retraction, which is achievable during the short HDR treatment sessions.

These different situations are summarized in Fig. 6, which shows schematically the equivalent number of HDR fractions required to replace an LDR regimen of 60 Gy to Point A in 72 hours. (Note that for the calculations used to derive the data in Fig. 6, the repopulation parameter kT in eq. (1) has been ignored. Hence, these data apply strictly only if the overall time for the course of treatment (teletherapy and brachytherapy) is unchanged when converting from LDR to HDR. The left half of Fig. 6 represents the situation where the repair rate constants, $\mu$, for both tumor and normal tissue cells are identical, specifically 0.46 $h^{-1}$, corresponding to repair half-times of 1.5 h, whereas to the right, the half-time for repair for tumor cells is changed to 0.5 hours (repair rate constant of 1.4 $h^{-1}$). As shown, for equal repair rates, 17 fractions (of about 3.5 Gy) are needed if the tumor and normal tissue doses are equal, as determined by Dale.[4] If the average normal tissue dose (e.g., to rectal and/or bladder tissues) is 72% of that to Point A for *both* HDR and LDR, equivalent to that reported in a survey of LDR data,[16,17], fractions are still required. But if there is some additional sparing of normal tissues such that this ratio is reduced to an average of 63% for HDR, as shown in the same survey,[16] the number of HDR fractions is reduced to only five.

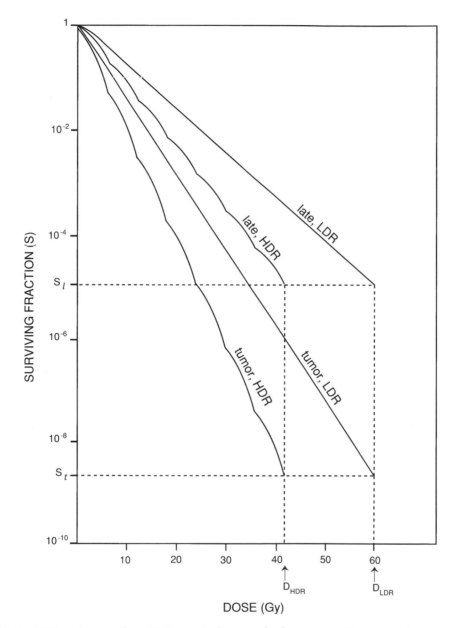

**Fig. 5.** LDR and equivalent HDR survival curves for late responding normal tissue cells (l) and tumor (t) when the doses to normal tissues and tumor are the same and more rapid repair of tumor cells is assumed. Assumed values: $(\alpha/\beta)_t = 10$ Gy, $(\alpha/\beta)_l = 2.5$ Gy, $\alpha_t = 0.3$ Gy$^{-1}$, $\alpha_l = 0.08$ Gy$^{-1}$, $\mu_t = 1.4$ h$^{-1}$, $\mu_l = 0.46$h$^{-1}$. Note that equivalence to a 60 Gy LDR regimen is achieved with an HDR dose of 42 Gy in seven fractions.

If different repair rates are assumed (right side of Fig. 6), then the three conditions above lead to significantly reduced numbers of HDR fractions of 7, 5, and 1, respectively. For example, for a reduction in total dose from 60 Gy to 42 Gy, 7 HDR fractions give the same tumor and normal tissue cell survivals as LDR. This is the situation illustrated in Fig. 5.

The actual numbers in Figs. 5 and 6 should not be taken too seriously since they are based upon assumed values of $\alpha$, $\beta$, and $\mu$, none of which is known accurately for any tissues. These figures are only presented here to illustrate the concept that LDR can be replaced by HDR with respect to both tumor and normal tissue effects. There is reason to suppose that HDR brachytherapy can be as good as, or even better than, conventional LDR, provided that an adequate number of fractions can be delivered and that the appropriate dose/fraction can be determined. It should be noted, however, that in this analysis it has been assumed that all tumor cells have the same radiation sensitivity, and that cellular sensitivity does not change during the course of therapy. Both of these assumptions are likely to be oversimplifications. Some tumor cells may be hypoxic and hence radioresistant, and these may or may not reoxygenate during treatment. Furthermore, with LDR therapy, as the dose rate is reduced there may be a certain limited range of dose rates for which the inverse dose-rate effect prevails, this being caused by cells accumulating at a block in G2, a

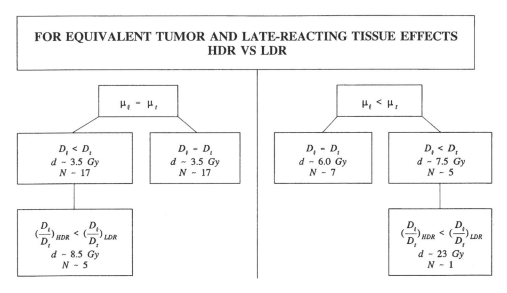

**Fig. 6.** HDR regimens that are equivalent to a tumor dose of 60 Gy in 72 h (at LDR) according to the L-Q model in various situations: left side $\mu_l = \mu_t = 0.46$ h$^{-1}$; right side $\mu_l = 0.46$ h$^{-1}$, $\mu_t = 1.4$ h$^{-1}$. HDR tumor dose per fraction (d) and the number of fractions (N) depends upon the relative doses to tumor (t) and late-reacting normal tissues (l). Assumptions: $(\alpha/\beta)_t = 10$ Gy, $(\alpha/\beta)_l = 2.5$ Gy, physical sparing of normal tissues when $D_l < D_t$ is 28%, extra sparing for HDR when $(D_l/D_t)_{HDR} < (D_l/D_t)_{LDR}$ is 13%. Note that the equivalences in this figure are based only on sublethal damage repair concepts. Other phenomena, such as reoxygenation, need to be considered when assessing an HDR scheme.

sensitive phase of the cell cycle.[21] Hence, in this dose-rate range, cells might actually *increase* in sensitivity as the dose rate is reduced. This inverse dose-rate effect has rarely been observed in radiobiological experiments, and so it is reasonable to ignore it in comparisons of LDR and HDR, which is fortunate since it would be very difficult to model mathematically. As far as potential reoxygenation is concerned, it has been suggested that, even though the L-Q model analysis predicts, under certain conditions, as low as a single fraction of HDR might be equivalent to LDR, it appears expedient to consider treating with about five fractions in order to avoid impairment of tumor control caused by inadequate reoxygenation.[19] Even then, if five fractions are used, this does not ensure that the HDR schedule is both an effective and safe replacement for LDR because the appropriate dose/fraction still needs to be determined. If the L-Q model is used to calculate this dose, the value determined depends upon the relatively poorly-known parameters assumed. Hence, the L-Q model should only be used to estimate roughly what HDR dose/fraction to employ. This then needs to be fine tuned by clinical observations, such as Phase I/II dose-escalation trials. On the other hand, it is important to recognize that the L-Q model is being used here only to compare treatment regimens. Such comparisons are far less sensitive to choices of parameters than absolute calculations of effect.

**Pulsed Brachytherapy**

With pulsed brachytherapy (PB), a source with activity intermediate between that employed for HDR or LDR is used to deliver a series of short exposures of duration 0.2–0.5 h, for example, every hour or so, to approximately the same total dose and overall time as with LDR.[12] The rationale is to simulate LDR remote afterloading but with several of the advantages of HDR, such as single stepping source, optimized dose distributions, no radiation exposure to personnel, etc. But is this really equivalent to LDR, or is it more closely related to intermediate dose rate or even HDR?

This problem has been addressed in several articles, each using the L-Q model to calculate cell survival.[9,10,12] As would be expected, the L-Q model predicts that how closely PB simulates LDR depends on the pulse repetition frequency and also on the dose rate in the pulses. Generally, these studies have shown that, for pulses delivered every hour, the biological difference between PB and LDR should be clinically insignificant. However, by decreasing the number of pulses such that pulses are delivered only once every few hours, the dose/pulse becomes so high that there is a significant decrease in repair such that PB becomes more damaging than LDR, and the result is an increased risk of complications. This could be alleviated by a concomitant reduction in the total dose. However, application of the L-Q model shows that this would probably cause a significant reduction in tumor-control probability compared with LDR for the same late normal-tissue complications, which means a decrease in therapeutic ratio. Fowler and Mount[12] show this graphically in terms of the ratio of late/tumor damage, as defined by the ratio of BEDs (Fig. 7).

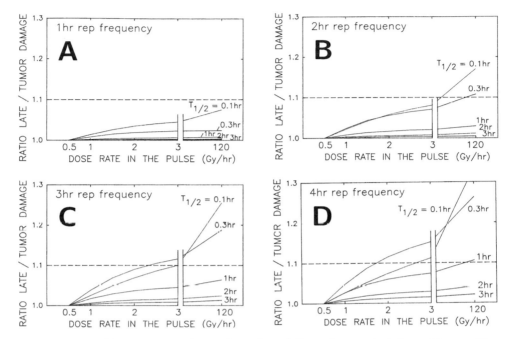

**Fig. 7.** Ratio of late to tumor BEDs for pulses delivered every 1, 2, 3, or 4 hours. The dashed line is drawn arbitrarily where the damage ratio has risen 10% above the level traditionally accepted in continuous LDR of 0.5 Gy/hr. In the PB region, to the left of the graph break, no ratio exceeds the 10% extra level for pulses repeated every 1 or 2 hrs (A and B). However, for pulses repeated every 3 hr (C), the 10% increase level might be exceeded if tissues have $T_{1/2}$ values below about 0.5 hr. For pulses repeated every 4 hr (D) this is more likely, but if $T_{1/2}$ values exceed 1 hr, it is still unlikely. The curves to the left of the break apply to PB. To the right of the break we illustrate HDR (from Fowler JF and Mount M[12]).

Figure 7 shows that, for constant tumor effect, late effects increase as (a) the dose rate in the pulse increases (i.e., the length of each pulse decreases); (b) the pulse repetition frequency decreases; and (c) the half-time for repair decreases.

It should be noted that hourly pulses appear to be always relatively safe, regardless of the repair rate or the length of each pulse. With such a schedule, because each fraction will normally last less than 0.7 hours, this corresponds to hyperfractionated HDR, with incomplete repair between pulses. For a constant BED to tumor, the BED to normal, late-reacting tissues does not increase more than 10% with pulses delivered every 2 hours, for whatever repair rates are assumed. However, with pulses repeated less often than this, this arbitrary 10% limit could be exceeded, especially if cells are repairing rapidly. These pulsed brachytherapy calculations have assumed that the repair rates for normal and tumor cells are equal. If, by chance, tumor cells repair faster than late-reacting normal cells, this will be to the advantage of PB, and lower pulse repetition frequencies will be safe. However, this is all theory and, as with HDR, only careful clinical observations can provide definitive answers to these questions.

## Conclusions

From radiobiological considerations, HDR can safely be used to replace LDR with respect to both tumor control and late effects, provided enough fractions are delivered and the total doses are reduced appropriately. If repair kinetics of tumor and late-reacting tissue cells are similar, the required number of fractions will be quite high, probably more than 15, unless some additional physical sparing of the normal tissues can be incorporated. But if tumor cells repair faster than normal cells, only about six fractions will be needed, and this might be reduced even further if some geometrical sparing occurs. Under these circumstances, theoretical predictions indicate that even as low as one fraction might be sufficient. However, it is important to stress that, unless palliation is the only objective, the use of single fractions is not recommended because other radiobiological phenomena, such as reoxygenation or reassortment, require at least several fractions.

Pulsed LDR brachytherapy, which is similar to hyperfractionated HDR, appears to be a safe and effective replacement for conventional LDR provided the pulse repetition frequency is high enough. With fewer than one pulse every two hours it is possible that a greater than 10% increase in BED to normal tissues might be necessary in order to keep the same probability of tumor control. Hence, unless clinical data should prove to the contrary, it is unwise at this point to deliver pulses less often than once every hour or so.

---

## REFERENCES

1. Stitt JA, Fowler JF, Thomadsen BR, et al. High dose rate intracavitary brachytherapy for carcinoma of the cervix: the Madison System. 1. clinical and radiobiological considerations. Int J Radiat Oncol Biol Phys 24: 335-348, 1992.
2. Hall EJ. Radiobiology for the Radiologist, 3rd ed. Philadelphia, Pa: Lippinott; 1988, 244.
3. Barendsen GW. Dose fractionation, dose rate and iso-effect relationships for normal tissue responses. Int J Radiat Oncol Biol Phys 8:1981-1997, 1982.
4. Dale RG. The application of the linear-quadratic dose-effect equation to fractionated and protracted radiotherapy. Br J Radiol 58:515-528, 1985.
5. Fowler JF. The linear-quadratic formula and progress in fractionated radiotherapy. Brit J Radiol 62:679-694, 1989.
6. Fowler JF, Lindstrom MJ. Loss of local control with prolongation in radiotherapy. Int J Radiat Oncol Biol Phys 23: 457-467, 1992.
7. Withers HR, Taylor JMG, Maciejewski B. The hazard of accelerated tumor clonogen repopulation during radiotherapy. Acta Oncol 27:131-146, 1988.
8. Thames HD. Effect-independent measures of tissue responses to fractionated irradiation. Int J Radiat Oncol Biol Phys 45:1-10, 1984.
9. Brenner DJ, Hall EJ. Conditions for the equivalence of continuous to pulsed low dose rate brachytherapy. Int J Radiat Oncol Biol Phys 20:181-190, 1991.
10. Fowler JF. Why shorter half-times for repair lead to greater damage in pulsed brachytherapy. Int J Radiat Biol 26: 353-356, 1993.
11. Dale RG, Huczkowski J, Trott KR. Possible dose rate dependence of recovery kinetics as deduced from a preliminary analysis of the effects of fractionated irradiations at varying dose rates. Br J Radiol 61:153-157, 1988.

12. Fowler JF, Mount M. Pulsed brachytherapy: the conditions for no significant loss of therapeutic ratio compared with traditional low dose rate brachytherapy. Int J Radiat Oncol Biol Phys 23: 661-669, 1992.
13. Orton CG. Recent developments in time-dose modelling. Australas Phys Eng Sci Med 14:57-64, 1991.
14. Fowler JF. Potential for increasing the differential response between tumors and normal tissues: can proliferation rate be used? Int J Radiat Oncol Biol Phys 12:641-645, 1986.
15. Orton CG. High and low dose rate remote afterloading: a critical comparison. In: R. Sauer, ed. International Radiation Therapy Techniques—Brachytherapy. Berlin, Germany: Springer-Verlag; 1991, 53-57.
16. Orton CG, Seyedsadr M, Somnay A. Comparison of high and low dose rate remote afterloading for cervix cancer and the importance of fractionation. Int J Radiat Oncol Biol Phys 21: 1425-1434, 1991.
17. Lambin P, Gerbaulet A, Kramar A, et al. Phase III trial comparing two low dose rates in brachytherapy of cervix carcinoma: report at two years. Int J Radiat Oncol Biol Phys 25: 403-412, 1993.
18. Dale RG. What minimum number of fractions is required with high dose-rate remote afterloading? Br J Radiol 60:301-302, 1987.
19. Brenner DJ, Hall EJ. Fractionated high dose rate versus low dose rate regimens for intracavitary brachytherapy of the cervix. Br J Radiol 64:133-141, 1991.
20. Dale RG. The use of small fraction numbers in high dose-rate gynecological afterloading: some radiobiological considerations. Br J Radiol 63:290-294, 1990.
21. Hall EJ. Radiobiology for the Radiologist, 3rd ed. Philadelphia, Pa: Lippincott; 1988, 122.

**Chapter 3**

# Design and Implementation of a Program for High Dose Rate Brachytherapy

*Pavel V. Houdek, Glenn P. Glasgow,
James G. Schwade, and André A. Abitbol*

## Criteria for HDR Brachytherapy Program Design

The design of a high dose rate (HDR) brachytherapy program is commonly determined by the current commitments and future intentions of the institution involved concerning the delivery of comprehensive care to cancer patients. It is recognized that a successful high-volume HDR brachytherapy program requires the full cooperation and rapport of surgical and medical oncologists, interventional radiologists, anesthesiologists, and other specialists essential to this treatment modality. Furthermore, the program is defined by the previous brachytherapy history of the radiation oncology department considering expansion. Funds and space available for the project are other important factors that have to be considered in the process of designing an HDR brachytherapy program.

Before any true planning can commence, it is essential to collect all institutional and departmental data describing the spectrum of cancers and anatomical sites commonly treated using brachytherapy, the number of cancer patients seen per year at the institution, the average number of brachytherapy applications per year, and a list of new treatment protocols that might be implemented at the HDR brachytherapy facility when it becomes available. Some initial conclusions to guide the planning process may be drawn from data concerning the estimated number of brachytherapy procedures, which is one of the most important parameters in determining the scope and proportions of any proposed program.

It is noted that approximately one half of all cancer patients seen at most institutions receive radiotherapy at some time during the course of their disease. Of these, 5 to 15% may require brachytherapy treatment. It should also be noted, when the number of HDR brachytherapy patients is being estimated, that the average number of brachytherapy procedures per patient

From: Nag, S. (ed.): *High Dose Rate Brachytherapy: A Textbook*, Futura Publishing Company, Inc., Armonk, NY, © 1994.

is not the same for low dose rate (LDR) and HDR modalities. Generally, HDR brachytherapy is delivered over a larger number of applications than LDR treatment. For example, LDR intracavitary brachytherapy of cervical cancers is usually delivered in 1 or 2 applications, whereas commonly used HDR protocols for the same site call for 4 to 12 treatment sessions.

The design of the program is greatly affected by the availability of radiology and surgical oncology services. The presence or absence of dedicated interventional radiology special procedures rooms and fully equipped operating rooms also affects HDR program design. These factors, together with the previously estimated number of brachytherapy procedures, then determine the equipment and amount of space that need to be acquired and allocated for the HDR brachytherapy program, in addition to that needed solely for the installation of the HDR remote afterloading unit itself. This data also helps decide if the duplication of already existing institutional facilities and/or equipment can be justified.

Budgetary and space restrictions are, of course, always present. Consequently, the objective of the planning process is to design an optimal HDR brachytherapy program that takes patient, institutional, and departmental needs into consideration, yet can be implemented within existing constraints. Thus, the accuracy and rapidity of HDR brachytherapy treatment delivery, as well as the overall cost effectiveness of the operation, are major criteria used in the development of a suitable program.

## Implementation of an HDR Brachytherapy Program

### General Considerations

The selection of an HDR remote afterloading unit is one of the first steps in establishing an HDR brachytherapy program. Currently available units use similar technology and are associated with similar capital equipment costs. Differences exist, however, in the selection and/or availability of HDR brachytherapy treatment planning systems and treatment applicators. It should be noted that without a dedicated computer system to automatically program the afterloader according to an optimized treatment plan, the HDR unit cannot be used efficiently. The ability of the system to compute dose distributions is not the primary reason substantiating this statement but rather the system's proficiency in rapid and accurate programming of the afterloading unit and its ability to optimize treatment plans. This makes the system indispensable in the clinical setting.

The availability and cost of special brachytherapy accessories necessary for HDR techniques, as, for example, gynecologic applicators, needs to be taken into consideration during the equipment selection process. It is also important to evaluate the versatility and limitations of the remote afterloading unit as applied to its use in special HDR brachytherapy techniques and in the treatment of a large number of different anatomical sites.

Furthermore, the cost of annual service contracts and the price of high-activity Ir-192 replacement sources have to be examined. Typically, four source changes are required every year. The commitment of the manufacturer to HDR technology, the number of satisfied users, and the safety record of the afterloading unit should also be considered.

The next step in the process of program implementation is actual installation of the selected HDR equipment. Since instantaneous dose rates around HDR units with 370 GBq (10 Ci) sources preclude their use in conventional rooms, HDR afterloading machines require special HDR facilities. Three different examples of specialized HDR facilities are reviewed below. They are presented in order of increasing cost.

### Installation of HDR Equipment in an Accelerator Room

Most existing teletherapy vaults possess adequate shielding for the 370 GBq (10 Ci) Ir-192 sources that are commonly used in HDR units at present. The definition of adequate shielding stipulates that it provide sufficient radiation protection for a maximum projected workload determined by (1) maximum amount and type of radioactive material to be used at any one time, (2) duration of its use, (3) the number of brachytherapy applications, and (4) length of the treatment sessions.

Satisfactory radiation protection specifies that dose equivalents in adjacent unrestricted areas must be (1) less than 0.02 mSv (2 mrem) in 1 hour and (2) less than 1 mSv (100 mrem) annually for members of the general public continuously (frequently) exposed to radiation, the latter recently adopted by the United States Nuclear Regulatory Commission (USNRC).[1] The older standard of 5 mSv (500 mrem) annually to members of the general public may still be allowed in specific license applications if appropriate justification is provided.[1]

The use of an HDR unit in an accelerator room is the least desirable HDR facility from the point of view of both patient and staff. It represents a satisfactory solution only if a very small number of simple HDR procedures are carried out per week (typically no more than two). Delivery of HDR brachytherapy treatments in such a facility is difficult because all schedules, including those for exam, simulator, and accelerator rooms must be adjusted. This problem is often further accentuated when the adjusted schedule is not followed because surgical and/or other procedures preceding treatment (e.g., catheter insertion for endobronchial implants) are done elsewhere and hence, are not under the full control of radiotherapy staff. Consequently, the HDR procedure then becomes a major inconvenience to both patients and personnel, even if it is completed uneventfully. It should also be noted that sometimes HDR treatments are delivered to cachectic patients and in such cases further complications that can be even more disruptive to the ordinary radiotherapy environment may be expected.

Since only minor construction (cable runs, additional safety lights, etc.) is usually required when an HDR unit is installed in an accelerator room, the capital cost of HDR program implementation is minimal. It is determined by the cost of the HDR equipment and initial source(s), associated accessories including the treatment planning system, HDR applicators, catheters, for example, and by installation costs. If patient vital-signs monitoring systems including, for example, ECG, pulse oximeter ($SpO_2$(percentage of saturated oxygen)), and noninvasive blood pressure (NIBP) monitors, are not already available in the department, they also need to be acquired.

Thus, the total capital cost of HDR program implementation for this type of facility would be about $300,000 ± $50,000 in 1992. The annual cost of maintaining the program is essentially determined by the cost of a service contract that usually also includes the cost of four new sources per year. Presently, service contracts cost about $30,000 per year. Since the HDR facility described here would almost always be a small volume operation, it would involve very little, if any, additional personnel costs. A realistic estimation of annual revenues generated by such an HDR program should assume that about 100 ± 50 procedures would be performed per year, depending on the number of cancer patients seen at the institution, referral patterns, and quantity of other radiotherapy equipment available in the department (i.e., number of accelerators and simulators).

## Dedicated HDR Brachytherapy Suite/Operating Room

Figure 1 gives an example of a dedicated HDR facility designed for a large volume HDR brachytherapy program at the University of Miami's Sylvester Comprehensive Cancer Center. The HDR facility is a part of the new Radiation Oncology Department[2] inaugurated in 1992. It consists of a shielded operating room (OR) and control, recovery, storage, and scrub areas and occupies a space of approximately 24 ft. × 24 ft. The OR dimensions are about 18 ft. × 18 ft. The 2-foot thick OR walls are fabricated from concrete and have a specific density of approximately 147 $lb/ft^3$. Radiotherapy simulators equipped with fluoroscopic and computed tomography (CT) accessories are installed in adjacent rooms.

The simulators mentioned above are used for all radiographic and fluoroscopic procedures required for treatment planning purposes, as well as for final verification of catheter/applicator positioning. Treatment planning is carried out at a nearby computer network area that houses all departmental treatment planning systems. Direct image transfer between the simulator and treatment planning areas is a valuable time-saving feature of the simulator/treatment planning system implementation.

Occasionally, the simulator rooms are also used as procedure rooms. More often, however, catheter and/or applicator placement is carried out in an appropriately equipped examination room. A radiolucent trauma board and standard stretcher are used to facilitate patient transfers.

The dedicated HDR suite was constructed in compliance with operating room and radiation safety building codes and regulations. Consequently, a va-

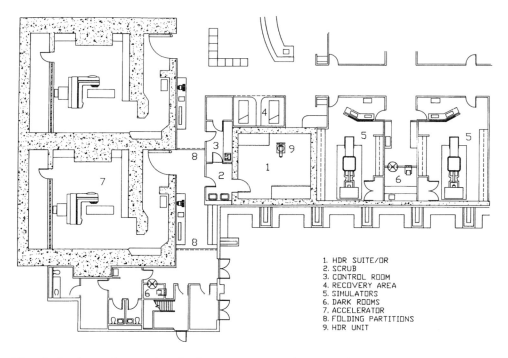

1. HDR SUITE/OR
2. SCRUB
3. CONTROL ROOM
4. RECOVERY AREA
5. SIMULATORS
6. DARK ROOMS
7. ACCELERATOR
8. FOLDING PARTITIONS
9. HDR UNIT

**Fig. 1.** Dedicated HDR brachytherapy suite and OR at the University of Miami's Sylvester Comprehensive Cancer Center. Note that this suite can also be used for intraoperative radiotherapy procedures.

riety of special equipment has been installed in the OR and/or in the supporting space. This equipment includes two anesthesia columns housing emergency power, medical gases, and vacuum, standard OR lights, patient monitoring equipment (ECG, $SpO_2$, NIBP) with remote displays, a patient support assembly, an isolation transformer, emergency power and lights, equipment for visual/audio communication with the patient, radiation detectors, warning lights, visible and audible alarms, an electrically operated shielded door with positive action interlocks, and of course, the HDR unit itself. A list of commonly required equipment is presented in Table 1.[3]

Although the vast majority of HDR procedures can be carried out in this facility, bronchoscopy or esophageal, cervical, and other applicator/catheter placement procedures are often completed in special procedure/operating rooms located outside of the department. This practice has been adopted for two reasons: (1) to minimize facility costs by avoiding equipment and/or space duplication, and (2) to minimize the inconvenience that the HDR procedure may represent to other professionals involved. It is necessary to emphasize that implementation of this HDR program is a relatively simple project, compared to the task of sustaining a high volume of procedures once HDR brachytherapy becomes routine, and is no longer a novel treatment modality in the institution.

The dedicated HDR suite/OR shown in Figure 1 was designed and built as a part of the Sylvester Comprehensive Cancer Center. Since this was a multi-

---

**Table 1**

**Equipment List for HDR Suite/IBU**

---

HDR unit, control console, HDR unit storage

Patient procedures table

Audio/visual patient communication systems

In-room and remote radiation detector and indicators; door interlock(s)

Operating room/procedure light(s), emergency lighting

Anesthesia area: medical gases and vacuum, designated location and
electrical power for patient monitoring equipment, remote displays

Sink/scrub area

Storage area/cabinets; applicators/catheters; positioning and/or fixation
clamps; medical supplies

Emergency-off buttons at console, in maze, and in room

Emergency power for selected equipment: audio, video, anesthesia,
patient monitoring, lighting, radiation detectors and indicators,
remote afterloader

Optional R/F imaging equipment, overhead track or isocentrically
mounted track; x-ray generator location; x-ray control console

Optional dedicated scrub area/change room; sterile environment;
pass-through barrier (containment area)

Optional treatment-planning workstation networked to imaging equipment

---

million dollar project,[2] it is difficult to provide the reader with accurate accounting concerning the cost of the HDR facility alone. It can be estimated, however, that in 1992, the funds required to build a 600 sq. ft. facility of this type would be about $300,000 ± $50,000, considering both construction (about $350 per sq. ft.) and equipment costs. The funds needed for acquisition of the HDR remote afterloader, HDR treatment-planning system, and patient monitoring equipment have already been estimated at $300,000 ± $50,000. The total capital costs associated with program implementation in the form of a dedicated HDR facility are thus approximately $600,000 ± $100,000. Annual operating expenses are determined by the service contract ($30,000) and personnel costs. Additional staff (i.e., one full-time equivalent at $50,000) may be required if a large volume of procedures is continuously sustained (i.e., more than three procedures per week).

It is important to realize, however, that capital costs can be kept to such a minimum only if the duplication of medical equipment available elsewhere in the institution (i.e., diagnostic x-ray machines) is avoided. This is only possible, however, if at least two fully equipped radiotherapy simulators are available in the department. The reason for this is that it is not practical or possible to sustain a high-volume HDR brachytherapy operation (typically one or more procedures per day) and at the same time satisfy departmental demands related to target localization and/or treatment technique simulation for all teletherapy patients using only a single radiotherapy simulator.

The dedicated suite may be designed in such a way that it also serves as an intraoperative radiotherapy facility.[4] Usually, program cost justification is simplified when the HDR suite is of a multipurpose design. As seen from Fig. 1, by

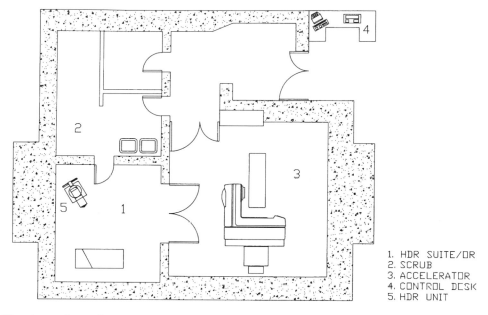

**Fig. 2.** Dedicated intraoperative radiotherapy facility at the Regional Cancer Center at Baptist Hospital of Miami. This facility is also used as an HDR suite.

utilizing a set of folding partitions (8), a sterile environment may be established and maintained within the area of the HDR suite (1) and accelerator room (7) that was also designed for intraoperative radiotherapy. An alternate configuration is offered in Fig. 2, which shows the existing intraoperative facility at the Regional Cancer Center of the Baptist Hospital in Miami that is also used as an HDR suite. It is noted that the facility design presented in Fig. 1 permits independent use of the HDR unit as well as the linear accelerator.

In summary, it might be of interest to note that the capital costs of HDR program implementation, using a dedicated HDR facility, are about twice as great as those associated with program implementation using an existing teletherapy vault. Similarly, annual operating costs double when the dedicated HDR suite concept is implemented. The revenues generated are determined by the number of procedures carried out. Three to five procedures per week would probably be the minimum number of procedures necessary to justify the capital and operating expenses associated with the program. The maximum number of procedures (i.e., the dedicated HDR suite capacity) would depend upon the complexity of the procedures involved. In general, however, suite capacity is usually not a limiting factor affecting the scope of the program.

As an example, if the department sees about 1,000 thousand cancer patients per year and HDR brachytherapy is indicated for 10% of them, then the number of HDR treatments delivered per year would most likely be between 200 and 500, assuming that 2 to 5 HDR fractions are commonly given to each patient. It follows that only one to two procedures will be carried out each day at the HDR facility, whereas easily twice as many treatments could actually be delivered there. Thus, the maximum number of procedures carried out at the dedicated HDR facility, and hence the maximum revenue generated by the HDR program, are determined by the number of cancer patients seen at the department and not by the treatment capacity of the HDR suite.

## Integrated HDR Brachytherapy Unit

If permitted by financial and space constraints, the HDR program can be implemented using the concept of an integrated brachytherapy unit (IBU). This unit is, in fact, a dedicated HDR suite/OR equipped so that all procedures associated with HDR brachytherapy treatment delivery may be completely carried out there. This approach to HDR program implementation, however, necessitates the duplication of medical equipment that may already be available elsewhere (i.e, that required for bronchoscopy or esophageal, cervical, and other applicator and/or catheter placement). It follows that equipment selection and installation within the unit must be done in close cooperation with the other departments that ordinarily provide these services to satisfy their requirements for the IBU.

In order to fully integrate the process of HDR brachytherapy, the IBU must also be equipped with a radiographic/fluoroscopic (R/F) x-ray machine, preferably furnished with digital imaging capabilities. An image network should be established within the IBU that provides for direct image transfer between x-ray equipment and the treatment planning system, which would also be a part of this facility. A list of equipment that may be required for IBU operation is presented in Table 1.[3]

Although an integrated HDR brachytherapy suite has been described in the literature[5] and is shown schematically in Fig. 3, the authors of this chapter are not aware of any publicly available financial analyses for fully functioning IBUs in the United States. Consequently, the financial analysis that follows is rather speculative and based on the authors' experience of HDR brachytherapy program operation using both of the other previously described alternatives.

Although the consolidation of all diagnostic, surgical, and treatment procedures in one space, the IBU, is ideal, especially from the patient's point of view, a detailed financial assessment should be performed before this very expensive choice for HDR program implementation is selected.

In view of the fact that R/F equipment has to be installed in the IBU and also that the supporting space needs to be at least as large as that associated with the dedicated suite, it follows that an IBU requires up to 50% more floor space than a dedicated HDR suite. Because of these space requirements, construction costs for an IBU would be about $450,000, and the cost of imaging and other associated medical equipment about $500,000. Since acquisition of an HDR afterloader with accessories requires about $300,000, the total capital costs of HDR program implementation, using the IBU concept, are at least $1.25 million. Annual program operating costs would also likely be significantly greater than the annual expenses associated with a dedicated HDR suite be-

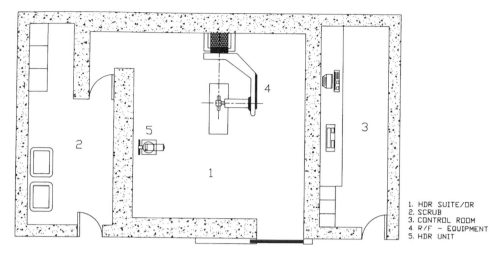

**Fig. 3.** Integrated brachytherapy unit (from Van't Hooft E[5]).

cause of profound increases in personnel costs necessitated by having the IBU in operation at least 8 hours each day, and hence having staff assigned to it.

The capacity of an IBU, however, in terms of patient throughput, cannot be greater than the capacity of a dedicated HDR suite because the patient occupies the unit for the entire time period required to complete the HDR procedure. Thus, it is unlikely that more than three to five procedures can be completed in an IBU in any given day. It may be possible to carry out a conservative projection of the revenues generated on the basis of the assumption that four procedures are completed each day in an IBU. It may also be noted that additional revenues can be generated by making the unit available for ancillary procedures performed as part of, but not necessarily required strictly for, HDR brachytherapy treatment.

In summary, the IBU concept is suitable only for large institutions or departments that can consistently sustain a high-volume brachytherapy operation. Assuming that four brachytherapy procedures are carried out every day, and that each patient receives four HDR fractions on average, a department has to see approximately 2,500 cancer patients per year, and HDR brachytherapy has to be the treatment of choice for 10% of this population. There are very few, if any, radiation oncology departments in the United Staters that see this many patients per year.

## Radiation Safety Policies and Procedures

### General Considerations

Purchasers of remote afterloading units must apply for a license or license amendment with the appropriate regulatory agency—either an "agreement" state agency or the USNRC for nonagreement states and for federal (Veteran

Affairs) hospitals. Radiation safety policies and procedures must be developed prior to application for, or revision of, a nuclear materials license. Issues that should be addressed are (1) safety features inherent in the remote afterloading unit and in the facility design, (2) an initial radiation survey of the facility and subsequent "per patient" surveys, (3) routine precautions required during normal use and during source exchanges, (4) emergency procedures, and (5) training and retraining of personnel with respect to unit operation, routine safety, and radiation emergency procedures.

### Safety Features: HDR Unit and Facility Design

The safety features of HDR units include, but are not limited to, (1) a backup battery system to prevent loss of computer data during power failures (ideally this will also allow for continuation of treatments that have been interrupted due to power failures, (2) a button on the control console allowing resumption of treatment after planned interruptions, (3) a simulation mode that employs a dummy source to test source guide tubes and applicator clearances immediately prior to each treatment, (4) console indicators that show when the source is "in" and "out" of the safe and when the room access door is closed or open, and (5) a last-resort mechanical system for manually returning the source to the safe in the event that all electric source return mechanisms fail.

The facility design safety features include a positive-action door interlock that retracts the source when the door is opened and does not allow the source to leave the shielded device until the proper reset sequence is completed. Other features within the vault include warning lights, audible alarms, a radiation detector independent of the HDR unit, a closed circuit video camera and communication devices for monitoring, listening to and speaking to patients. A clearly visible warning light above the entry door should be in place outside of the vault. A trough or wormhole for dosimetry cables is also very useful. If the HDR unit and teletherapy unit share a vault, special care is required to ensure that one unit cannot be turned on while a procedure is underway on the other unit. Usually this can be achieved by electrical interlocks. Alternatively, operating keys for both units may be placed on a single key ring with no duplicate keys available within close proximity to the treatment area.

### Radiation Surveys: Facility and Patients

After installation of the remote afterloading unit and source in the treatment facility, a radiation survey must be performed under conditions that yield maximum exposure rates in adjacent areas, as assumed in the license application. This confirms that instantaneous exposure rates around the unit do not produce dose equivalents that exceed values projected in the license application. For routine use of HDR units, measurement of exposure rates outside the treatment facility and in adjacent areas "per treatment" is unnecessary if the license application has established alternate procedures to prove that exposure rates in unrestricted areas comply with regulatory standards. This is much preferred to carrying out surveys during each treatment.

Documentation of radiation surveys performed on patients prior to their exit from the HDR suite is generally required for licensure, depending on the regulatory agency and license application content. Such surveys confirm that no sources have been lost in the patient. An independent, visible radiation detector is generally required inside of the room and may serve as the exit survey device. However, it must have sufficient sensitivity to respond to the smallest individual radioactive element used in the HDR source at the maximum possible distance from it. An additional posttreatment survey with a hand-held Geiger-Müller counter is good practice in documenting the absence of any radiation source within the patient.

## Precautions: Routine Use and Source Exchange

Routine radiation safety procedures include, but are not limited to, having an emergency container available in the treatment room, as well as long-handled forceps for retrieving the source in case it breaks from the drive mechanism or fails to return to the primary safe. The emergency container should be placed close to the patient and be large enough to accept the entire applicator assembly used for any particular patient in the event that it becomes necessary to remove the entire applicator containing an intact source. Medical supplies and associated devices to assist with emergency applicator removal should be readily available. A small metal tool chest, having drawers organized and labeled much like a cardiac "crash cart," provides for optimum emergency preparedness. Table 2 lists suggested contents and the organization of such an HDR brachytherapy emergency kit. A radiation survey meter must also always be available, as well as a sign "DANGER—DO NOT ENTER—OPEN SOURCE," for immediate posting if required.

Radiation monitors (whole body) are required for all personnel operating the unit or working in the HDR facility. The use of ring-badge radiation monitors for personnel operating HDR units is a good practice. Although incidents such as having a source jammed in an applicator are unusual and infrequent, ring badges provide an additional measure of dose equivalent received by personnel exposed during such emergencies.

The frequency of source exchange is largely at the discretion of the institution. Source changes must be carried out only by qualified and properly trained personnel as defined in the license application. Ideally, the transfer of sources between the safe and shipment container, and vice versa, should be completed remotely from the control console outside the room or from a properly shielded area inside of the room. Policies and procedures for handling radioactive sources of remote afterloaders are conceptually the same as those for conventional brachytherapy sources.

They usually include, but are not limited to, (1) establishing a procedure for receiving and returning sources (with adequate time after source exchange

**Table 2**

**HDR Brachytherapy Emergency Kit**

Drawer 1: Radiation dose minimization/monitoring of personnel
2 high-dose pocket dosimeters with spare batteries
1 stopwatch

Drawer 2: Removal of source from applicator/catheter in patient
1 pair of wire cutters
1 pair of conventional pliers
1 pair of needle-nose pliers
2 pairs of long forceps
1 magnifying glass with a long handle
1 small magnet with a long handle

Drawer 3: Removal of "live" applicator/catheter from patient
1 suture-removal kit
Set of prepackaged betadine swabs
Set of prepackaged sterile swabs
Set of disposable scalpels
Prepackaged sterile 4 × 4 gauze pads
Wound-dressing tape
1 pair scissors
1 suturing kit consisting of 4-0 silk sutures on atraumatic needles, 4-0 gut
sutures on atraumatic needles, or 4-0 gut sutures and needles; tissue pick-ups;
1 needle holder; steri-strips

to prepare and ship the decayed source); (2) establishing a regular frequency for leak testing—usually every 6 months (if sources are retained for shorter periods of time, the user may rely on the manufacturer's leak test, provided it is sufficiently recent); (3) establishing a regular frequency for inventory checks (since remote afterloading sources are self-contained, it is possible to devise alternate procedures for licensure that substitute for a physical inventory); and (4) specifying the type of radiation surveys to be made with each source exchange in order to (a) ensure that all sources are either in the safe of the remote afterloader or in the shipment container, (b) determine the exposure rate at specific points around the HDR unit safe—these rates must be within the limits set by the regulatory licensing agency, and (c) confirm that maximum exposure rates at points outside the treatment vault, identified in the license application, are within the limits set by that agency.

In the case of a patient receiving multiple fractions who is under treatment when a source change occurs, it is especially important to confirm that the new source activity is used for calculation of subsequent treatment times.

**Emergency Procedures**

It is important to have separate procedures established for electrical (power-loss) emergencies, fire emergencies (involving the treatment facility or remote afterloading device), and radiation emergencies. For the last event, typical complications include (1) the source failing to seat in the applicator and aborting the treatment, (2) potential interruption of treatment because the source dislodges from the applicator, an applicator dislodges from the patient, or a source guide tube becomes loose or ruptures, (3) clock or timer failure during therapy, (4) failure of a source to retract at the end of therapy, and (5) the source capsule or individual sources within breaking away from the guide wire and spilling radioactive material in the room.

The ultimate emergency would be losing a source in the patient, for example, some accident in which the applicator fails, the source breaks loose, and lodges in the patient. Some advance consideration must be given to the actions required if this occurs. We emphasize that separate procedures must be thought out for each category of emergency, and these procedures must provide alternate actions to take if the first emergency response fails. These procedures must not only be posted but practiced by those operating the HDR unit.

**Training of Personnel**

As part of the purchase price, the vendor should include a training course to be attended by personnel who will use and operate the equipment—usually medical physicists, engineers (if applicable), dosimetrists, technologists, health physicists, and attending physicians. The course should thoroughly review available applicators and their proper use, the functions and operation of the unit under normal conditions, the functions and operation of the unit under emergency conditions, all safety features, radiation protection procedures, suggested quality assurance procedures, and all aspects of the dose calculation (treatment planning) system, if applicable.

The medical physicist and engineer should also receive detailed instructions concerning source exchange procedures, if allowed. These individuals cannot be considered qualified to exchange sources until they have met the necessary requirements established by the regulatory agency for persons allowed to exchange sources. Generally, this issue must be addressed in the license application. Proper documentation of the contents of this training and attendance records of those present are required by regulatory agencies.

In general, the written license identifies the individual physicist, safety officer, or other individuals who are responsible for instructing the remaining staff members who operate the unit. The identified individual, usually the medical physicist or health physicist, is responsible for providing instruction on radiation safety procedures to all personnel caring for patients treated with the remote afterloader. This includes retraining at intervals specified in the license.

---

## REFERENCES

1. United States Regulatory Commission. Federal Register 56, No. 98, Tuesday, May 21, 1991; 10 CFR 20;1301 (a) (1) and (2), 23398.
2. Houdek PV, Schwade JG. New criteria for radiotherapy department design. In: Chiesa A, Gasparotti R, Maroldi R, eds. Planning Considerations in Diagnostic Imaging and Radiation Therapy. Brescia, Italy: Clas International S.R.L.; 1988, 515.

3. Glasgow GP, Bourland JD, Grigsby PW, et al. Remote afterloading technology. American Association of Physicists in Medicine Report No. 41. New York, NY: American Institute of Physics; 1993, 27.
4. Schwade JG, Houdek PV, Serago CF, et al. The impact of intraoperative radiation therapy on the planning of radiation oncology departments. In: Chiesa A, Gasparotti R, Maroldi R, eds. Planning Considerations in Diagnostic Imaging and Radiation Therapy. Brescia, Italy: Clas International S.R.L.; 1988, 479.
5. Van't Hooft E. The concept of an integrated brachytherapy unit. In: Mould RF, ed. International Brachytherapy. Veenendaal, The Netherlands: Nucletron International B.V.; 1992, 139.

# Chapter 4

# High Dose Rate Remote Afterloading Equipment

*Glenn P. Glasgow and Lowell L. Anderson*

## Introduction

Delivery of a high dose rate (HDR) remote afterloading treatment requires a radioactive source, a source-drive mechanism with an operating console (microprocessor), an isodose computation computer, source transfer tubes, and an applicator. A radiation oncologist, in selecting equipment, must clearly know what anatomical sites are to be treated since no one combination of these items can treat all anatomical sites. We will review the basic physical properties of radioactive sources used in HDR units, identify the most common features of HDR remote afterloaders and the functions of these features, review specific features of four commercial HDR units, and describe some applicators used to treat the most common anatomical sites.

## Brachytherapy Physics Concepts

Radionuclide beta decay generally produces both beta rays and gamma rays. In brachytherapy sources beta rays (usually with energies less than 3 MeV) are prevented from producing an undesirable, excessive, absorbed dose to immediately adjacent tissue by being absorbed in the metallic encapsulation of the source. Most radionuclide decay yields a spectrum of gamma rays with maximum energies often exceeding 1.0 MeV. The average gamma-ray energy is a useful parameter for comparing brachytherapy radionuclides.

The radioactive decay of a radionuclide is characterized by its decay constant or transformation constant. Each radionuclide exhibits the property that the activity, or the rate at which atoms decay, is proportional to the number of atoms ($N$) present with the potential to decay. The fractional decay rate per unit time is a constant, $\lambda$ (transformation constant), defined by $\lambda = -(\delta N/N/\delta t)$ with units of reciprocal time (e.g., seconds$^{-1}$, days$^{-1}$, years$^{-1}$).The half-life, $T_{1/2}$, expressed in seconds, hours, days, or years, is the time in which some initial number of atoms, $N$, decays to one half of that number, $N/2$. Hence, $T_{1/2} = 0.693/\lambda$.

The traditional unit of activity of a radionuclide is the curie (Ci). Historically, the curie was defined as the number of alpha particles emitted by radon

From: Nag, S. (ed.): *High Dose Rate Brachytherapy: A Textbook*, Futura Publishing Company, Inc., Armonk, NY, © 1994.

in secular equilibrium with 1 g of radium; a curie is $3.7 \times 10^{10}$ disintegrations per second. In the International System of Units, the unit of activity is the becquerel (Bq), one disintegration per second. Hence, 1 Bq equals about $2.7 \times 10^{-11}$Ci.

The apparent activity of an encapsulated source is the activity of an unencapsulated source that produces the same air-kerma rate at a known distance as that produced by an encapsulated source at the same distance on the source's transverse (perpendicular) axis. Because of source self-attenuation, the true activity, or content activity, in the encapsulated source generally is greater than the apparent activity of the source.

The air-kerma rate constant, $\Gamma_\delta$, is a measure of the ability of photons from the radionuclide to transfer energy to air and is given by the quotient of $l^2(dK/dt)$ by A where $(dK/dt)$ is the air-kerma rate due to photons of energy greater than $\delta$ at a distance l from a point source with an activity A. Defined for an ideal unencapsulated point source, it includes all photon radiation, both nuclear and non-nuclear in origin, with energies greater than $\delta$ where $\delta$ often is 11.3 keV (non-nuclear photons are the characteristic x-rays and bremsstrahlung radiation arising from conversion electrons).

When a radioactive source is encapsulated in metal, some of the less-penetrating radiation (e.g., beta rays, low-energy gamma rays, and x-rays) are removed by filtration. The air-kerma strength of such a source is given by $S = l^2(dK/dt)$, where the kerma rate is determined on the transverse axis of the source at a distance of l, sufficiently large that the inverse square law is obeyed. Air kerma strength is the quantity recommended by the American Association of Physicists in Medicine to describe brachytherapy source strength.[1] Air-kerma strength has units of cGy cm² hr⁻¹ for low dose rate (LDR) sources and units of cGy cm² sec⁻¹ for HDR sources. Convenient abbreviations for these units are $U_h$ and $U_s$, respectively. Although both air-kerma strength and apparent activity quantify photons emerging from the source, air-kerma strength is more closely related to the quantity of primary interest, that is, dose rate in water. To obtain the transverse-axis dose rate in air, one simply divides the air-kerma strength by the square of the distance (for brachytherapy sources, dose and kerma may be considered the same); the dose rate to (a small mass of) water at the same point in air is obtained by multiplying this result by the ratio of the mean-mass energy absorption coefficients for water and air. For photon energies between 180 keV and 4 MeV, this ratio is almost constant at 1.11. The air-kerma strength of a given source may be obtained by multiplying the apparent activity by the air-kerma rate constant.

The penetrability of brachytherapy sources is commonly expressed by stating their half-value layer (HVL) or tenth-value layer (TVL) in lead or water. When these thicknesses of specified substances are placed in the path of the radiation coming from the source, the air-kerma rate at some point of measurement is reduced by one half and one tenth, respectively. Higher energy gamma-ray sources have higher HVLs and TVLs.

The specific activity of a radionuclide is the activity per unit mass and is inversely proportional to the atomic mass, M, and half-life, $T_{1/2}$. Radionuclide-containing materials with higher specific activity (lower atomic mass and shorter half-life) and higher density permit brachytherapy sources of smaller dimensions.

## Most Common Features of HDR Remote Afterloaders

A typical HDR treatment requires data (planned source positions, dwell times, isodose curves) from the radiotherapy planning computer for entry into the operating console. As treatment begins, a radioactive source attached to a drive cable moves from the HDR unit by way of the transfer (source-guide) tube attached to the HDR unit and the applicator with quick connectors. The HDR unit contains (1) a safe to shield the radioactive source, (2) the drive mechanism or stepping motor, (3) the emergency motor, (4) the indexer, for moving the source to selected catheters, (5) indexer motor, (6) emergency mechanical retraction system, (7) source position monitoring system, (8) backup batteries, and (9) the simulated (dummy) source and cable and other related electronic components.

The three radionuclide sources historically used in HDR units are $^{60}$Co, $^{137}$Cs, and $^{192}$Ir, and Table 1 lists some of their more important physical properties. Cobalt 60 is produced from neutron capture in $^{59}$Co, which has a high cross section for thermal neutrons, and the subsequent decay to $^{60}$Ni releases two highly energetic gamma rays (1.17 MeV and 1.33 MeV); $^{60}$Co has a relatively long half-life (5.26 years), a desirable feature for an HDR brachytherapy source. Cesium-137, a fission product, has a 30-year half-life; its single gamma ray (0.66 MeV) is less penetrating (HVL$_{Pb}$ = 0.65 cm) than $^{60}$Co gamma rays (HVL$_{Pb}$ = 1.1 cm). Iridium-192 is produced by thermal neutron capture in $^{191}$Ir.

### Table 1

### Physical Properties of Radionuclides Used in HDR Remote Afterloading Devices

| Parameter | Symbol | Units | $^{60}$Co | $^{137}$Cs | $^{192}$Ir |
|---|---|---|---|---|---|
| Half-life | $T_{1/2}$ | (day, year) | 5.26 yr | 30 yr | 73.8 day |
| Air-kerma rate constant—ideal unencapsulated point source | $\Gamma_{\delta)k}$ | ($\mu$Gy.m$^2$/h/MBq) | 0.3085 | 0.0773 | 0.111 |
| Beta-ray energies (maximum) or range of energies | $E_\beta$ | (MeV) | 0.313 | 0.514, 1.17 | 0.24–0.67 |
| Gamma-ray energies or range of energies | $E_\gamma$ | (MeV) | 1.17 1.33 | 0.662 | 0.136–1.062 |
| Average gamma-ray energy | $E_\gamma$ | (MeV) | 1.25 | 0.662 | 0.38 |
| Half-value layer in water | HVL$_w$ | (cm) | 10.8 | 8.2 | 6.3 |
| Half-value layer in lead | HVL$_{Pb}$ | (cm) | 1.1 | 0.65 | 0.30 |
| Specific activity + | A* | (Ci/g) | 200 | 10 | 450 |
| Physical density | $\rho$ | (g/cm$^3$) | 8.9 | 1.873 | 22.42 |

+ Approximate values for practical sources.

It has a 73.8 day half-life and low-energy gamma rays (average gamma-ray energy, 0.38 MeV, $HVL_{Pb}$ = 0.3 cm) and is widely used as a source for HDR units.

$^{60}$Co and $^{137}$Cs have longer half-lives but lower specific activities than $^{192}$Ir, sources of which typically have specific activities of over 400 Ci/g. Hence, $^{60}$Co and $^{137}$Cs sources are used in HDR devices designed for intracavitary treatment with applicators that have larger inner lumens that accommodate the larger diameter (3 to 4 mm) $^{60}$Co and $^{137}$Cs sources, but such sources are less popular now. Higher activity 370 GBq (10.0 Ci) $^{192}$Ir sources with smaller diameters (0.6 to about 1 mm) are best for intraluminal and interstitial HDR treatments. However, the 73.8 d half-life of $^{192}$Ir necessitates 3 to 4 source changes yearly at an annual cost of $15,000 to $26,000. Despite the cost, $^{192}$Ir is used in most HDR remote afterloaders.

Cylinders or pellets of radioactive material are sealed inside a thin-wall metal source capsule designed to absorb undesired beta rays. Depending on design, the source capsule can contain a single pellet or multiple pellets. The length of the source capsule determines the minimum radius of curvature through which the source can turn; the smaller the length of the capsule, the smaller the radius of curvature. Source capsule lengths vary from 5 mm to 14 mm.

Source drive cables usually are stainless steel less than 1.2 mm in diameter. The source capsule is welded (electron beam, laser, argon-arc, or other method) to the end of the cable. The length over which the source drive cable travels determines how far the source can extend from the machine; typical distances are 900 mm to 1500 mm.

Transfer tubes (source-guide tubes) generally feature quick connectors or standard (Luer) connectors for applicators. With some systems the length of the transfer tube is critical, and the connectors may be adjustable to maintain a calibrated length. Generally, HDR units have self-testing mechanisms (optical verifier) to test applicator connectors. If the applicator connector fails, the source either will not leave the HDR unit or, if it is out of the unit, it will automatically retract.

The HDR unit usually consists of a mobile base (casters and locking brakes) that supports an enclosure for the necessary electrical components, together with the source container (often called the projector or source safe). Units typically weigh 100 kg to 250 kg and have a base area of about 1.5 m². Ease of mobility may be particularly important if multiple treatment vaults are to be used. The height of the projector often is adjustable over a few decimeters; in some units the projector can rotate about the base. The projector contains a radioactive source shield (safe) of tungsten or depleted uranium designed to shield one or two 370 GBq (10.0 Ci) or 444 GBq (12.0 Ci) sources and to keep surface air-kerma rates to 1 μGy/hour at 1 meter from the surface of the source safe.

The source drive mechanism (stepping motor or similar device) moves the source, or a simulated (dummy) source, in a few seconds from the HDR unit to the applicator, and then moves it through the applicator in a prescribed manner. The times of movement between adjacent dwell points are fractions of a second. A source-position monitoring system checks the source movement for prescribed accuracy. Two source movement designs are used. With the "step-forward" design, the source is pushed forward to the desired positions; with a "step-backward" design, the source goes first to the distal end of the applicator or some reference point and then is pulled backward to the desired locations. Either system produces a source position accuracy of ± 1 mm.

A simulated (dummy) source or cable is used to confirm proper applicator connections and to test if the source can travel through the transfer tube and applicator without obstructions. The real source cannot be used if this test fails. The simulated source can also be used under fluoroscopy to confirm that the real source is programmed to travel to the prescribed positions in the applicator.

On multiple channel units, an indexer motor moves the indexer to prescribed channel or catheter locations to perform multiple channel treatments.

An emergency system generally relies on a backup battery to permit either retaining programmed computer data in memory or actually completing treatment and retracting the source in the event of an alternating current power failure. An emergency source retraction system usually consists of an emergency motor for use in case of primary motor failure and, additionally, a mechanical manual retraction system (e. g., a one-way hand crank) to retract the cable and source. A radiation detector and alarm system in the HDR unit is a desirable feature; it alerts the user if the source fails to return to its fully shielded position in the safe.

The remote control unit outside of the treatment vault generally is a dedicated microprocessor that controls the HDR unit and the source movement. In some cases, it is a freestanding microprocessor, either detached from the isodose planning computer or communicating with it through a serial port. In other cases these two functions are performed by the same computer system. One unit features a programming card that is prepared at the isodose planning computer and is then transferred to the freestanding controller to perform the treatment.

In the freestanding design, the remote control unit is a dedicated microprocessor with a small display window and a thermal-tape printer. The control unit usually is turnkey operated with status lights (source in/out, door open/closed, alarm on/off lights, etc.) to indicate the status of various functions; dedicated push buttons and a numeric key pad allow programming data regarding source travel distances, positions, dwell times, skipped positions, and other treatment information. Interrupt, cancel, emergency off, and other special function push buttons are prominently positioned.

Some units feature the ability to store, in memory, standard treatments or specific patient treatments for recall. Most units feature automatic source decay correction by an internal clock, permitting treatments to be planned as if the source retained its original activity; dwell times are increased automatically as the source decays to compensate for the source decay. Thermal printers often are used to document treatments by supplying printouts of pertinent data or error codes. Systems that perform isodose computations usually feature a state-of-the-art IBM compatible or equivalent computer with large (20 megabytes or greater) memory, a high-quality color monitor, a printer, a keyboard for data entry, and a digitizing tablet for entering film data. The isodose (brachytherapy, radiotherapy, etc.) planning computer either will be a dedicated unit marketed by the manufacturer of the HDR unit or a conventional radiotherapy planning computer with a brachytherapy planning menu offering a HDR option. The former will likely offer more features specific to HDR brachytherapy planning than the latter.

Dedicated HDR planning computers now offer user-friendly menu-driven software typical of those found on most state-of-the-art external beam radiotherapy planning computers. Data entry is generally by the keyboard and/or with a film digitizer. Some units may feature the ability to enter and use computer tomography scans for planning. Options for source-position reconstruction data entry often include orthogonal films or oblique films or isocentric, stereo shift, or variable angle films obtained with the aid of a localization box. Rapid reconstruction algorithms, screen magnification of regions of interest, point-dose calculations, variable isodose curve selection, and multiple view reconstructions and displays are only a few of the many features now available with most HDR brachytherapy planning systems. Optimization of isodose curves within constraints (e.g., boundary conditions established by assigning limiting doses at selected anatomical points) is a desirable feature for HDR isodose planning systems. Often, multiple optimization algorithms (nonlinear regression analysis, singular value decomposition, etc.) are menu selectable. Hard copy display (life-size or magnified) by printers, plotters, and color copiers all are available. Dose-volume histograms and similar analytic features are also making an appearance.

## Specific Features of HDR Remote Afterloading Units

Table 2 compares some specific features of four commercially available remote afterloaders that use $^{192}$Ir sources. A recent monograph, *Remote Afterloading Technology*,[2] contains a more extensive list of remote afterloaders with other designs. Remote afterloading is a rapidly developing field, and new features may well have been added to these units by the manufacturers prior to the publication of this book.

Report 38 of the International Commission on Radiation Units and Measurements (ICRU)[3] notes that *high* denotes dose rates greater than 12.0 Gy/h (0.20Gy/min). *Pulsed* remote afterloading, which is under active development, uses up to a 37. GBq (1.0 Ci) $^{192}$Ir source for 10 to 30 minutes of every hour, yielding average dose rates of 1.0 Gy/h (0.017 Gy/min) to 3.0 Gy/h (0.05 Gy/min). Since pulsed dose-rate units are attempts to simulate (radiobiologically) LDR treatments, their features are not considered in Table 2.

The Curietron 192 (Fig. 1) is a 20-channel unit. The source is a 99% pure $^{192}$Ir cylinder 0.7 mm in diameter and a 4-mm-long argon arc welded in a 14-mm-long stainless steel capsule 1.2 mm in outside diameter. The capsule is welded to a 2-m-long stainless steel cable of 1.2 mm diameter. The minimum

**Table 2**

**Specific Features of High Dose Rate Remote Afterloading Devices**

| Manufacturer or Vendor | Curietron 192 Oris (CIS-US) (France) | microSelectron (HDR) Nucletron Engineering BV (Netherlands) | GammaMed 12i ISOTOPEN-TECHNIK Dr. Sauerwein GmbH (Germany) | OMNITRON 2000 OMNITRON Corporation (United States) |
|---|---|---|---|---|
| 1.(a) Number of sources and container maximum storage activity | 2 × 10 Ci $^{192}$Ir | 1 × 10 Ci $^{192}$Ir | 1 × 20-Ci $^{192}$Ir | 1 × 12-Ci $^{192}$Ir |
| (b) Physical size (capsule) | 1.2 mm OD × 14 mm L | 1.1 mm OD × 5.0 mm L | 1.1 mm OD × 6.5 mm L | 0.59 mm OD × 10 mm L |
| 2. Smallest outside diameter of applicators | 4.7 mm | 1.4 mm | 1.6 mm | 0.89 mm |
| 3. Method of source attachment | Source silver soldered to steel drive cable | Source laser welded to drive cable | Source welded to steel drive cable using a special weld technique | Source permanently connected to platinum wire |
| 4. Maximum source extension | 1,500 mm | 1,500 mm | 1,250 mm | 1,500 mm |
| 5. Number of applicator channels | 20 | 18 | 24 | 10 |
| 6. Method of source movement | Step-forward; 30 steps over last 800 mm of catheter | Step-forward; 48 steps of 2.5 mm over 12 cm length; 5 mm over 24 cm | Step-back; 40 steps to 400 mm length; 1 mm to 10 mm steps | Step-back in 11 mm increments over 20 cm |
| 7. Source arrangements and dose calculations | Point source at 30 positions, dwell times from 1 sec. to 999.9 sec.; size of step: 4, 5, 6, 7 . . . mm | Point source at 48 positions, 2.5 mm apart, dwell times to 999 sec. in 0.1-sec. increments | Stepping source and dwell times to 999 sec. in 1-sec. increments | Step/dwell times used to achieve desired dose distribution |
| 8. Method of source retraction in the event of failure | Backup battery and winch | Dual monitors and backup battery; emergency hand crank | Hand crank, backup battery | Backup battery; mechanical crank |
| 9. Control unit and isodose planner system | Separate control unit and isodose planning system | Separate control unit and isodose planning system | Integral control unit and isodose planning system | Integrated control unit and isodose planning system |
| 10. Dose optimization | Yes | Yes, 300 optimization points | Yes; 60 optimization points | Yes |
| 11. Special features | Can use 2 sources simultaneously | Memory storage—99 standard treatments | Memory storage of all planned and treated patients | Small source size; allows use of 20 gauge interstitial needles |

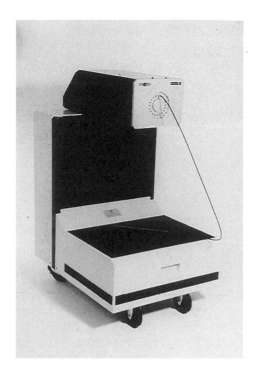

**Fig. 1.** Curietron 192 HDR Unit. (Courtesy of Christian Sumeghy, CIS Bio International, Cedex France)

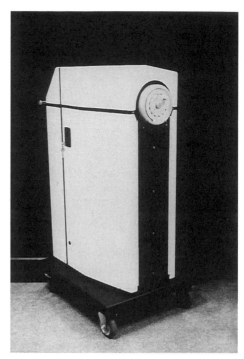

**Fig. 2.** microSelectron HDR Unit. (Courtesy of Miles Mount, Nucletron Corporation, Columbia, Maryland)

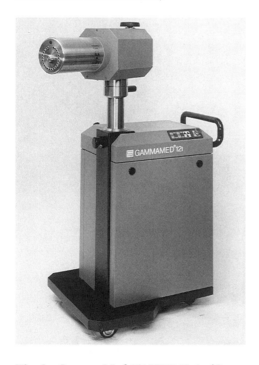

**Fig. 3.** GammaMed 12i HDR Unit. (Courtesy of Steve Woodruff, Frank Baker Associates, Pequannock, New Jersey)

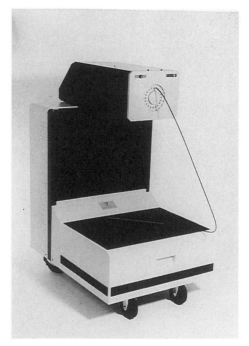

**Fig. 4.** Omnitron 2000 HDR Unit. (Courtesy of Tony Bradshaw, Omnitron International, Inc., Houston, Texas)

radius of curvature is 50 mm. Transfer tubes 500 mm to 1,200 mm long feature quick connectors at one end and Luer connectors for the applicators. The device can use two sources simultaneously in two adjacent channels. The maximum length of the applicator is 640 mm and that of the transfer tube is 1,500 mm. Thirty different positions spaced 4 mm to 20 mm apart in 1-mm increments over the last 800 mm of the catheter can accept dwell times from 1 second to 999 seconds. The unit uses the "step-forward" principle; transfer times are 0.2 seconds between positions separated by 5 mm. The unit contains Geiger-Müller counters on either side of the shielding safe, a backup drive mechanism, backup batteries, and a mechanical winch for emergency source retraction. Although available in Europe, the unit has not been marketed in the United States.

The microSelectron HDR (Fig. 2) is an 18-channel unit. The source is a $^{192}$Ir pellet 0.7 mm in diameter and 4 mm long inside a source capsule 5 mm long with a 1.1-mm outside diameter. The capsule is laser welded to a stainless steel drive cable of the same outer diameter. The minimum radius of curvature is 1.5 cm. The source is moved in a "step-forward" manner through an applicator up to 120 mm long. As many as 48 positions separated by 2.5-mm increments or as many as 24 positions separated by 5-mm increments can accept dwell times up to 999 seconds in 0.1 second increments. Recently, the manufacturer retrofit all units to convert from a 1,000-mm maximum source extension (from the projector face) to a maximum extension of a 1,500-mm cable. The transfer tubes are a standard length for each type of applicator. The unit features dual radiation monitors, backup batteries, and an emergency hand crank for emergency source retraction. The microprocessor control unit is separate from the isodose planning computer but can be programmed using a computer. Up to 99 standard plans can be recalled from memory. The dose optimization algorithms on the isodose planning computer allow up to 40 user-specified dose limiting points.

The GammaMed 12i (Fig. 3) is a 24-channel unit. The smallest $^{192}$Ir source pellet is 0.6 mm in diameter by 3.5 mm long and is in a capsule 6.5 mm long with a 1.1-mm outside diameter. Other source designs are available. Although the source safe is designed to shield up to a 740-GBq (20.0 Ci) source, the 370-GBq (10.0 Ci) source is commonly used. The source capsule is welded to the stainless steel drive cable of the same diameter. The source progresses on the "step-back" principle, traveling first to the most distal end of the applicator, which is a fixed reference distance, and then is pulled backward. The stepping motor allows 40 positions over 40-cm lengths with increments between steps of 1 mm to 10 mm in 1 mm increments; dwell times to 999 seconds in 1.0 second increments are allowed. The source head is adjustable to a 150-cm height and can rotate about the base. Transfer tubes of different lengths are designed for use with applicators of specific lengths so the total distance of transfer tube plus applicator is 1,300 mm. The unit features a radiation detector, backup batteries, and a one-way hand crank for emergency source retraction. One integrated computer system serves as the unit controller and the isodose planning station. The dose optimization algorithm allows 60 user-specified dose points;

a patient management system allows storage and recall of treatment parameters used for patients.

The Omnitron 2000 (Fig.4) is a 10-channel device. The source consists of two pellets of $^{192}$Ir 0.3 mm in diameter and 5 mm long in a nickel and titanium alloy capsule only 0.59 mm in diameter and 10 mm in length; it is the smallest-diameter commercially available HDR source. The source is at the end of an ultrathin (0.59 mm diameter) nickel-titanium alloy wire and is an integral part of the wire. The maximum extension of the source is 1,500 mm, and the source is stepped in 11-mm increments over a 200-mm distance that can be set anywhere in the 1,500-mm length. A "step-back" design is used. Applicator wire lengths are checked after each use to confirm that the entire wire was retrieved with no breaks. The source housing is designed to shield a 444 GBq (12.0 Ci) source. Transfer tubes are of specific lengths for use with applicators of specific lengths. The device has backup batteries and a manual retraction handle for emergency source retraction. An integrated computer system serves as both source controller and isodose computation computer.

All of the four systems described have some other features in common. Simulated (dummy) sources or cables are used for pretreatment tests to confirm that no obstructions exist in the transfer tubes and applicators. Source positional accuracy is stated as ± 1 mm. Self-diagnostic tests are performed to confirm that applicator connectors are secure, that positional accuracy is maintained, and that the source returns to the fully shielded position inside the source safe.

Ancillary equipment often is needed for radiation emergencies, quality assurance, and source calibration. An emergency container (Fig. 5), with long-handled forceps or other source-retrieval system, must be available for retrieving and storing the source in the event the source fails to retract into the safe, separates from the drive cable, or ruptures, releasing the radioactive pellet or pellets. Vendors generally offer source position verification devices (Fig. 6) that use either remote visual observation of the source or radiographs of simulated sources in coincidence with autoradiographs of the radioactive source. High dose rate well-ionization chambers (Fig.7) are now available for confirmation of the stated source activity or other certificate-stated parameter and confirmation of the subsequent decay of the source.

## Applicators and Accessories

Manufacturers of HDR units have been very responsive to customer requests for applicators with specific design features. Two applicator catalogs each list over 15 HRD applicators identified either by city, hospital, physician, anatomical site, or a combination thereof. Many popular manually afterloaded applicators designs are now available for HRD remote afterloading. Readers are cautioned to remember that conventional manual afterloading applicators cannot be used with HDR remote afterloaders since these applicators require special connectors to attach to the HDR units.

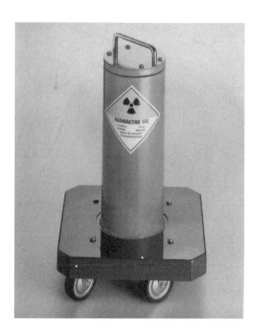

**Fig. 5.** Emergency source container. (Courtesy of Felix Mick, Mick Radio-Nuclear Instruments, Inc., Bronx, New York)

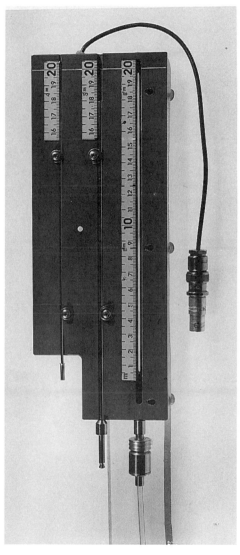

**Fig. 6.** Source position verification device. (Courtesy of Jerome Meli, Yale University, New Haven, Connecticut)

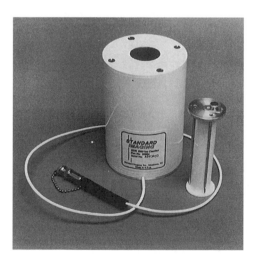

**Fig. 7.** HDR well-ionization chamber. (Courtesy of Ed Neumueller, Standard Imaging, Middleton, Wisconsin)

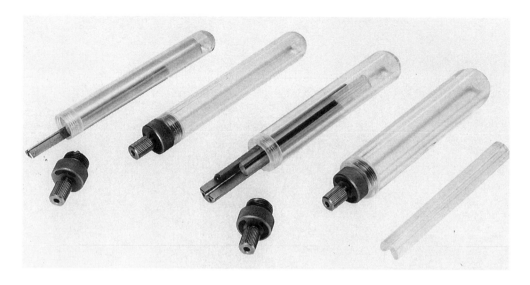

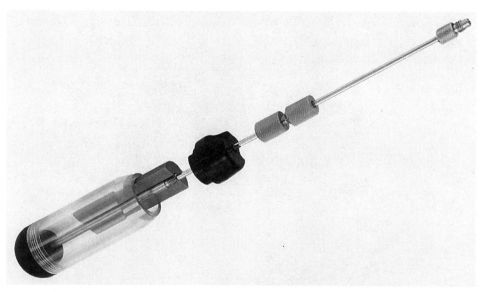

**Fig. 8.** (top) Vaginal cylinder applicator with segmented shields. (bottom) Rectal applicator with segmental shields (Courtesy of Felix Mick, Mick Radio-Nuclear Instruments, Inc., Bronx, New York)

Cylindrical applicators (Fig. 8), 20 mm to 40 mm in diameter, without or with removable segmental quadrant shields, are used for vaginal and rectal treatments. Intrauterine tandems (Fig.9a), which approximate the design of some LDR applicators used to treat cancer, are available. They are either straight or have 15°-, 30°-, or 45°-end angulation and are used with either unshielded or shielded ovoids with diameters of 20 mm, 25 mm, or 30 mm. Fixa-

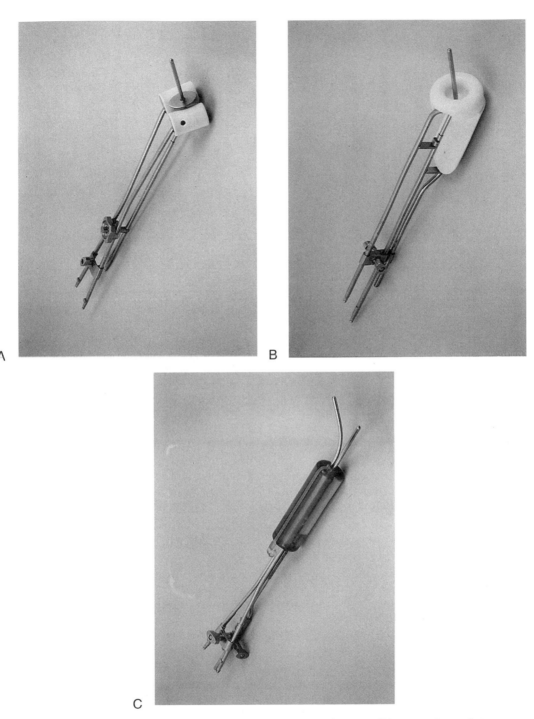

**Fig. 9.** (a) Fletcher-Suit-Delcios-style gynecology applicator. (b) gynecological ring applicator with rectal retractor. (c) endometrial applicator. (Courtesy of Miles Mount, Nucletron Corporation, Columbia, Maryland)

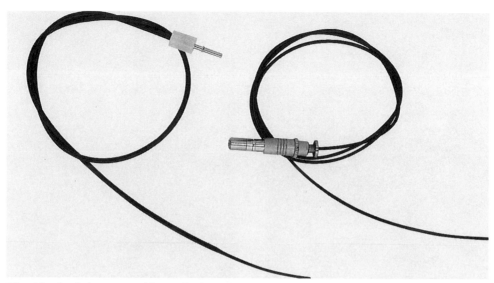

**Fig. 10.** (right) open-end bronchial applicator. (left) closed-end esophageal applicator. (Courtesy of Felix Mick, Mick Radio-Nuclear Instruments, Inc., Bronx, New York)

tion mechanisms are used to secure the relative position of the ovoids to the intrauterine tube. The microSelectron HDR features a ring applicator (Fig. 9b) derived from the Stockholm box with a rigid intrauterine tube technique, popular in Austrian, German, and Scandinavian hospitals. Endometrium applicators (Fig. 9c) feature two 3.2-mm diameter tubes with 15 angled ends; a locking mechanism allows the position relative to the anatomy to be maintained during treatment.

Bronchial applicators (Fig. 10, right) as long as 1 m and as small as 1.7 mm in diameter (5 French Gauge) can be introduced into a bronchoscope with a 20-mm diameter channel. The GammaMed open-ended bronchial applicator has a tapered tip so that a sealing plug can be inserted into the applicator after the bronchial guide wire is removed but before the radioactive source is inserted. Closed-end esophageal applicators (Fig.10, left) are designed for insertion into an outer tube placed in the esophagus.

GammaMed also features a centering intraluminal applicator that prevents the radioactive source from seating against the side of the tube and keeps it on the central axis of the tube. Nasopharynx and oropharynx applicators are available as well.

Numerous apparatuses are available for performing HDR interstitial implants. Flexible interstitial implant tubes of 1.9 mm diameter are available for use with the microSelectron; this tubing is slightly larger than the 1.7-mm diameter tubing used for many manual afterloading interstitial implants. Steel interstitial needles 80 mm to 200 mm long, with a variety of trocar points, are available, as are Celcon (plastic) (Radiation Therapy Resources, Inc., Valencia, Calif.) needles. Needles are available individually or in combination with rectal (Fig. 11) and perineal (Fig.12) applicators.

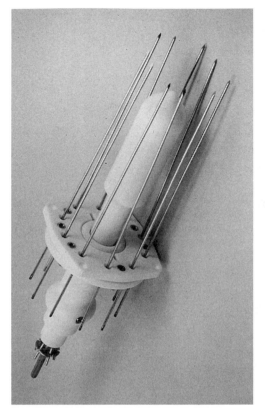 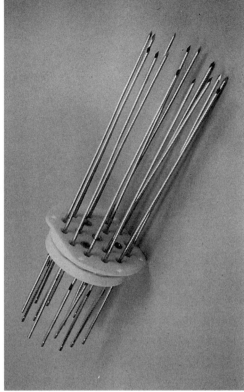

**Fig. 11.** Manchester Rectal Applicator. (Courtesy of Miles Mount, Nucletron Corporation, Columbia, Maryland)

**Fig. 12.** Porter Perineal Applicator. (Courtesy of Miles Mount, Nucletron Corporation, Columbia, Maryland)

For HDR units designed for the source to travel a fixed distance, interstitial needles must be used with matched source guide tubes so that the guide tube plus needle is a fixed length. Mixing of needle lengths and source guide tubes is not allowed; in planning equipment purchases, thought must be given to the interstitial needle lengths to be used most commonly.

Numerous elegant templates designed for breast, perineum, and rectum implants are available. Again, as the diameter of HDR interstitial needles often is 0.1 mm to 0.2 mm larger than needles used for manual interstitial implants, templates designed to hold the smaller-diameter needles may not work with the larger-diameter HDR needles. Special blunt-tipped needles designed for interstitial brain implants also are available.

A host of applicator clamps, base plates, and other accessories are available to position and hold applicators. Standard inactive (dummy) source strands are available to aid with determining, through x-rays and autoradiography, that the radioactive source is positioning accurately and moving to preselected positions in an applicator. All of the applicators and interstitial needles

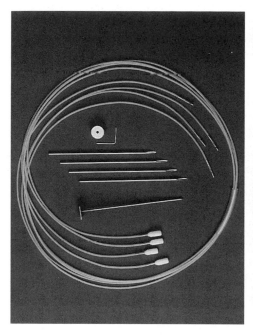

**Fig. 13.** OmniCath. (Courtesy of Tony Bradshaw, Omnitron International, Inc., Houston, Texas)

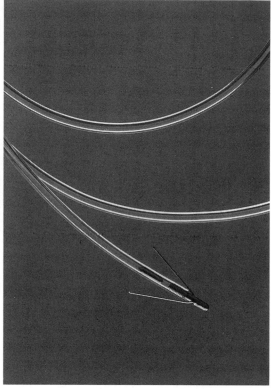

**Fig. 14.** The PulmoCath. (Courtesy of Tony Bradshaw, Omnitron International, Inc., Houston, Texas)

described can be cleaned and sterilized using conventional procedures normally used with manual afterloading applicators.

The Ominitron 2000 features several new catheter designs. The OmniCath (Fig. 13), a special catheter, has a releasable stainless steel marker that can be sutured in place. Sealed access posts on the distal end of the catheter allow fractionated HDR treatments for periods as long as 3 weeks. When the catheter is removed, the proximal stainless steel marker is released and remains at the implant site. Another catheter, the PulmoCath, (Fig. 14) features a flexible metal "grappling hook" at the end that can anchor the catheter at a desired position in the lumen into which it has been inserted. It has a quick release feature that allows it to be easily retracted.

These are only a few of the many special applicators developed for use with HDR remote applicators. These applicators allow new HDR treatment regimens to be developed for numerous anatomical sites; other soon-to-be-developed applicators will expand the role of HDR remote afterloading brachytherapy in cancer therapy.

# Conclusion

This chapter has presented the basic brachytherapy physics aspects of HDR sources and equipment and has described the most common features of HDR remote afterloaders and specific features of four HDR devices. It has also described a few of the many applicators available for HDR remote brachytherapy. HDR remote afterloading technology is changing rapidly, and new developments and methods of treatments are constantly being introduced by those who see the promise that these technical innovations bring to brachytherapy

## REFERENCES

1. Nath R, Anderson LL, Jones D, et al. Specification of brachytherapy source strength. American Association of Physicists in Medicine Report 21. New York, NY: American Institute of Physics; 1987, 21.
2. Glasgow GP, Bourland JD, Grigsby PW, et al. Remote afterloading technology. American Association of Physicists in Medicine Report 41. New York, NY: American Institute of Physics; 1993.
3. International Commission on Radiation Units and Measurements. Report 38: Dose and volume specification for reporting intracavitary therapy in gynecology. Bethesda, Md.: ICRU; 1985, 5.

# Chapter 5

# Calibration Principles and Techniques

*Larry A. DeWerd, Gary A. Ezzell, and*
*Jeffrey F. Williamson*

## Introduction

Often in the past, hospital personnel responsible for the clinical use of brachytherapy sources have assumed that the manufacturer's stated source activity is correct. This assumption can result in errors. As an example, the 3M Co.[137]Cs sources manufactured in the early 1970s were discovered by the Radiological Physics Center and the Centers for Radiological Physics to have an activity 7% lower than the stated activity. The problem was officially declared by 3M to be a 5% error. This is a clear example of the need to independently verify vendor calibration values. In addition, source strength in the past has typically been specified in terms of equivalent mass of radium or activity, whereas the treatment is specified in terms of dose (Gy or rads). Conversion from activity to dose can also result in systematic errors. These two procedures and the potential errors inherent in them justify the importance of this chapter.

Historically, the strength of sealed radioactive sources has been specified using a variety of physical quantities and units. Radium tubes and needles have traditionally been specified in terms of the actual mass of [226]Ra they contain, whereas sources utilizing radium substitutes such as [137]Cs and [192]Ir are usually specified in terms of an equivalent mass of radium. The quantity "apparent" or "effective" activity has been widely used for [125]I and [198]Au dosimetry. The actual activity contained in the source remains in use for radiation protection and regulatory purposes. A clear understanding of these various quantities and their relation to absorbed dose in medium is essential to assure a meaningful and accurate calibration of high intensity [192]Ir sources used in single-stepping source remote afterloading devices as well as accurate dose calculation in clinical treatment planning. Like their low dose rate (LDR) counterparts, high dose rate (HDR) source vendors use a variety of source-strength specification quantities. However, unlike commonly used LDR sources,[1-3] the National Institute of Standards and Technology (NIST) has no standard against which such sources can be calibrated. Consequently, HDR source vendors use a variety of often poorly documented secondary source strength standards and experimental calibration techniques whose relationship to existing NIST ex-

From: Nag, S. (ed.): *High Dose Rate Brachytherapy: A Textbook*, Futura Publishing Company, Inc., Armonk, NY, © 1994.

**Table 1**

**Ratios of Activity Certified by Manufacturer and Measured at University of Wisconsin**

| Source Number | Measurement Date | Manufacturer's Activity | Measured Activity | Ratio |
|---|---|---|---|---|
| 243 | Jan. 27, 1990 | 7.27 Ci | 7.52 Ci | 1.034 |
| 356 | May 12, 1990 | 7.27 | 7.14 | 0.982 |
| 460 | Aug. 20, 1990 | 5.13 | 5.28 | 1.029 |
| 591 | Nov. 6, 1990 | 6.08 | 6.61 | 1.087 |
| 745 | Dec. 6, 1990 | 6.70 | 7.18 | 1.072 |
| 886 | Apr. 9, 1991 | 6.80 | 6.40 | 0.941 |

ternal beam or LDR source air-kerma standards is often obscure. The calibration quantity endorsed by the American Association of Physicists in Medicine (AAPM) is air-kerma strength.[4] This quantity was chosen because of its direct relation to dose in a patient.

This chapter begins with a brief discussion of the need for accurate calibration. Next, source-strength specification quantities and standards applicable to HDR $^{192}$Ir sources will be reviewed. Procedures for measuring air-kerma strength in a free-air geometry will then follow. Finally, the use of re-entrant chambers for routine HDR source calibration will be discussed.

## The Need for Institutional Calibration

End-user calibration of HDR sources is necessary not only to check vendor-stated calibration but to ensure traceability to national standards. Definitions of traceability and standards are discussed later in the section on the definition of standards. Since no national laboratory, such as the NIST, has a standard for HDR $^{192}$Ir sources, vendors assign large uncertainties to their stated calibration values. Mallinckrodt Diagnostica, for example, assigns an uncertainty of ±10% for its activity values for an HDR $^{192}$Ir source. Table 1[5] illustrates the agreement of the manufacturer-stated source activity with the measured activity for a number of sources. This data was obtained using a re-entrant chamber specifically designed for HDR measurements (see the section on re-entrant well-ionization chambers). From this data note that all vendor calibrations for the source activity lie within the stated ±10% limit. However, the range of measured values extends from +8.7% to −7.5%. This illustrates the importance of users measuring their own calibration value, as is done for $^{60}$Co teletherapy sources. This is also the recommendation of Task Group 41 of the AAPM.[6] Good clinical practice dictates the necessity of calibrating these sources since it is very important to be able to specify the radiation dose better than ±10%.

## Calibration Concepts and Quantities

In this section, the various historically-used source-strength specification quantities will be defined and their relationship to air-kerma strength, $S_K$, will be developed with special reference to HDR brachytherapy sources. In addition, the relationship between absorbed dose and source strength will be discussed. Air-kerma strength is a source-strength quantity developed and endorsed by Task Group 32 (TG-32) of the AAPM[4,7] and is consistent with the quantity reference air-kerma rate endorsed by many European and international advisory bodies,[8-11] including the American Endocurietherapy Society (AES).[12]

Abandoning traditional source-strength quantities in favor of air-kerma strength, which is applicable to all neutral particle-emitting sources, has many advantages. Conceptual confusion is avoided since air-kerma strength explicitly defines source strength in terms of the quantities used to experimentally standardize the output of the most-common brachytherapy sources. In contrast, equivalent mass of radium and apparent activity are defined by misleading references to activity, which obscure the relationship between source strength and the experimental basis of source calibration. Use of the air-kerma strength formalism in dose computation eliminates nonfunctional or "dummy" constants, such as the exposure-rate constant, $(\Gamma_\delta)_x$, from the equations relating source strength to absorbed dose in medium which, in turn, eliminates a potential source of significant dosimetric error.

## Source-Strength Calibration Quantities

Source description quantities fall into one of two categories: measures of source output and measures of radioactivity actually contained in the source. The most commonly used source-strength specification quantities, equivalent mass of radium and apparent activity, are source-output quantities. Reference exposure rate, reference air-kerma rate, and air-kerma strength also fall into this class. Each of these quantities is equivalent or traceable to a measurement of source output in free space along the transverse bisector of the source at a large distance relative to the dimensions of the source and detector. As illustrated by Fig. 1, the detector is an ion chamber or other instrument, the response of which is proportional to air kerma or exposure over the range of photon energies encountered. Some output quantities describe output directly in terms of exposure rate or air-kerma rate at a reference point, whereas others, such as equivalent mass of radium, specify output relative to that of a standard source. The qualifier "free in space" entails that output must be specified as if the source pictured in Fig. 1 were suspended in a vacuum of infinite extent, necessitating corrections for absorption and scattering in any medium, for example, air or ionization chamber walls actually present in the calibration geometry. In contrast, source strength specifications using measures of contained radioactivity are traceable to counting experiments or other direct measures of the radioactivity contained in the source, without regard to self-absorption or reduction of source output by its encapsulation. The quantities activity and mass of radium fall into this category.

Air-kerma strength ($S_k$) is defined as the product of air-kerma rate[13] in free space, $\dot{K}(d)$, measured along the transverse bisector of the source, and the square of the measurement distance, d,

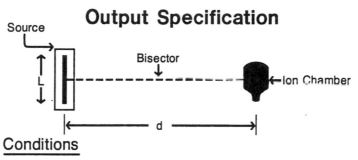

## Output Specification

**Conditions**
1. Large distance d >> source and detector dimensions
2. Free in space
   - measured in air
   - corrected for air attenuation
   - corrected for scattering from air, walls, etc.

**Fig. 1.** Schematic showing experimental setup used to define brachytherapy source output standards, which are the basis of source specification in terms of apparent activity, equivalent mass of radium, reference exposure rate, reference air-kerma rate, and air-kerma strength ($A_{app}$, $m_{eq}$, $R_x$, $R_K$, and $S_K$). The measurement distance d need not be the same as used in the definitions of reference exposure rate or reference air-kerma rate.

$$S_k = \dot{K}(d) \cdot d^2 \tag{1}$$

The geometric relationship between the point of output determination and an arbitrary filtered source is illustrated in Fig. 1. The distance d must be large enough that both source and detector may be treated as mathematical points. Such standardization measurements are performed in air using room-scatter corrections if needed. If kerma, time, and distance are assigned units of $\mu Gy$, h, and m respectively, $S_k$ will have units of $\mu Gy \cdot m^2 \cdot h^{-1}$ as recommended by the Task Group 32 report. In this paper, these units are denoted by the symbol $U_h$, that is,

$$1 U_h = 1 \text{ Unit of Air-kerma strength}$$

$$= 1\ \mu Gy \cdot m^2 \cdot h^{-1}$$

$$= 1\ cGy \cdot cm^2 \cdot h^{-1} \tag{2}$$

The symbol $U_h$ was introduced by the AES[12] to distinguish LDR source strength (which uses time units of hours) from the HDR case, where time is quantified in units of seconds. AES recommended the special symbol, $U_s$ for HDR source-strength specification:

$$1\ U_s = 1 \text{ Unit of Air-kerma strength for HDR sources} \tag{3}$$

$$= 1 \ \mu\text{Gy}\cdot\text{m}^2\cdot\text{s}^{-1}$$

$$= 1 \ \text{cGy}\cdot\text{cm}^2\cdot\text{s}^{-1}$$

where $1 \ U_h = 3600 \cdot U_s$.

The reference exposure rate was introduced by the National Commission on Radiation Protection and Measurements (NCRP)[8] in 1974 to replace relative output quantities such as equivalent mass of radium. NCRP recommended that "the specification of gamma-ray brachytherapy sources *should* be in terms of the exposure rate at one meter from, and perpendicular to, the long axis of the source at its center." More specifically, the reference exposure rate, $R_x$, is defined as

$$R_x = \dot{X}_0 \cdot d_0{}^2 \tag{4}$$

where $\dot{X}_0$ is the exposure rate in free space on the transverse bisector of the source at a reference distance, $d_0$, from its center. The distance $d_0$ is usually specified to be 1 meter, and $X_0$ is given units of roentgen/hour (or some multiple thereof) resulting in units of $R \cdot m^2 \cdot h^{-1}$ for reference exposure rate, $R_x$. Notice that the reference distance, $d_0$, need not be equal to the measurement distance, d. The reference exposure rate is related to air-kerma strength by the following equation:

$$S_k = R_x \cdot \left(\frac{W}{e}\right) = \dot{X}_0 \cdot d_0{}^2 \cdot \left(\frac{W}{e}\right) \tag{5}$$

where (W/e) is the average energy required to produce an ion pair in dry air and has the value[14] 33.97 J/C = 0.876 cGy/R. Equation 5 assumes that the correction for radiative loss by charged particles released by photons having the lower energies commonly used in brachytherapy is negligible. At higher energies, the value of $S_k$ would be divided by the quantity $(1 - g)$, where g is the fractional energy lost to Bremsstrahlung, having the value 0.0032 for $^{60}$Co gamma rays, 0.0016 for $^{137}$Cs gamma rays, and zero for photons below 300 keV.[15] Thus, the values would be 0.879cGy/R for $^{60}$Co and 0.878 cGy/R for $^{137}$Cs.

Reference air-kerma rate, the European counterpart to air-kerma strength, is very similar to the reference exposure rate, except that exposure rate is replaced by air-kerma rate. Reference air-kerma rate, $R_k$, can be defined as the product of air-kerma rate, $\dot{K}_0$, in free space and the square of distance on the transverse bisector of the source at distance $d_0$ from its center. The distance, $d_0$, is usually specified to be 1 meter. If $\dot{K}_0$ is assigned units of $\mu\text{Gy}\cdot\text{h}^{-1}$, then the reference air-kerma rate has the commonly assigned units $\mu\text{Gy}\cdot\text{m}^2\cdot\text{h}^{-1}$. Air-kerma strength is numerically equal to reference air-kerma rate at 1 meter:

$$S_k = R_k = \dot{K}_0 \cdot d_0{}^2 \tag{6}$$

The quantity equivalent mass of radium, $m_{eq}$, is widely used to describe the strength of sealed sources of $^{137}$Cs, $^{192}$Ir, and other radium substitutes by vendors, physicists, and radiation oncologists. It is also widely used as prescription parameter in intracavitary therapy (mgRaEq·hr). It is that mass of $^{226}$Ra, encapsulated by 0.5 mm of platinum (Pt), that has the same air-kerma strength as the given source. Intuitively, it is that mass of $^{226}$Ra that has the same output on its transverse bisector as the given source. Equivalent mass of radium, $m_{eq}$, must be carefully distinguished from mass of radium, $m_{Ra}$, which is applicable only to $^{226}$Ra sources and is not necessarily numerically identical to $m_{eq}$. The unit of $m_{eq}$ is mg, although the 'unit' mgRaEq is often used in the clinical literature. These quantities are related to air-kerma strength by the following equation:

$$S_k = m_{eq} \cdot (\Gamma_\delta)_{x,Ra,t} \cdot \left(\frac{W}{e}\right) \tag{7}$$

where $(\Gamma_\delta)_{x,Ra,t}$ is the exposure rate constant for $^{226}$Ra filtered by the thickness, t, of platinum in units of $R \cdot cm^2 \cdot mg^{-1} \cdot h^{-1}$. In general, the exposure rate constant is defined as the exposure rate in free space at 1 cm from a bare 1 mCi point source. All gamma rays, characteristic x-rays, and internal Bremsstrahlung x-rays having energies greater than $\delta$ are included. Classically, $(\Gamma_\delta)_x$ is considered to be a universal property of the radionuclide so that all phenomena associated with finite source size and packaging, that is, reduction of output by self-absorption and attenuation by its encapsulation, are specifically excluded. By historical accident, $^{226}$Ra is the only radionuclide that is universally treated as having filtration-dependent exposure-rate constants. Thus, we use the special symbol $(\Gamma_\delta)_{x,Ra,t}$ to denote the exposure-rate constant for $^{226}$Ra. The widely-used value of 8.25 $R \cdot cm^2 \cdot mg^{-1} \cdot h^{-1}$ for t = 0.5 mm Pt is based upon measurements by Attix and Ritz.[16] The quantity apparent activity, $A_{app}$, is a description of relative output analogous to equivalent mass of radium. It is the activity of an unfiltered point source of the given radionuclide that has the same air-kerma strength as the given encapsulated source. In contrast, activity, A, is the rate at which spontaneous nuclear transitions occur inside the source and contains no corrections for self-absorption, filtration, or other factors that determine output. It plays no useful role in brachytherapy dosimetry and is used only to inventory radionuclides for radiation safety purposes. Both quantities take units of mCi, MBq($10^6$ Bq), or Bq for LDR sources, whereas units of Ci and GBq ($10^9$ Bq) are used for HDR sources. Air-kerma strength is related to these quantities by the following equations:

$$S_k = A \cdot (\Gamma_\delta)_x \cdot E(d) \cdot \left(\frac{W}{e}\right) \tag{8}$$

$$S_k = A_{app} \cdot (\Gamma_\delta)_x \cdot \left(\frac{W}{e}\right) \tag{9}$$

In equation 8, the effects of absorption and scattering of radiation in the source material and the encapsulation are taken into account by the dimensionless factor, E(d). It is defined as the ratio of reference air-kerma rate, including the effects of self-absorption by the source material, filtration by the source casing, and geometric distribution of the source, to the reference air-kerma rate from an unfiltered point source of the same contained activity as the given source. For a point source of activity A encapsulated by a spherical filter of radius, t, E(d) is given by

$$E(d) = e^{-\mu t} \tag{10}$$

where $\mu$ is the effective attenuation coefficient of the filter material. This expression is a valid approximation[17] for sources that can be modeled as filtered line sources for which the point of calibration is located in the transverse plane at a distance, d, that is much larger than the source active length.

Since both apparent activity and equivalent mass of radium are relative measures of source output and are only indirectly related to the amount of activity contained in the given source, the $(\Gamma_\delta)_x$ values in equations 6 and 9 are dummy constants. That is, the accuracy of the calculated absorbed dose rate in the medium is independent of the value assigned to $(\Gamma_\delta)_x$ so long as both vendor and user assume the *same* value. Vendors using apparent activity or equivalent mass of radium to report source strength in essence convert a statement of source output, for example, $S_k$, into $A_{app}$ or $m_{eq}$ by dividing $S_k$ by an assumed value of the exposure-rate constant. To calculate absorbed dose in medium around such sources, users must multiply the vendor-supplied $m_{eq}$ or $A_{app}$ value by the same $(\Gamma_\delta)_x$ value. For example, Mallinckrodt Diagnostica (supplier of Nucletron sources) utilizes a $(\Gamma_\delta)_x$ value of 4.66 R·cm²·mCi⁻¹·h⁻¹ to relate apparent activity and reference air-kerma rate on its calibration certificates. Should their calibration value specified in Ci be used for treatment planning (not a choice endorsed by the authors), any other value of $(\Gamma_\delta)_x$ in the dose calculation algorithm will lead to dosimetric error. It is essential that users employ the same $(\Gamma_\delta)_x$ values as the manufacturer for dosimetric calculations rather than more physically accurate or definitive values taken from the recent literature.

Although $(\Gamma_\delta)_x$ is a meaningful physical concept, it has no meaningful physical role in the dosimetry of output-calibrated sources. Continued use of such dummy constants constitutes a significant potential source of dosimetric error since the user may choose the wrong $(\Gamma_\delta)_x$ value. In contrast, the E(d) and $(\Gamma_\delta)_x$ values appearing in equation 8, which relates A to $S_k$, are not dummy values. These constants describe physical processes that define the physical relationship between amount of radioactivity in the source and output produced.

## Absorbed Dose and Air-Kerma Strength—Filtered Point Source

The role of air-kerma strength in minimizing dosimetric uncertainty and the use of dummy constants in dosimetry is made strikingly clear by the equations relating absorbed dose rate in water (or any medium) to source strength for geometrically simple source configurations. A widely used dose calculation model in HDR treatment planning consists of an isotropic point source of activity A encapsulated in a spherical filter of radius, t, surrounded by water. Absorbed dose rates (in cGy/h or cGy/s, depending on choice of units $U_h$ or $U_s$) at distance r from the source per unit contained activity, apparent activity, and air-kerma strength, respectively, are given by

$$\dot{D}(r) = A \cdot (\Gamma_\delta)_x \cdot \left(\frac{W}{e}\right) \cdot E(r) \cdot \overline{(\mu_{en}/\rho)} \, _{air}^{med} \cdot \frac{T(r)}{r^2} \tag{11}$$

$$\dot{D}(r) = A_{app} \cdot (\Gamma_\delta)_x \cdot \left(\frac{W}{e}\right) \cdot \overline{(\mu_{en}/\rho)} \, _{air}^{med} \cdot \frac{T(r)}{r^2} \tag{12}$$

$$\dot{D}(r) = S_K \cdot \overline{(\mu_{en}/\rho)} \, _{air}^{med} \cdot \frac{T(r)}{r^2} \tag{13}$$

The factor T(r) accounts for scattering and attenuation by the medium and is defined by

$$T(r) = \frac{\text{Dose in medium}}{\text{Medium kerma in free space}} \left.\right\} \begin{array}{l} \text{at distance} \\ \text{r from a} \\ \text{point source} \end{array}$$

and $\overline{(\mu_{en}/\rho)}_{air}^{med}$ = ratio of average mass energy absorption coefficients in medium to that in air. The mass energy absorption coefficients for air and for water are averaged over the energy-fluence spectrum in free space. The quantity $(W/e) \cdot \overline{(\mu_{en}/\rho)}_{air}^{med}$ is often denoted by the symbol $f_{med}$.

When air-kerma strength is adopted as the basis of dose computation (equation 13), dose rate is inferred explicitly from measured output in free space resulting in unambiguously well-defined physical roles in the dose computation process for each term of equation 13. The term $\overline{(\mu_{en}/\rho)}_{air}^{med}$ in all of the equations converts air kerma in free space at 1 cm to medium kerma in free space, whereas the $r^{-2}$ term relates medium kerma rate at 1 cm to the same quantity at distance r. The factor T(r) accounts for photon scattering and attenuation in the medium, allowing the absorbed dose rate in the medium to be estimated from the medium kerma rate in free space at that point. In the contained activity case, each of the additional terms of equation (11) also have well-defined physical roles. $(\Gamma_\delta)_x$ allows exposure in free space arising from the radioactive material, in the absence of self-absorption or filtration, to be inferred from the rate of nuclear transformation in the source. (W/e) converts exposure to air kerma, E(r) accounts for photon attenuation in the source capsule, and the remaining quantities function as just described. However, the accuracy of the absorbed-dose estimate is directly influenced by the accuracy with which the values assumed for $(\Gamma_\delta)_x$, (W/e), and E(r) correctly describe actual physical processes,[18] whereas when air-kerma strength is utilized, these error sources are irrelevant. In contrast, the $(\Gamma_\delta)_x$ term in the apparent activity equation (12) functions simply as a dummy factor to 'undo' the initial and unnecessary conversion of air-kerma strength to $A_{app}$ performed by the physicist at calibration as expressed by equation (9). Although the same symbol, $(\Gamma_\delta)_x$, is used in equations (11) and (12), it is not used in the apparent activity model, equation (12), to describe a physical process. The absolute dose rate in the medium is in-dependent of the values assigned to the dummy constants, so long as the same values are used for source-strength specification and dose computation.

Equations (12) and (13), which are almost universally used in clinical HDR treatment planning, are both based on the theoretical relationship between output in free space and the absorbed dose in the medium. *Only if the $S_K$ value used for dose calculation accurately represents the true air-kerma strength of the source will any theoretical method of dose calculation, including the point source model, yield accurate absolute dose rates in the medium.* If the experimental measurements underlying the user's HDR source calibration standard fail to accurately realize the definition of air-kerma strength, dose calculation error will result no matter how recent and accurate the dosimetric data selected for implementing the dose-calculation algorithm. Conversely, HDR dose rate measurements must be evaluated critically to ensure that the data are normalized to an air-kerma strength standard based upon a sound experimental realization of its definition.

## Clinical Calibration Problems

Physicists responsible for calibrating HDR brachytherapy sources face a task that is in some ways familiar and in others less so. The fundamental principle underlying the calibration procedure is identical to those involved in calibrating cobalt teletherapy units: measurement of exposure or air kerma at a reference point using an appropriately calibrated ionization chamber, and then calculation of the absorbed dose using well-documented conversion factors.[19] In the teletherapy context, the measurement is carried out at a distance from the source, which is typical of patient treatment and which is large compared to the dimensions of the detector. The radiation field to be measured is collimated to a narrow beam, and it is not difficult to support an effectively pointlike detector in order to make an in-air measurement of the primary radiation for the source with positional uncertainties, which are very small.

The move to uncollimated brachytherapy sources and very short treatment distances carries the physicist into less familiar territory. At "treatment distances" ranging from millimeters to a few centimeters conventional ionization chambers can no longer be considered pointlike, and errors in positioning lead to dramatic changes in the measurement. Although corrections for the finite size of idealized chambers can be found in the literature,[20,21] they become uncomfortably large for distances less than 5 cm. Additionally, any device used to rigidly support the chamber at a fixed distance from the source will contribute unwanted scatter to the readings. Again, corrections for scatter can be determined (see the section on Calibration of HDR $^{192}$Ir Source), but they should be minimized, and doing so unavoidably increases positional uncertainty. Moving the calibration point farther away from the source mitigates these concerns but diminishes the fluence of primary radiation at the detector, and consequently reduces the signal in relation to room scatter and to leakage currents in the dosimetry system.

Choosing a calibration distance, therefore, requires balancing these competing effects. Figure 2 demonstrates one such analysis for a particular Farmer-type ionization chamber used to calibrate a 10 Ci $^{192}$Ir source. The correction factors, expressed as percentages, for chamber size, positional uncertainty, room scatter, and leakage current have been combined in quadrature in order to determine a range of distances for which the combined corrections are minimized. The combined curve demonstrates a broad minimum centered on about 16 cm, with only small increases between 10 and 20 cm.

Various authors[22,23] have described calibration apparatuses called jigs designed to support an ionization chamber 10–20 cm from a source holder. Each design unavoidably compromises mechanical rigidity in order to minimize scattering, and so it is desirable to be able to check the distance from the source to the chamber at the time of measurement. One possibility is to radiograph the chamber and a dummy source at a well-defined magnification. Another technique used to reduce the positional uncertainty is to have dual source holders opposite a chamber midway between them. Averaging the readings obtained from each source position allows the source-to-chamber distance to be taken as half the source-to-source distance. If one assumes that the distance of measurement is subject to some absolute uncertainty such as 0.5 mm, then doubling the distance measured improves the relative precision of the measurement.

However clever the jig design, some positional uncertainty and scatter, even from the surrounding room, will affect the measurement. Goetsch et al.[23] describe a method to account for errors in setup distance and scatter. This method is used for the interim calibration for HDR $^{192}$Ir sources and is further described in the following section.

Another correction to be considered is the exposure to the chamber during the transit of the source to and from the measurement position. This can be accomplished by using an externally-triggered electrometer to collect charge during a timed interval after the source has stopped moving[23] or simply by subtracting two readings taken for differing intervals, thus eliminating the transit exposure common to both. Another method would be to take a current reading if the signal is large enough; this is the case with the re-entrant chambers. Note that the transit exposure can be treated as a "timer error" correction, as is commonly done for cobalt teletherapy, but its magnitude strongly depends on the source-to-detector distance. This transit exposure is significant at calibration distances. The effect of transit exposure under clinical circumstances is the subject of a recent article[24] that indicated that the transit dose can contribute 200 cGy under certain clinical circumstances. The importance of electrical

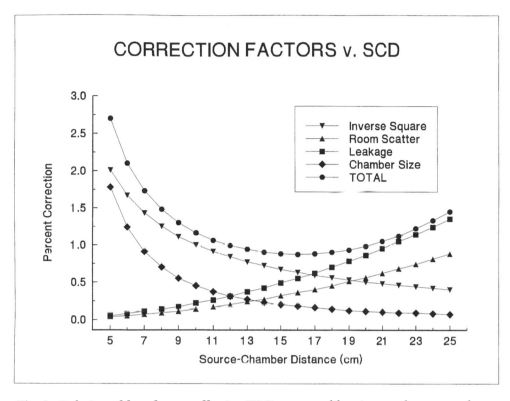

**Fig. 2.** Relation of four factors affecting HDR source calibrations to the source-chamber distance (SCD). The chamber is assumed to be of a Farmer-type design. The inverse square factor reflects an assumed positional uncertainty of 0.05 cm. The room scatter correction is typical for an in-air calibration condition. The electrical leakage correction assumes $5 \times 10^{-14}$ A leakage. The chamber-size correction is from Kondo and Randolph.[21] Combining the four factors in quadrature provides a means of selecting an optimal source-chamber distance for in-air calibrations.

leakage currents in the individual dosimetry system should be evaluated since the signal levels are typically 50 to 100 times less than usually encountered in teletherapy measurements.

An in-air calibration procedure will, therefore, produce a dosimeter reading per unit time at a reference distance, with that reading being corrected for scatter, transit irradiation, electrical leakage, and the finite size of the chamber. Converting the dosimeter reading to the quantity-exposure strength (or air-kerma strength), requires that the system be calibrated for the energy spectrum of the source. Two isotopes are currently used for HDR brachytherapy, $^{60}$Co and $^{192}$Ir. Calibrations for $^{60}$Co are readily available, but to date no national standard for $^{192}$Ir has been determined. $^{192}$Ir is problematic because its emissions fall in an energy gap between the standards that have been established at NIST: free air ionization chambers for kilovoltage x-ray spectra and graphite cavity chambers for $^{60}$Co and $^{137}$Cs.

# Interim Calibration Technique

Until such time as an $^{192}$Ir primary standard is established, an interpolative technique proposed by Goetsch et al.[23] has been accepted by the AAPM as an interim standard. The method has two general procedures associated with it: determination of an $^{192}$Ir calibration factor for the ionization chamber and determination of the source strength using this chamber factor. AAPM Task Group 41 recommends the use of the air-kerma strength as the unit of choice.

## Definitions of Standards

This section includes definitions for the terminology used for traceability and standards. The use of these terms indicates the accuracy of the calibration to national standards.

*Calibration:* The comparison of a measurement system or device of unknown accuracy to another measurement system or device with a known accuracy to detect, correlate, and report any variation in the accuracy of the instrument being compared.

*Primary Standard:* A standard that has the highest metrological qualities in a specified field, typically national standards, calibrated by NIST.

*Reference Standard:* A standard, generally of the highest order in a calibration system, that establishes the basic accuracy values for that system.

*Transfer or Secondary Standard:* A standard that has a value derived from the primary standard. The quantity is to be derived under consistent and precise methods as outlined in protocols. This can be designated measuring and test equipment used in a calibration system as a medium for transferring the basic value of reference standards to lower echelon transfer standards or other measuring and test equipment. In some cases a transfer standard may be used as a working standard.

*Working Standard:* A standard within an institution that has been calibrated at a secondary laboratory, such as the Accredited Dosimetry Calibration Laboratory (ADCL).

*Traceability:* The ability to relate individual measurement results to national standards or nationally accepted measurement systems through an unbroken chain of comparisons.

*Consensus Standard:* A process that is used as a de facto standard by agreement of the community when no recognized U.S. national standard is available. Presently, the HDR $^{192}$Ir standard is a consensus standard.

From the definitions above, the ion chambers at an institution would be termed working standards having at best a tertiary traceability, that is, three steps removed from NIST standards.

## Determination of Chamber Calibration Factor

The HDR $^{192}$Ir spectrum consists of a number of gamma energies. It is different from the pure unencapsulated $^{192}$Ir spectrum in that the lower energy emissions are absorbed in the encapsulation. The spectrum of an HDR $^{192}$Ir encapsulated source can be exposure weighted to approximate the effective energy as being 397 keV. This energy falls approximately halfway between the $^{137}$Cs gamma-ray energy of 662 keV and the effective energy (146 keV) for a 250 kVcp medium filtration x-ray beam (HVL = 3.2 mm Cu). NIST traceable air-kerma calibration factors are available for both of these latter beam qualities. The chamber must be fitted with a buildup cap of at least 0.3 g/cm$^2$, thick enough to block all electrons emanating from the source or capsule, and thick enough to provide charged-particle equilibrium (CPE) for the highest-energy secondary electrons present in either the $^{137}$Cs reference beam or the $^{192}$Ir source. The chamber should be calibrated at $^{137}$Cs and 250 kVp orthovoltage energies, which bracket the $^{192}$Ir effective energy using the same chamber-wall thickness at each energy. Thus, the $^{192}$Ir calibration factor may be interpolated by averaging the other two $N_x$ factors (exposure factors) or $N_k$ (air-kerma factors) and multiplying by an attenuation correction depending on the thickness of the wall and cap. $N_x$ or $N_k$ is the calibration factor given by NIST. These calibration energies are also available from two ADCLs, the University of Wisconsin and K & S. Some physicists have calibrated their chambers at $^{60}$Co and the 250 kVcp x-ray beam. This interpolation technique will still work, within 1%, taking into account that the $^{60}$Co beam has an energy of 1.2 MeV. The closest energy beam is $^{137}$Cs and thus is recommended. The pertinent equation is

$$(A_wN_x)_{Ir} = [(A_wN_x)_{x\text{-ray}} + (A_wN_x)_{Cs}]/2 \qquad (14)$$

or

$$(N_x)_{Ir} = [(A_wN_x)_{x\text{-ray}} + (A_wN_x)_{Cs}]/2(A_w)_{Ir} \qquad (15)$$

where $(N_x)_{Ir}$, $(N_x)_{x\text{-ray}}$, and $(N_x)_{Cs}$ are the exposure calibration factors for $^{192}$Ir, 250-kVcp x-rays, and $^{137}$Cs, respectively, and $(A_w)_{Ir}$, $(A_w)_{x\text{-ray}}$, and $(A_w)_{Cs}$ are the corresponding ratios of exposure inside the chamber to that at the same location in free space. If $(N_x)_{x\text{-ray}}$ and $(N_x)_{Cs}$ do not differ by more than 10%, which is usually the case, then the equation for $(N_x)_{Ir}$ can be written as

$$(N_x)_{Ir} = (1 + x) [(N_x)_{x\text{-ray}} + (N_x)_{Cs}] / 2 \qquad (16)$$

where x = 0.0037 (t/9.3 × 10$^{22}$) for a wall thickness of t electrons /cm$^2$. Once the $(N_x)_{Ir}$ value is determined, the chamber can be positioned in air in the presence of the HDR [192]Ir source to make measurements for an exposure or air-kerma value. This can be done using the jigs as previously described or using the method described in the following section. The Task Group No. 41 report[6] suggests that this method described be used. When jigs are used with the above interpolated factor, agreement within 2% between the old method of using the Co-60 $N_x$ factor with a cap and the 250 kVcp factor without a cap is found.[25]

## Calibration of the HDR [192]Ir Source

An in-air calibration geometry such as that shown in Fig. 1 or the use of standard jigs should be used in conjunction with an interpolated [192]Ir factor as described above. Distances should be large enough that the source appears to be a point source. Distances greater than or equal to 10 cm from the source are sufficient for this purpose. All sources of scatter should be minimized; thus, the holder should be constructed of low-density plastic. The source and chamber should be placed in the center of the room and well above the floor (at least 1 m from any wall or floor). In this location the room scatter should remain relatively constant with any changes in distance (from 10 cm to 40 cm) from the source; this has been shown to be the case.[23] Because the radiation fluence under these conditions generates low current in the standard 0.6 cc farmer chambers, larger-volume chambers such as 3 cc are preferable. Since long times are needed to integrate the charge, leakage effects can become significant and should be accounted for. In addition, the collection efficiency of the chamber should be measured and taken into account. This can be done in the usual manner by measuring the signal at full voltage (usually 300 V) and at half voltage (usually 150 V) and determining the ion collection efficiency using standard equations.[19] Because of the proximity of the source and the ionization chamber, a gradient correction, caused by nonuniform irradiation of the chamber walls, (the Kondo-Randolph[21] effect), should be included. Finally, corrections for the charge collected during source transit (end effect) need to be done, unless the signal is large enough to allow current measurements to be performed. This effect can be eliminated if the beginning of the charge collection is after the source is in place and the charge is collected for a given time period. Alternately, the charge collected, Q, for a time, t, can be taken as the difference between the charge collected for two timed measurements divided by the difference between the corresponding times. The subtraction of the two integrated charges removes the contribution from source transit because it is a constant. Therefore,

$$\frac{Q}{t} = \frac{Q(t_2) - Q(t_1)}{t_2 - t_1} \tag{17}$$

Thus, the equation used for a given measurement at distance, d, is

$$\dot{K}(d) = [(Q - Q_L) / t]*P_{ion}*C_{T,P}*A_{ion}*N_k*P_{grad}*(3600s/h) \tag{18}$$

where:

K(d) is the air-kerma rate in free space and has units of Gy/h at the distance, d, of measurement

Q is the charge collected in time t

$Q_L$ is the leakage charge collected in the time t

$P_{ion}$ is the correction for collection efficiency

$C_{T,P}$ is the correction for temprature and pressure

$N_k$ is the calibration factor (the exposure $N_x$ could also be used here)

$A_{ion}$ is the correction for the collection efficiency at the time of calibration

$P_{grad}$ is the gradiant or Kondo-Randolph correction

and 3600 is the conversion from seconds to hours.

The percentage of scatter signal versus measured signal increases with distance from the source since the measured signal becomes smaller. Therefore, the measured air-kerma rate, $\dot{K}(d)$, could be done at large distances, to eliminate distance setup errors, with an additional measurement for the scatter contribution, using a shielding block. This method of room-scatter correction is used by the K & S ADCL in implementing their consensus standard.

A less-difficult, although more time-consuming, method is to make measurements at several distances and determine distance setup variations and scatter corrections from deviations from the inverse square law; this is the method used by the University of Wisconsin ADCL. In this manner, the response is corrected for both room scatter and the effective distance between the source and chamber centers. A drive mechanism, such as a beam-scanning system or optical bench, can be used for accurate distance changes to maintain the error in setup distance. Thus, if the apparent source-chamber setup distance, d, is in error by the amount c (c can be positive or negative), then the true center-to-center source-chamber distance, d', is given by

$$d' = d + c \tag{19}$$

As explained above, the contribution from the room scatter radiation, $\dot{K}_s$, is included in the measured air-kerma rate, $\dot{K}(d)$. Then the signal from primary radiation only, $\dot{K}_p(d)$ is given by

$$\dot{K}(d) = \dot{K}_p(d) + \dot{K}_s \tag{20}$$

This model assumes that the room-scatter air-kerma rate contribution is independent of distance. This has been shown to be the case over distances of 10 cm to 40 cm.[23] Therefore, at each nominal distance, d, a constant, the air-kerma strength, $S_k$, can be written based on the inverse square law relationship.[23]

$$S_k = \dot{K}_p(d) * d'^2 = (\dot{K}(d) - \dot{K}_s) (d + c)^2 \qquad (21)$$

Three measurement groups at three distances can be made to determine the three unknowns, $S_k$, $\dot{K}$, and c, in this equation, or the unknowns can be overdetermined by doing measurements at more than three distances. The University of Wisconsin ADCL uses this technique with seven distances of 10, 15, 20, 25, 30, 35, and 40 cm. The seven distances above redundantly determine the scatter and error in distance since there are 3 unknowns with 35 solutions.[26] A computer-generated solution then can be used to average the solutions.

## Re-Entrant Well Ionization Chambers

The complexity and time involved for HDR source calibrations can be significantly reduced with the use of re-entrant ionization chambers specifically designed for this purpose.[23,27] These instruments, which are commercially available, must be calibrated against in-air measurements at ADCLs in the United States. DeWerd has performed a series of such transfer measurements using both Omnitron and Nucletron units having different [192]Ir source claddings. These measurements showed that the resultant re-entrant chamber factors agreed to within 2% for two different types of re-entrant chambers for both HDR units. An evaluation of the available re-entrant chambers[28] found that all were capable of long-term reproducibility of 0.5% or better (see Table 2). The chambers are well suited for both formal calibration of new sources and also spot checks of source strength on even a daily basis.

Two significant characteristics of re-entrant well chambers are the simplicity of repositioning the source within the well and the large signal produced. Each of the commercial chambers is provided with a guide tube, which holds a treatment catheter along the axis of the cylindrical well. The signal varies by less than 1% when the source is placed within a 1.5 to 6.0 cm long region, depending on chamber design. Considering the length of an HDR source, typically 0.4 cm, and the repositioning accuracy of the HDR unit, typically 1 mm, it is easy to obtain highly reproducible readings.

The high ionization currents produced in such chambers indicate the need to evaluate recombination losses. Two of the commercial chambers tested in the study required recombination corrections of 0.2% or less, whereas a third applied a 3–7% correction via software. One of the commercial chambers uses a collecting voltage of 500 V to reduce its recombination correction to 0.2%. Independently assessing the need for and accuracy of recombination corrections

### Table 2

### Characteristics of Re-entrant Ionization Chambers for High Dose Rate $^{192}$Ir Calibrations*

| Parameter | Re-entrant Chamber | | |
| | HDR-1000 | HDR-1 | ATOM LAB 44 |
| --- | --- | --- | --- |
| Length along chamber axis over which the relative response changes by less than 1% | 2.5 cm | 1.5 cm | 6.0 cm |
| Standard error of repeated measurements of HDR sources over the 90-day use cycle | 0.03% | 0.1% | 0.1% |
| Approximate sensitivity to $^{192}$Ir | 8.1 nA/Ci | 10.8 nA/Ci | 145 nA/Ci |

*Summarized from Ezzell GA[28].

should be an important part of dosimetry quality assurance. This can be accomplished in the usual manner of making measurements at full and half voltage.

To assure response constancy over time, these chambers should have a consistency check established for them upon receipt. This can be done using a radioactive source, such as $^{90}$Sr or $^{137}$Cs, which can be reproducibly positioned in the re-entrant chamber to monitor consistency with time. Alternatively, an external exposure using a $^{60}$Co source set at a given consistent distance and a given field size can be used. The response of the chamber should remain constant within ±0.5%.[27] Periodic verification of whether the chamber has remained vented (or sealed) should also be done. In addition, it is recommended that the chambers be recalibrated every 2 years at an ADCL.

Use of these chambers for calibration is a straightforward procedure. The chamber should be located in a "scatter free" location.[29] The catheter from the HDR unit, usually a endobronchial catheter, should be inserted into the well and fixed in position. The distance set on the HDR unit should be determined to place the source at the position of calibration, given in the ADCL calibration report. Either charge or current measurements can be made; some chambers have a readout device that is considered a part of the chamber. Unless the readout system for the re-entrant chamber only reads in units of apparent activity, calibration factors are given for air-kerma strength, exposure strength, and apparent activity. The users manual for the re-entrant chamber should be consulted for details. Assuming an air-communicating chamber calibrated at an ADCL, the following equation can be used for a current signal from the re-entrant chamber.

$$S_k = I * E * C_{T,P} * N_{Rk} * A_{ion} * P_{ion} \qquad (22)$$

where:

$S_k$ is the air-kerma strength of the $^{192}$Ir source
I is the current measured from the re-entrant chamber
E is the correction factor for the electrometer scale
$C_{T,P}$ is the correction for temperture and pressure
$N_{Rk}$ is the ADCL-provided air-kerma strength calibration factor for the re-entrant chamber
$A_{ion}$ is the correction for efficiency at the time of calibration
$P_{ion}$ is the correction for collection efficiency at the time of measurement.

Note that not all of these factors are for the various re-entrant chambers. For example, some chambers have $A_{ion}$ and $P_{ion}$ equal to 1.000 as discussed above, and others use a system factor.

These chambers can also be useful for other studies. One was used to investigate the thermal and scatter effects on the radiation sensitivity of chambers.[29] This paper showed that scatter effects were not significant if chambers are not located any closer than 25 cm from a wall. In addition, a study[30] on the half-life of $^{192}$Ir is easily performed with these re-entrant chambers.

## Conclusions

To summarize, calibrations of HDR sources are fundamentally based on in-air measurements of exposure or air kerma. Field calibrations are required since the manufacturer's source specifications cannot be accepted without verification. Experience has shown that calibrations with Farmer-type chambers and fixed-distance jigs are reproducible to a precision of at least 1.5% and with re-entrant well chambers to 0.5%. With the general acceptance of standard methodology, HDR brachytherapy source calibrations can be as consistent as external beam calibrations.

---

## REFERENCES

1. Loftus TP. Standardization of $^{125}$I Seeds used for brachytherapy. J Res Nat Bur Stand 89:295-303, 1984.
2. Loftus TP. Standardization of $^{192}$Ir gamma-ray sources in terms of exposure, J Res Nat Bur Stand 85:19-25, 1980.
3. Loftus TP. Standardization of $^{137}$Cs gamma-ray sources in terms of exposure units (roentgens). J Res Nat Bur Stand 74A:1-6, 1970.
4. American Association of Physicists in Medicine. AAPM report no. 21: specification of brachytherapy source strength. Report of task group 32. New York: American Institute of Physics, 1987.

5. Ezzell GA, Hicks J, DeWerd LA. Calibration & quality assurance: I.In: International Brachytherapy. Veenendaal, The Netherlands: Nucletron International, B.V.; 1992, chapter 54, 233-236.
6. American Association of Physicists in Medicine. AAPM report no. 41: remote after-loading technology. Report of task group 41. New York: American Institute of Physics, 1993.
7. Williamson JF, Nath R. Clinical implementation of AAPM task group 32 recommendations on brachytherapy source strength specifications. Med Phys 18:439-448, 1991.
8. National Commission on Radiation Protection and Measurements. Specification of gamma-ray brachytherapy sources. NCRP report no 41. Washington, D.C.: NCRP, 1974.
9. British Committee on Radiation Units and Measurements. Specification of brachytherapy sources. Br J Radiol 57:941-942, 1984.
10. Comite Francais Mesure des Rayonnements Ionisants. Recommendations pour la determination des doses absorbees en curietherapie. CFMRI report no. 1. Paris, France: Bureau National de Metrologie, 1983.
11. International Commission of Radiation Units and Measurements. Dose and volume specification for reporting intracavitary therapy in gynecology. ICRU report no. 38. Bethesda, Md: ICRU, 1985.
12. Williamson JF, Anderson LL, Grigsby PW, et al. American Endocurietherapy Society recommendations for specification of brachytherapy source strength. Endocurie/Hypertherm Oncol 9:1-7, 1993.
13. International Commission on Radiation Units and Measurements. Radiation quantities and units. ICRU report 33. Washington, D.C.: ICRU, 1980.
14. Boutilon M, Perroche-Rous AM. Re-evaluation of the W value for electrons in dry air. Phys Med Biol 32:213-219, 1987.
15. Schulz RJ, Almond PR, Kutcher G, et al. Clarification of the AAPM task group 21 protocol. Med Phys 13 (5):755-759, 1986.
16. Attix FH, Ritz VH. A determination of the gamma-ray emission of radium. J Res Nat Bur Stand 59:293-305, 1957.
17. Nath R, Gray L. Dosimetry studies in prototype [241]Am sources for brachytherapy. Int J Radiat Oncol Biol Phys 13: 897-905,1987.
18. Williamson JF, Morin RL, Khan FM. Monte Carlo evaluation of the sievert integral for brachytherapy dosimetry. Phys Med Biol 28: 1021-1032, 1983.
19. American Association of Physicists in Medicine, Task Group 21, Radiation Therapy Committee. A protocol for the determination of absorbed dose from high-energy photon and electron beams. Med Phys 10:741-771, 1983.
20. Dove DB. Effect of dosemeter size on measurements close to a radioactive source. Br J Radiol 62:202-204, 1959.
21. Kondo VS, Randolph ML. Effect of finite size of ionization chambers on measurements of small photon sources. Rad Res 13: 37-60, 1960.
22. Ezzell GA. Evaluation of calibration techniques for the microSelectron HDR. In: Mould RF, ed. Brachytherapy 2: Proceedings of the Fifth International Selectron User's Meeting. Leersum, The Netherlands: Nucletron International BV; 1989, 61-69.
23. Goetsch SJ, Attix FH, Pearson DW, et al. Calibration of [192]Ir high-dose-rate afterloading systems. Med Phys 18: 462-467, 1991.
24. Bastin KT, Podgorsak MP, Thomadsen BR. The transit dose component of high dose rate brachytherapy: direct measurements and clinical implications. Int J Radiat Oncol Biol Phys 26: 695-702, 1993.
25. Ezzell GA. The effect of alternative calibration procedures using the NEL 2505/3 ionization chamber: a brief communication. Selectron Brachytherapy Journal 5:42-43, 1991.

26. DeWerd LA, DeWerd SM, Attix FH. Solution to inverse square equations involving distance error and scatter correction. Wisconsin Medical Physics Report #197. Madison, Wisc.: University of Wisconsin, 1993.
27. Goetsch SJ, Attix FH, DeWerd LA, et al. A new re-entrant ionization chamber for the calibration of iridium-192 high dose rate sources. Int J Radiat Oncol Biol Phys 24:167-170, 1992.
28. Ezzell GA. Evaluation of new re-entrant ionization chambers for high dose rate brachytherapy calibrations. Endocurie/Hypertherm Oncol 9:233-238, 1993.
29. Podgorsak MB, DeWerd LA, Thomadsen BR, et al. Thermal and scatter effects on the radiation sensitivity of well chambers used for high dose rate Ir-192 calibrations. Med Phys 19 (5): 1311-1314, 1992.
30. Podgorsak MB, DeWerd LA, Paliwal BR. The half-life of high dose rate Ir-192 sources. Med Phys 20:1257-1259, 1993.

# Chapter 6

# Treatment Planning and Optimization

*Bruce R. Thomadsen, Pavel V. Houdek,*
*Rob van der Laarse, Gregory Edmunson,*
*Inger-Karine K. Kolkman-Deurloo, and A. G. Visser*

## Introduction

Treatment planning for high dose rate (HDR) brachytherapy follows the same patterns as for low dose rate (LDR) brachytherapy, but each step entails more details. The "payoff" for the intensified planning comes as improved therapy for the patient. As noted in Chapter 2 on radiobiology, HDR treatments carry the burden of a decreased therapeutic ratio compared to LDR. To overcome this handicap, the planning process needs to utilize the physical advantages afforded by the HDR system and procedure.

## Localization

The rise of HDR stimulated a rapid increase in the use of fluoroscopy associated with insertions. Part of the increase accompanies the increased number of fractions used with HDR. Some facilities, particularly those using a large number of fractions (e.g., 10), hope to avoid repetition of dosimetry at each session by positioning the application identically to the first treatment at each subsequent session through the use of fluoroscopy. The rapid change in anatomy accompanying the radiation course, as the tumors shrink and normal tissue loses its elasticity, complicates this approach. The appropriate application at the first fraction may well be inappropriate, or impossible, on subsequent insertions. Nonetheless, such an approach may simplify the proceedings in some cases.

Even for applications not attempting to duplicate previous treatments, fluoroscopy assists in correcting asymmetries in an application or in positioning the appliance so as to minimize the dose to sensitive structures. For either use of fluoroscopy, a ready, fixed biplane system greatly simplifies and speeds positioning.

There has been some progress toward using biplanar fluoroscopy images, captured by computer, directly for dosimetry. Such an approach cuts the localization time, but distortions in the television image and limited resolution

From: Nag, S. (ed.): *High Dose Rate Brachytherapy: A Textbook*, Futura Publishing Company, Inc., Armonk, NY, © 1994.

(usually on laterals) has hindered routine application of this method, although none of the problems lie beyond current state-of-the-art technology, only at the limits of medical economics.

Film remains the mainstay of brachytherapy localization. Other technologies that substitute for film in radiology, for example, photostimulable phosphors and digital radiography, also are finding their way into brachytherapy localization but with a several-year delay. As of this writing, no commercial dosimetry system uses localization other than film, except by direct entry of source coordinates.

Commercial dosimetry systems frequently allow users to choose between data entry using orthogonal films or shift films. At least one manufacturer allows anatomical structure entry using one method and source entry using the other. General triangulation using a frame around the patient containing opaque fiduciary markings in a fixed, known geometry gives great latitude in setting the orientation between the two nominally orthogonal films: something greatly appreciated if using a portable or standard radiographic unit. Radiotherapy simulators can provide the required accuracy for orthogonal or shift films. A fixed, orthogonal biplane C-arm unit simplifies the filming process and minimizes the time between films for patient movement. Generally, any of the methods, used carefully, suffices. The instructions for the computerized dosimetry system used will detail the film orientation and information required. Adams[1] gives an excellent discussion of errors involved in reconstruction based on radiographic images; the discussion applies equally to HDR as to LDR.

Notwithstanding the method of localization and reconstruction, two compelling reasons combine to render accurate reconstruction more important in HDR treatment than in LDR.

(1) As noted previously, when radiobiologically changing from LDR to HDR, irradiated normal structures increase in sensitivity relatively more rapidly than tumors. Often, treatments bring neighboring organs to the brink of tolerance. Accurate calculation of doses allows repositioning applicators if necessary to avoid complications.

(2) Geometrically, changes in application position can be made before treatment delivery more effectively than with LDR since the applicator and retractors maintaining distance from normal structures can be held in place during treatment.

The lack of immobilization of the applicator in LDR wasted high accuracy in reconstruction and dosimetry. The section "Execution of the Planned Treatment" discusses immobilization in more detail.

## Dose Specification and Prescription

As with any radiotherapy treatment, certain quantities must be specified.

(1) *The absolute dose to a reference location.* The reference location can be a visible anatomical structure, such as the trigone of the bladder contain-

ing contrast; an invisible (on a radiograph) anatomical structure with a location defined with respect to visible structures, such as the pelvic lymph nodes using Chassagne's pelvic-wall reference points;[2] or an invisible anatomical structure with a location defined with respect to visible parts of an applicator, such as Paterson's modification of the Manchester Point A.[3] The Paris Dosimetry System (PDS)[4,5] uses the "low-dose" positions between catheters (known as basal dose points) as reference locations (though defining the reference dose as a fraction of the dose at these locations). In most situations, the reference location should relate to the dose target, rather than regions of concern for normal tissues.

(2) *Relative doses to specified volumes.* Treating a target volume adequately requires delivering the dose to more than just a point. Often, in LDR brachytherapy, the distribution would be specified simply by stating the source loading and the treatment volume accepted as inferred from that loading. Practitioners frequently described tandem and ovoid applications or endobronchial treatments simply by quoting activities and lengths. This practice arose, at least in part, because of the limited ability to vary the activity distribution with a given inventory of radium or cesium sources or with iridium wire. As commented upon earlier, HDR planning sessions usually start with a desired dose distribution and calculate a time distribution for the source that produces that desired distribution.

(3) *Fractionation schema.* With LDR, the dose rate determines both the biological effectiveness of the application and the duration, given a prescribed dose. HDR applications use a high enough dose rate so that the time required to deliver any practical dose remains short compared to the half-time of radiation repair (about 1.5 hours), removing it as a variable for biological effectiveness. Instead, the dose per fraction and number of fractions enter into the calculation. The schema also spells out the relationship between brachytherapy and external beam treatments.

(4) *Limitations.* As stated before, brachytherapy prescriptions frequently treat normal structures to their tolerance. As such, these structures limit the maximum dose a given application can deliver. These limits serve as boundary conditions on the optimized weighting distribution.

Dosimetry "systems," such as the Manchester system[6] or the PDS, can still be used with HDR treatments, provided appropriate changes are made in the dose per fraction accounting for the different radiobiological effectiveness,[7] and, of course, changes from a fixed time with various activities to a fixed activity with various times. Often, the systems provide a basis with which to begin, but with the flexibility of the HDR stepping-source mechanism, dose distributions can be obtained with lower doses to normal tissues (for example, by keeping the dwells within the target volume) and improved dose homogeneity within the target volume. As an example of changes that should be made, consider a typical Paris-system volume implant, with the basal dose

(BD) taken as the average of the doses at the low-dose points between the catheters (basal dose points) and the dose given to the target, the reference dose (RD), specified as 85% of the BD. Because of uniform loading of such an implant, the doses at the interior-most basal dose points exceed the doses at the outer basal dose points. Assume that the lowest-dosed basal dose points deliver the minimum acceptable dose in the target volume and that the excessive doses at the remainder of the basal dose points, and over the remainder of the implanted volume as a whole, provide no increased benefit but may increase later complications (not a universally accepted assumption). Reducing through optimization the high-dose values at the inner basal dose points while keeping the outer basal dose points at their desired value lowers the BD. Thus, to deliver the same absolute dose, RD, to the same volume as before, a higher percentage of the BD must be used (e.g., 90%). Thus, the optimization results not only in a more uniform dose throughout the implanted volume (reducing the spread of doses at the basal dose points) but a more uniform dose throughout the target volume (by raising the percentage at the edge of the volume).

With a Manchester system implant, a similar change in dose may follow optimization. Although the Manchester system rules define a limited optimization (and often, very well), a stepping-source afterloader can improve the uniformity through the implanted volume. The Manchester system specifies the dose as a nominal dose ± 10%, that is to say, a nominal dose 11% above the minimum dose, with the maximum dose approximately 22% above the minimum. Reducing the variation to ± 5% effectively raises the minimum dose by approximately 5%. If the desire is to keep the same minimum dose in the implanted volume (i.e., hold tumor control constant while reducing complications), the nominal specified dose would have to decrease by 5%.

As discussed by Thomadsen et al.,[8] because the biological effectiveness increases with increased dose per fraction, to obtain the same differential in relative biological effectiveness between two dose levels as was obtained in LDR, for example, between the BD (100%) and the RD (90% in an optimized case), the differential with HDR must be moderated to some extent. Assuming that acute effects limit the maximum dose that can be delivered without complication in the implanted volume, and that the BD runs 111% higher than the RD (the isodose surface where the implant delivers the prescribed dose), by delivering 5 HDR fractions of 9.1 Gy each to achieve the same biological effect to the tumor as 70 Gy at 0.55 Gy/hr with a LDR implant, the relative biological effectiveness at the BD runs 113.5%. If late-responding tissues limit the maximum doses, the relative biological effectiveness at the BD increases to 116.6%. Thus, because the biological effectiveness changes more steeply with the dose for HDR than for LDR, designing optimized HDR implants to push both BD and RD tissues to their tolerances requires greater dose uniformity than with LDR, possibly using RD = 0.93 BD.

An example of modifications to a LDR system to adapt to HDR follows. The example ignores the biological effects and the required increase in uniformity to examine the changes accompaning optimization. To include these other effects, simply change the RD from 85% to 90% or 93% of the BD.

**The Stepping Source Dosimetry System as an Extension of the Paris Dosimetry System**

The Paris Dosimetry System (PDS) was designed for LDR implants of needles or flexible catheters, loaded with wires of equal linear activity or with regularly spaced pellets of equal activity.[9] For a given target volume, the Paris system specifies the spacing between the active lengths in the catheters and gives rules on how to implant a target volume V = L × W × T as a function of L, W, and T, with L the length, W the width, and T the thickness of the target volume.

The PDS can easily be adapted to HDR by applying equidistant dwell positions with equal dwell times. However, while the application of a stepping source appears so much like an iridium wire, the use of increased dwell times at the longitudinal ends of the implant (through optimization) keeps the active dwell positions inside the target volume. The extension of the PDS to include this optimization can be called the Stepping Source Dosimetry System (SSDS).[10]

*Summary of The Paris Dosimetry System*

The PDS uses the following parameters (see Fig. 1).

(1) S is the spacing between the catheters.
(2) In a single-plane implant the lateral margin, $M_l$, is the lateral distance between the reference isodose line and the outer catheters in the central transversal and longitudinal plane.
(3) In multiplane implants the safety margin, $M_s$, is the distance between the reference isodose line and the outer catheters in the central transversal plane.

The PDS implantation rules can be approximated as follows:

(1) The spacing S varies between 8–15 mm for short implants (L ≤ 3 cm, AL ≤ 4 cm) and 15–22 mm for long implants (L ≥ 7 cm, AL ≥ 10 cm).
(2) For a target thickness T ≤ 12 mm, single plane implants are used, with S ≈ T/0.6, which gives $M_s$ ≈ 0.35 × S.
(3) For T ≥ 12 mm double-plane implants are used. A double-plane implant with a catheter pattern in triangles must conform to S ≈ T/1.3, which gives $M_s$ ≈ 0.2 × S. For a double plane implant in squares S ≈ T/1.57, which gives $M_s$ ≈ 0.27 × S.
(4) The active lengths in the catheters for single-and double-plane implants are given by AL ≈ L/ 0.7 for iridium wires and by AL ≈ L/0.8 for iridium pellets spaced 5 mm apart. The active lengths extend outside the target to correct for the bending of the reference isodose surface in between the catheter ends.

As described above, basal dose points are defined in the central transversal plane through the implant and are located midway between the catheters,

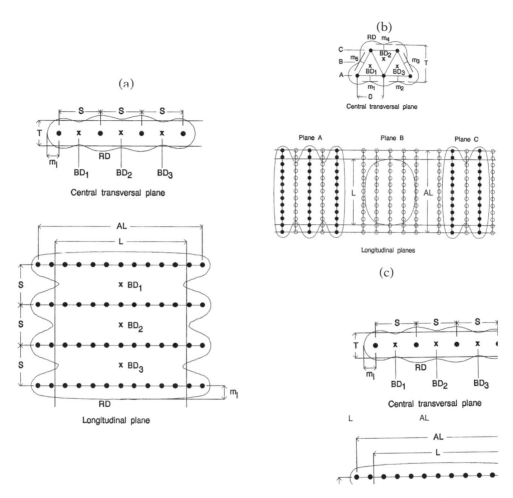

**Fig. 1.** Definitions of the parameters of the Paris Dosimetry System (PDS) for a (a) single-plane implant, (b) double-plane implant in a triangular pattern, and (c) double-plane implant in a square pattern, where ● = dwell position in the plane of dose distribution; ○ = dwell position either behind or in front of the plane of dose distribution; x = basal dose point, midway between the surrounding catheters; s = spacing between the catheters; T = thickness of the target volume; L = length of the target volume; AL = active length of the catheter; BD = the basal dose defined as the average dose in the basal dose points in the central transverse plane; RD = the reference dose isodose line, equal to 85% of BD; $m_l$ = lateral margin between the reference isodose line and the outer catheters in a single-plane implant; $m_s$ = safety margin, defined as the average margin between the reference isodose line and the outer catheters for multiplane-implants.

where the dose rate is lowest (see again Fig. 1). The BD is the mean of these dose points. The RD is taken as 85% of the BD. It defines an isodose surface extending 0.5 cm from the outer catheters (Fig. 2). This isodose surface will encompass the target volume T × W × L if the aforementioned rules are followed.

## *The Stepping Source Dosimetry System*

The Stepping Source Dosimetry System (SSDS) uses the same implant rules as the PDS, except that the active lengths in the catheters remains within 0.5 cm from the reference isodose surface. Thus, AL ≈ L − 1.0 cm. The dwell positions in the catheters are again taken equidistant. In SSDS dose points are defined between the catheters along the active lengths and thus through the whole target volume (Fig. 3). The dwell times are optimized such that practically the same dose is obtained in all dose points. The RD is taken as 85% of the mean dose in all dose points, as discussed above.

## *Differences Between SSDS and PDS*

(1) *Active lengths in catheters.* In a PDS implant the active wires or pellets must extend outside the target volume in order to compensate for the dose falloff at the ends of the implanted wires or catheters. For example, the extension for a target length of 7 cm, treated with a double-plane implant, is 1.5 cm at either end (see Fig. 2b).

In an optimized HDR stepping-source implant, the dwell times are such that the same dose is obtained in all dose points midway between the catheters over the whole length of the implant. This results in increased dwell times at the outer parts of the implant (see Fig. 3b). Contrary to the PDS-type implant, all dwell positions are now located inside the target volume. The RD isodose surface is encompassing the implant at a distance of 0.5 cm from the active dwell positions in the outer catheters.

(2) *Target volume and treated volume.* In a PDS implant the reference isodose dips deeply between the catheters at the outer ends of the implant owing to the linear source strength of the wire or the equal source strength of the pellets (Fig. 4b). Therefore, implants according to the PDS extend the active lengths outside the target. This results in an appreciable volume outside the target receiving a dose equal to or higher than the RD.

In an SSDS implant the increased dwell times at the outer ends of the catheters flatten the reference isodose surface in that area. As a result the outer active dwell positions should stay inside the target volume at 0.5 cm from the target surface (see Fig. 4b).

(3) *Dose homogeneity over the target volume.* In both implant systems the dose is quite uniform along the catheters in the central part of the implant. In the PDS the inner catheters have the same strength as the outer ones, resulting in a higher dose in the central part (Fig. 2). The differential volume-dose histogram (discussed later in this chapter) shows a peak at two dose values, each peak corresponding to a large volume (Fig. 5). The volume found at the lower dose is the volume between the outer

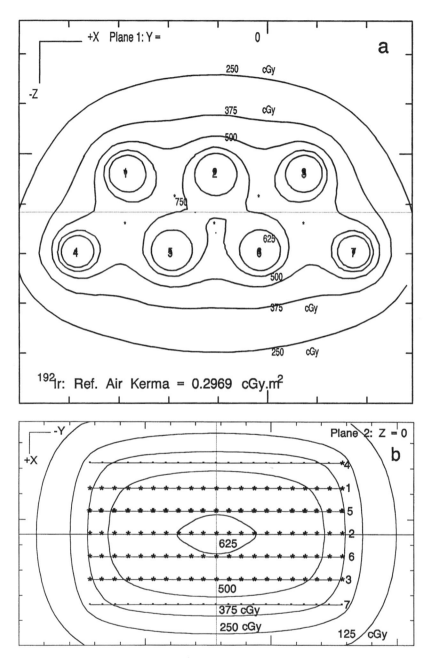

**Fig. 2.** Biplane breast implant according to the PDS. The dwell positions are equally spaced at 0.5 cm and are equally weighted. The reference dose, RD, is defined as 0.85 × mean dose in basal dose points in the central transverse plane. RD = 500 cGy. (a.) Central transversal plane· · · · · · · · indicates the central longitudinal plane. (b.) Central longitudinal plane· · · · · · · · indicates the central transversal plane.

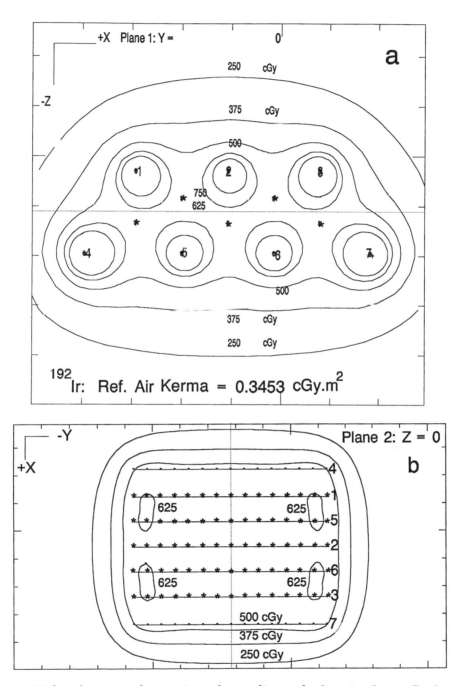

**Fig. 3.** Biplane breast implant optimized according to the Stepping Source Dosimetry System (SSDS). Active length of the catheters is 7 cm. The dwell positions are equally spaced at 0.5 cm. The dwell times are optimized to the same dose in all dose points. Reference dose, RD, is defined as 0.85 × best fit dose over all basal dose points in the central transverse plane. RD = 500 cGy. (a.) Central transversal plane· · · · · · · · indicates the central longitudinal plane. (b.) Central longitudinal plane· · · · · · · · indicates the central transversal plane.

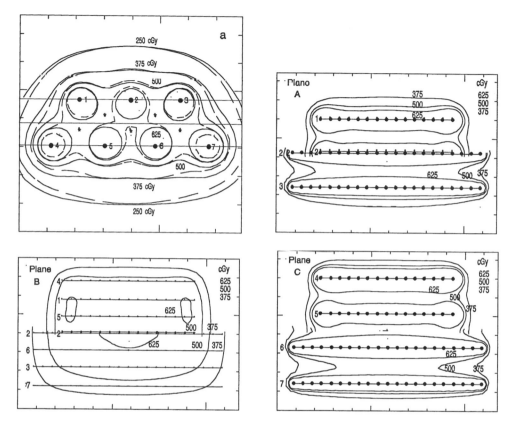

**Fig. 4.** Comparison of the resulting dose distributions with the PDS and the SSDS in Figs. 2 and 3. The upper left panel shows the central transverse plane: ——— indicates dose distribution optimized according to SSDS to the same dose in all dose points. Active length of the catheters is 7 cm. The RD (85% of the mean of all dose points) = 500 cGy. - - - - - - indicates dose distribution according to the PDS. The RD (85% of the mean of all basal dose points in the central transverse plane) = 500 cGy. Both reference isodose lines coincide except around the outer catheters where the PDS RD line bends inward to the implant. The SSDS distribution is the more homogeneous. The other panels compare the doses in the longitudinal planes: Plane A: the plane through catheters 1, 2, and 3 in Fig. 4a. Plane B: the central longitudinal plane. Plane C: the plane through catheters 4, 5, 6, and 7 in Fig. 4a. The upper part of each dose distribution is given by the SSDS implant and the lower part by the PDS. Note the more regular shape of the 500 cGy isodose line with the SSDS implant.

catheters 1, 4, and 5, and between 3, 6, and 7. The volume found at the higher dose corresponds to the volume between catheters 1, 2, 5; 2, 5, 6; and 2, 3, 6 in Figure 2a.

In SSDS the optimization of the dwell times of the stepping source leads to the same dose in all dose points in the inner regions and also in the outer regions of the implant. As is clearly seen in the differential volume-dose histogram, Fig. 6, a single large peak now appears, corresponding to a much larger volume under the peak dose. This is due to the optimization process that aims at obtaining the same dose in all dose

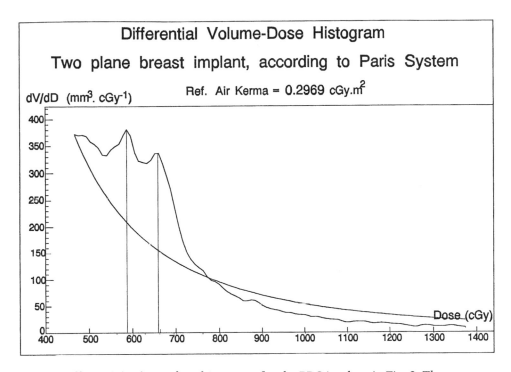

**Fig. 5.** Differential volume-dose histogram for the PDS implant in Fig. 2. The curve underlying the histogram is given by a point source in the center of the implant, indicating the influence of the inverse square law on the histogram. The peak at 660 cGy is caused by the volumes between the inner catheters (1, 2, 5; 2, 5, 6; and 2, 3, 6), and the peak at 580 cGy is caused by the volumes between the outer catheters (1, 4, 5; and 3, 6, 7).

points placed between the catheters and results in a large volume with that dose (see Fig. 3).

(4) *Reference dose (RD).* In PDS and SSDS the RD is the prescribed dose value on an isodose surface encompassing the target volume. In the Paris system the RD is based on the mean value of the basal dose points in the central plane only. In SSDS the RD is based on the mean dose over all dose points in the implant. As the dwell times are optimized to obtain the same dose in all dose points, the mean dose over all dose points is practically equal to the mean dose over the dose points in the central plane only. This explains why the reference isodose of both systems practically coincides in the central plane, except around the outer catheters.

This is demonstrated in Fig. 4a by catheters 4 and 7. In SSDS the outer catheters 4 and 7 are more heavily weighted than the inner catheters in order to compensate for the lack of dose from surrounding catheters and to prevent the inward bending of the 500 cGy reference isodose line around catheters 4 and 7, as occurs in the PDS.

In the volume-dose histogram of the SSDS implant (see Fig. 6), the dose under the peak, thus the dose with maximum volume-dose

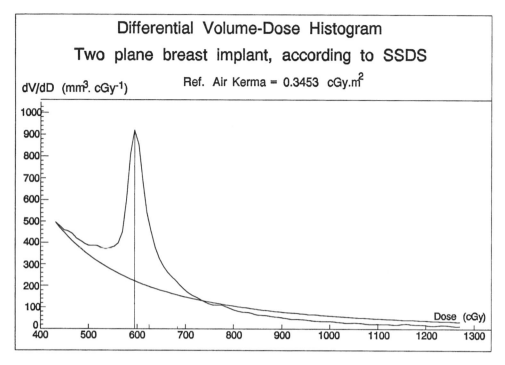

**Fig. 6.** Differential volume-dose histogram for the SSDS implant in Fig. 3. Again, the curve underlying the histogram is given by a point source in the center of the implant, indicating the influence of the inverse square law on the histogram. The large volume under the peak at 590 cGy corresponds to the volume around the dose points between the catheters, which are optimized to the same dose. Note that 85% of 590 cGy is 501.5 cGy, which is very close to the RD of 500 cGy in Fig. 3, the difference being caused by the voxel size of the histogram.

gradient, dV/dD, is equal to the mean dose in all dose points. So the reference dose is also equal to 85% of the peak dose in the differential volume-dose histogram.

(5) *Dose distribution.* The difference between the dose distribution according to the PDS and the SSDS is presented in Fig. 4. The RD of the PDS-type implant is taken as 85% of the mean dose in the dose points in the central plane only, and the RD of the SSDS-type implant is taken as 85% of the mean dose in all dose points over the implant. The RD in both cases is 500 cGy. The dotted lines in Fig. 4a are the isodose lines obtained with the PDS. The solid lines are the isodose lines obtained by SSDS, thus optimized to the same dose in the dose points placed midway between the catheters along the whole length of the implant.

Figure 4b compares the dose distribution of SSDS and the PDS in the planes through needles 1, 2, 3, through needles 4, 5, 6, 7, and in the longitudinal midplane. The upper half of the dose distribution of each plane is given by the SSDS implant, the lower half by the PDS-type implant. It is clearly shown that the SSDS implant gives a more homogeneous dose coverage of the target volume than does the Paris implant. The RD isodose line extends in the transversal planes 0.5 cm outward and in the longitudinal planes to at least 0.25 cm outward.

## Comparison with Geometric Optimization

A stepping source dose distribution obtained by geometrical optimization[11] (discussed later in this chapter) has a homogeneity over the target, which lies between the one obtained with optimization on rows of dose points and the one according to the PDS. Preliminary results show that by taking the active length in each catheter equal to the corresponding target dimension, thus AL ≈ L, the reference isodose surface again encloses the target volume completely.

## Dose Calculation

### Dose to a Target From a Dwell Position

For the most part, HDR dose calculations follow the same procedures and use the same algorithms as LDR calculations. This topic receives adequate coverage in more basic radiotherapy physics texts, so only aspects particularly pertaining to HDR planning will be covered here.

In nearly all clinical situations, points of interest will be far enough (more than about 7mm) from source dwell positions that the very small iridium-192 sources (or cobalt-60 pellets) used in HDR remote afterloading may be considered point sources for calculational purposes, according to Quimby's criterion (distance to a point of interest > 2 · source length).[12] The basic equation for the dose, ignoring the effects of heterogeneities in the surrounding medium, would be

$$\text{Dose} = (\text{Air-kerma rate* @ 1 m}) \, (\text{time}) \, k \, (\mu_{en}/\rho)_{tissue}/[(\mu_{en}/\rho)_{air} \, r^2] \qquad (1)$$

where k = the ratio of the dose in an infinite water phantom to that in air, and

$$\left(\frac{\mu_{en}}{\rho}\right)^{tissue}_{air} = 1.10$$

for both $^{192}$Ir and $^{60}$Co.[13] The time in the equation explicitly must be very short compared to the half-life of the source material (t $<<$ T$_{1/2}$), a stipulation always satisfied with HDR treatments by definition. Older computer systems often only allow source strength entry in terms of activity, usually in mCi, or radium equivalent (mg Ra eq.). This "activity" is derived by dividing the measured air-kerma rate by the air-kerma rate constant (Γ) for the isotope (for "activity") or for radium (for radium equivalent). Although considerable effort has gone into

---

*In conventional dosimetry using exposure rate instead of air-kerma rate, the equation becomes Dose = (exposure rate @ 1 m) f (time)/r², where f = dose/exposure factor.

establishing correct values for the air-kerma rate constant, in practice, the actual value used may be irrelevant, or, what is worse, may lead to error. The first step in a typical dose calculation using activity finds the activity from the air-kerma rate at 1 m by dividing by $\Gamma$ at the time of calibration. The second step calculates the air-kerma rate at 1 m by multiplying the activity by $\Gamma$ at the time of dose calculation. If the same value for $\Gamma$ is used in both steps, the effect of the multiplication merely is to cancel the result of the earlier division. The use of a different value in each of the two steps (e.g., if the dose-calculation computer has a built-in value different from that selected by the calibrating physicist from the assorted values in the literature) results in an error.

The attenuation of the capsule surrounding the source is often ignored. The calibration procedure usually just yields an air-kerma rate at 1 m for the source as a whole: radioactive material and capsule. The dose computation implicitly assumes that the attenuation in tissue of the radiation from the source unit behaves as that from iridium sources for which the attenuation factors were measured, that is, that differences in the filtration of the jacket produce no important change in the spectrum. Measurement in-phantom of just the source and naked capsule in a stainless steel tandem showed no difference, indicating that any effects due to the applicators can be ignored (M. Podgorsac, Ph.D., personal communication, 1993).

The effect of the tissue attenuation and scattering usually is modeled using an empirical formula, such as a Meisberger polynomial,[14]

$$K = a + b\,r + c\,r^2 + d\,r^3 \qquad (2)$$

where K = dose in waterlike medium/dose in air or van der Laarse's variation on van Kleffens and Star's formula.[15,16]

$$K = e(1 + f\,r^2)/(1 + g\,r^2) \qquad (3)$$

With the distance in cm, the values for the coefficients can be taken as

|   | $^{192}$Ir | $^{60}$Co |
|---|---|---|
| a | 1.0128 | 0.9942 |
| b | $5.019 \times 10^{-3}$ | $-5.318 \times 10^{-3}$ |
| c | $-1.178 \times 10^{-3}$ | $-2.610 \times 10^{-3}$ |
| d | $-2.008 \times 10^{-5}$ | $1.327 \times 10^{-4}$ |
| e | 1.018 | 0.994 |
| f | 0.00 | $1.00 \times 10^{-2}$ |
| g | $6.00 \times 10^{-4}$ | $1.41 \times 10^{-2}$ |

Within 9 cm of the sources, either formula works well. Beyond 9 cm, the Meisberger polynomial diverges from measured values.

None of the commercially available software packages corrects the calculated dose for nonunit density tissue inhomogeneities. At the time of writing, this aspect of dosimetry is just developing.[17,18]

Although the capsule jacket is assumed not to change the tissue effects, the jacket and source construction does produce a marked anisotropy. Cerra and Rodgers[19] measured the anisotropy for a Gamma Med IIi, and several investigators have reported on the anisotropy for a microSelectron.[20-22] The factors usually apply as multiplicative corrections as a function of the angle the ray to the target point makes with respect to the perpendicular bisector or the source axis since the calibration usually follows the same perpendicular bisector. Because the calculational algorithm assumes a point source dose function, the entry of the source position information usually only consists of one set of source coordinates marking the center of the source, rather than the two ends of the source, as would be done if using a linear source calculation model. In order to utilize the anisotropy factors, an axis is usually taken as the line between the source and the previous dwell position or a line parallel to a line connecting the previous and subsequent possible dwell positions. In applications with significant curvature between dwell positions, this approach can introduce spurious distortions in the calculated dose distributions, and the operator should consider not using the correction factors.

One source of error between the planned and delivered dose distributions comes from rounding the calculated dwell times to the minimum digit available. On one unit, the minimum time setting is 0.1 second. After the optimization process, the computer calculates the dose distribution using the idealized dwell times and then rounds the times to the nearest 0.1 second. Any plan with dwell times of the same order as this minimum time will contain some rounding error in the delivered dose distribution: the smaller the times, the greater the relative error. The solution for such a problem is simply to do the rounding first and then use the rounded times in the dose calculations.

## Dose During Transit for a Stepping-Source Unit

### General Considerations

During a typical HDR treatment session, the source moves rapidly from the afterloader safe to the first dwell point in a given catheter, where it stays for a predetermined duration. The source then moves, somewhat less rapidly, to the next dwell point, remaining stationary at this location for a preset period of time. The process is repeated for all dwell points in the catheter. The source then is rapidly retracted into the HDR afterloader safe and sent, through the indexer, to the first dwell point of the next catheter channel. This procedure is repeated in all catheters that are utilized during a particular treatment session. Unlike LDR brachytherapy techniques that usually deliver the prescribed dose in one or two applications, HDR brachytherapy doses are almost always given over several fractions, and hence the entire procedure described here is repeated many times.

It follows that the HDR brachytherapy technique of dose delivery, particularly when considering frequent source motion and the number of applications involved, differs significantly from that of LDR brachytherapy. Consequently, dosimetric factors that may prudently be neglected in standard LDR brachytherapy must be accounted for in HDR brachytherapy treatment calculations.

## Dosimetric Considerations

To begin with a typical LDR treatment example, consider an intracavitary gynecological application: the overall treatment time per insertion is usually somewhere between 48 and 72 hours. The time that the radioactive sources spend in transit, meaning the time required to insert and remove the sources from the applicator, is not longer than a few minutes and hence negligible in comparison with the total application time. Additionally, no more than two such applications are ordinarily given as part of standard therapy regimens.

Consequently, in standard LDR brachytherapy, the total dose delivered to any arbitrary point when the radioactive sources are in motion can always be neglected. It is, therefore, customary to compute the total dose to a given point as the sum of doses delivered by all sources used in the application while the sources are stationary at sites determined from the insertion's associated x-ray films.

In contrast with the simple dose calculation concepts outlined above, dose calculations in HDR brachytherapy should account for the fact that the time period during which the high activity source is in motion is not negligible, compared with the period of time when it is stationary at the application's individual dwell points. In addition, the HDR algorithm also needs to acknowledge that the dose delivered by the moving source is proportional to the number of brachytherapy treatment sessions. It is thus no longer possible to use simple LDR conventions when calculating dose distributions administered with the HDR treatment modality.

## Dynamic Dose Determination in HDR Brachytherapy

The total dose ($D_T$) delivered to the prescription and/or any other point of interest consists of two components: the dose delivered when the source is stationary ($D_S$) at a given dwell point and the dose delivered when the source is in motion inside, as well as outside, of the patient's body ($D_M$). Thus, for a single HDR application the total dose delivered to a given point P is defined by equation (4).

$$D_T(P) = D_S(P) + D_M(P) \tag{4}$$

This concept concerning HDR dose determination can be illustrated using a gynecological ring applicator (without tandem) as an example (Fig. 7). Assuming that the ring circumference is 10 cm, the source moves with a constant velocity of 5 cm/s, the dose delivered to point P in 1 second is D, and the dose prescribed at P is 2D. Consider two dwell points, A and B, with equal dwell times of 1 second.

Using the established LDR algorithm, that is, $D_T(P) = D_S(P)$, the dose delivered at P after completion of the treatment session is equal to the prescribed dose, 2D. In reality, however, the source first dwells for 1 second at point A and delivers a dose D at point P. The source then moves to point B. During this transition, which takes 1 second, the dose delivered to P is again D. Subsequently, point P receives dose D when the source dwells at B and dose D while the source is retracted from B to A. By using the HDR algorithm described by eq.(4), a significantly different result is obtained since the total dose delivered to point P is now

$$D_T(P) = 2D + 2D = 4D. \tag{5}$$

Hence, the true dose delivered to point P exceeds the prescribed dose by 100%, even if the source transit from the afterloader safe to point A and back to the safe upon completion of treatment is neglected.

Furthermore, consider a multifraction treatment example where the dose prescribed to point P is again 2D but is delivered in five fractions. Using LDR principles, the dwell time at each dwell point would be reduced from 1 second to 0.2 seconds, and the total dose delivered in five fractions would be as prescribed, i.e., equal to 2D. The true dose delivered to point P during each fraction, however, is

$$D_T(P) = 0.4D + 2D \tag{6}$$

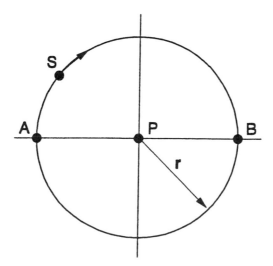

**Fig. 7.** Schematic of the gynecologic ring, $r = 5/\pi$.

And thus the total dose delivered in five fractions is $5 \times D_T(P) = 12D$ because the total dwell time remains constant at 2 seconds, but the total travel time increases by a factor of five. It may be noted, however, that the magnitude of error in determination of the total dose in this example is affected by the parameters used in the assumptions employed, specifically those concerned with source velocity, the number of dwell points, the total dwell time as determined by source activity and prescribed dose, and finally, the number of HDR fractions. To assess the magnitude of error, the most important parameters will now be discussed in more detail.

## Source Speed

The speed of the source is a function of the distance traveled, as described in the literature.[23] In general, as distance increases so does the average speed. Catheter length is commonly 1 meter, and the source travels this distance in about 2 seconds. A maximum measured source speed is 49.9 cm/s.[24] A minimum speed of 22.7 cm/s has been observed for a source traveling between dwell points spaced at 0.25 cm intervals (which is the highest resolution attainable in source position for this particular afterloading machine). The published measured average source speeds, applicable for dwell times of 0.1 s, 0.3 s, and 0.5 s, are presented in Table 1.

## Number of Dwell Points

HDR technology permits the meaningful optimization of brachytherapy dose distributions by offering a wide range of source dwell times (typically 0.1–999.9 s) and fine resolution in source positioning (0.25 cm). The combination of a large number of dwell points and the variability in dwell time that in LDR

### Table 1

#### Average Source Speed

| Distance (cm) | Speed (cm/s) |
| --- | --- |
| 0.25 | 22.7 |
| 0.50 | 27.1 |
| 1.00 | 30.3 |
| 2.00 | 32.3 |
| 3.00 | 32.7 |
| 5.00 | 33.1 |
| 10.0 | 34.5 |
| 99.5 | 49.9 |

terms would correspond to the number of sources and their activities makes the optimization process practical. Thus, if the objective of HDR brachytherapy is to produce a dose distribution that conforms tightly to the target, and hence provides for maximal sparing of surrounding normal tissues, then it is almost always advantageous to use a large number of dwell points and correspondingly short dwell times.[25] This is demonstrated in Fig. 8, which contrasts dose distributions optimized for maximum homogeneity around a gynecological ring applicator programmed with a minimal (2) and maximal (40) number of dwell points.

Since source speed is a function of the distance traveled, using a large number of dwell points always increases the magnitude of the moving source dose component. By using the example illustrated in Fig. 7 and data from Table 1, a 1-second dwell time at each of points A and B, and a prescribed dose of 2D at point P the total dose delivered is at least

$$D_T(P) = 2D + (5.00/33.1)D + (5.00/49.9)D = 2.26D \qquad (7)$$

If, however, 40 dwell points are used because a more-uniform dose distribution around the ring is required (as demonstrated in Fig. 8), the total dose delivered is

$$D_T(P) = 2D + 39 \times (0.25/22.7)D + (9.75/49.9)D = 2.62D \qquad (8)$$

Consequently, the prescribed dose of 2D is exceeded by 31% (13%) when 40 (2) dwell points are used.

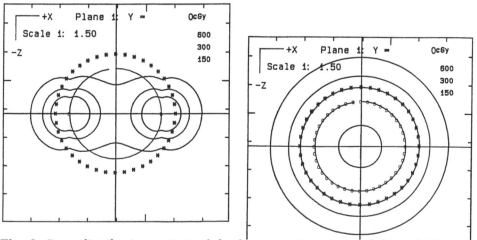

**Fig. 8.** Dose distribution optimized for homogeneity using 2 (left) and 40 (right) dwell points.

## Source Activity, Prescribed Dose, and Number of Fractions

Typically, a new $^{192}$Ir HDR source has an activity near 370 GBq. Such a source provides a dose rate of approximately 12 cGy/s at a distance of 1 cm, that is, a dose rate of approximately 4.7 cGy/s at the center, P, of the ring shown in Fig. 7. It follows that the magnitude of the dynamic dose component $D_M(P)$ is directly proportional to source activity.

Since all current HDR algorithms compute dose only as the sum of a series of stationary dose points, this dose component is considered to be numerically equal to the prescribed dose. Hence, the ratio $D_T(P)/D_S(P)$ can be used as an indicator of the dosimetric error that results from neglecting the dynamic dose component, $D_M(P)$. Because $D_M(P)$ is constant for any given implant geometry and is independent of the prescribed dose, the dosimetric error is inversely proportional to the prescribed dose specified by $D_S(P)$. Thus, smaller dosimetric errors occur for higher prescribed doses when expressed as a fraction of the total delivered dose. Conversely, the magnitude of dosimetric error increases with the number of fractions prescribed, given the same prescribed dose.

## Dynamic Dose Component—General Solution

The simple example of a gynecological ring has been used to convey the basic principles of dose determination in HDR brachytherapy. It is now necessary to describe how the dynamic dose component can be derived for more complex implant geometries. First, the general algorithm will be discussed, and then solutions for some particular situations will be offered.

The position of a source S that moves in space can be described by the three functions, $x = f_1(t)$, $y = f_2(t)$, and $z = f_3(t)$. The dose D delivered to point P in Fig. 9, when the source S travels during time interval

$$t = t_2 - t_1 \tag{9}$$

is

$$D(P) = C \int_{t_1}^{t_2} F(t) \, dt \tag{10}$$

Constant C represents the radiation emission parameters of S, and function $F(t)$ describes the attenuation of radiation between S and P at instant t. C is equal to the product of the specific dose rate constant and source strength. The numerical value of C is available in the literature.[26-28] $C = 4.33 \times 10^4$ cGy cm$^2$ h$^{-1}$ is used in these examples.

Assuming that $\mathbf{r}$ is the position vector of S and, furthermore, that only inverse-square attenuation is involved, then function $F(t)$ can be defined as

$$F(t) = 1/\mathbf{r}^2. \tag{11}$$

The distance between S and P, that is, the magnitude of the position vector $\mathbf{r}$ is

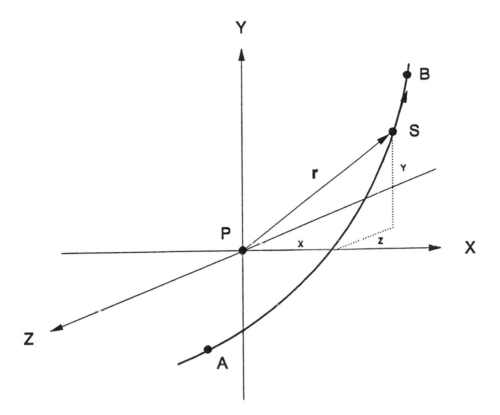

**Fig. 9.** Source S moving in space from point A to point B.

$$r = (x^2 + y^2 + z^2)^{1/2}. \tag{12}$$

The velocity vector **v** is defined by d**r**/dt, and its magnitude, that is, the source-instantaneous velocity **v** can be written as

$$v = [(dx/dt)^2 + (dy/dt)^2 + (dz/dt)^2]^{1/2} \tag{13}$$

Solutions of eq. (10) for three particular HDR applications are presented herein. More detailed derivations can be found in the literature.

Assume that the source S is moving with a constant velocity **v** along the path c (Fig. 10) from point A $(x_1, a, 0)$ to point B$(x_2, a, 0)$. Then the solution of eq.(10) yields the dynamic dose component delivered at point P.

$$D_M(P) = (C/av) \, [\arctan(x/a)]_{x_1}^{x_2}. \tag{14}$$

If the source S moves along a circular path (Fig. 11) with constant angular velocity $\Omega$ from point A $(r, \alpha_1, 0)$ to point B $(r, \alpha_2, 0)$, the moving dose component at point P is

$$D_M(P) = (C/r^2\Omega) \, [\alpha]_{\alpha_1}^{\alpha_2}. \tag{15}$$

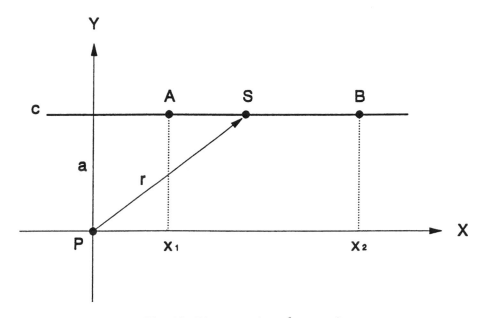

**Fig. 10.** Linear motion of source S.

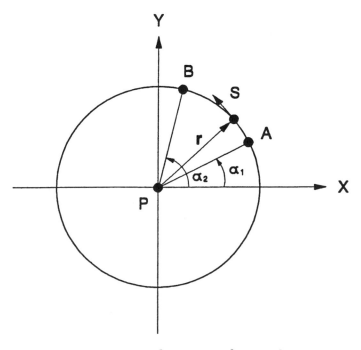

**Fig. 11.** Circular motion of source S.

Finally, if the source S is stationary at any point Q (x,y,z), then the magnitude of the position vector **r**, that is, $r = (x^2 + y^2 + z^2)^{1/2}$, is constant with respect to time and the solution of eq. (10) for period $t = t_2 - t_1$ gives the stationary dose component

$$D_M(P) = (C/r^2)\,[t]_{t_1}^{t_2}. \tag{16}$$

Presently employed HDR algorithms use this last solution for determination of the dose delivered to point P by source S dwelling at point Q over time period t. A correction for tissue absorption is usually provided, and correction for source anisotropy is optional.

## *Distribution of the Dynamic Dose Component*

The insert of Fig. 12 shows a 3 × 3 × 3 cm cube implanted with 16 catheters, each having 13 dwell points, spaced at 0.25 cm intervals. The distribution of the dynamic dose component along the line that transects the center of the cube and is parallel with the catheters is presented by the uppermost curve of Fig. 12. It is seen that the maximum value of $D_M$ is about 22 cGy for a 10 Ci $^{192}$Ir source. The second curve is representative of the dynamic dose component delivered along lines that are 1 cm away from the center of the cube and are parallel with the implant catheters. It is important to note that although the implant is symmetric about the origin, the distribution of $D_M$ is not. Consequently, if the dynamic dose component is not considered, two errors are always committed. First, the dose prescription point will always be overdosed because the true dose delivered is higher than the computed dose. Second, the computed relative dose distribution will always be skewed because the omitted dynamic dose component is not uniformly distributed throughout the implant volume.

## *Clinical Example*

Look again at the implant shown in Fig. 12. This implant is representative of several clinical situations, such as HDR conformal brachytherapy of the prostate, for example. The dose distribution has been optimized to deliver 300 cGy within the center of the implant (2 × 2 × 2 cm cube) and 200 cGy on its periphery (i.e., around the 3 × 3 × 3 cm cube), as shown in Fig. 13. This dose distribution was obtained using a commercial HDR brachytherapy treatment-planning system. It is interesting to note that the described optimization resulted in dwell times of 0.1 s at more than 35% of all dwell points. This confirms that the shortest-possible dwell time is often encountered through optimization.

Assume that the prescribed dose is the dose used in the optimization process (i.e., 300 cGy/200 cGy). Such a prescription would be similar to one presented at a recent symposium.[29] The prostate treatment protocol provided

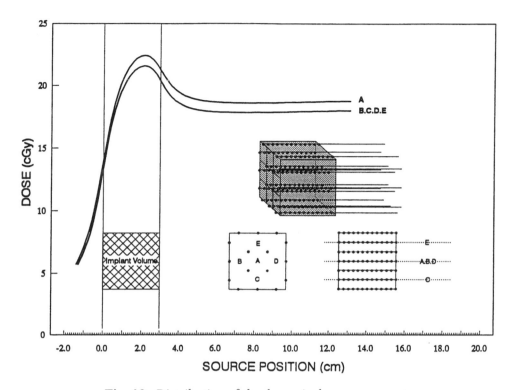

**Fig. 12.** Distribution of the dynamic dose component.

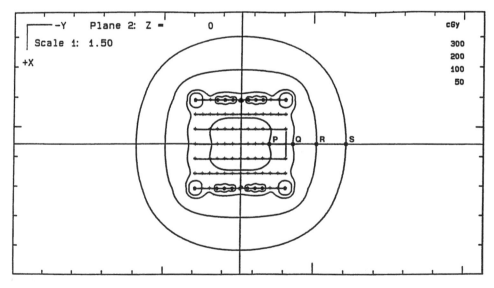

**Fig. 13.** Sagittal view of the optimized dose distribution for the implant shown in Fig. 12.

as an example here calls for 4 HDR brachytherapy fractions to be given over 40 hours, with each fraction delivering a 300-cGy matched peripheral dose.

Since the dynamic dose component delivers about 22 cGy per fraction inside of the cube and about 20 cGy on the catheter entrance side of the implanted volume, the dosimetric errors of the dose distribution presented in Fig. 13 are about 7% at points on the surface of the $2 \times 2 \times 2$ cm cube (point P), 10% outside of the $3 \times 3 \times 3$ cm cube (point Q), and 19% and 38% at points R and S, respectively. It is interesting to note that the dose delivered by the moving source to normal tissue inferior to the prostate gland is approximately 70–80 cGy (point R) when summating over all four fractions. Additionally, the errors are different on opposite sides of the cube because the distribution of the dynamic dose component is asymmetric (Fig. 12).

Although other examples may be presented in which the error might be significantly smaller, the opposite is also possible. For example, by changing the catheter spacing from 1 cm to 0.5 cm or by using pulsed HDR techniques that call for a much larger number of fractions, the error will be significantly larger.

## Implications For Patient Planning

At least one manufacturer runs a clock with a period of 0.1 s to count time for the source in a dwell position. The system only releases a source from a dwell position at the tick of the clock. If the source occupies a dwell position at the tick of the clock, the programs counts that the position was occupied for the entire preceding 0.1 s. In this way, part of the travel time from one dwell position to the next becomes incorporated in the latter's dwell time. If the dwell positions are sufficiently close, the dosimetric error in assuming that the source resides at the end of travel for all of the 0.1 s becomes negligible. If the source remains in transit at the tick of the clock, the time interval is not counted, and the dose contribution from the source during that clock period is ignored. Since the source can travel approximately 3 cm in the 0.1-s interval, the time for movement between one dwell position and any of the next 12 possible positions is counted in the first 0.1 s of the terminal dwell. In practice, as stated above, minimizing the separation between dwell positions (such that the interdwell distance remains at or below 5 mm) minimizes the interdwell dynamic component both because the transit time forms a smaller proportion of the clock period and because the distance varies less from that used in the treatment plan. In an application with many dwell positions, the dose error due to the difference in source position during interdwell transit may be negligible, whereas for the same difference in an application with few dwell positions and at points close to the catheter, the errors in dose can become large. However, as pointed out above again, a large application with many catheters increases the transit dose during the return of the source at the end of the treatment. Incorporation of algorithms such as those presented here into commercially available HDR dose calculation software would eliminate the discrepancy between the calculated and delivered dose distributions.

# Optimization

The use of the term "optimization" implies varying some parameters of the treatment in order to achieve as close as possible to the desired dose distribution. LDR treatments present a very limited number of options, for example, usually the choice of one of four source strengths for each of the four-to-six positions used in a gynecological applicator. HDR using a stepping source allows the use of relative weighting factors (i.e., comparative dwell times) spanning four orders of magnitude. Instead of the normal dosimetry problem of calculating the dose given a source and a target, optimization begins with the desired dose distribution and requires the calculations of the relative weighting factors for each dwell position.

## General Optimization

Van der Laarse[30] has discussed the fundamental principles involved in optimization for HDR brachytherapy. The desired dose distribution is described by placing optimization points at positions with respect to the applicator catheters or the patient and specifying the dose that those points should receive. The dose to an optimization point comes from each of the dwell positions in each catheter, and an equation expresses that dose as a composite of all of the dose components. In its most straightforward form, optimization entails solving the set of simultaneous equations for the doses to the optimization points with the dwell times as the unknowns. Depending on the number of optimization points (i.e., number of equations) and the number of dwell positions (i.e., number of unknowns), the system of equations falls into one of three cases.

Case 1. *More optimization points than dwell positions (overdetermined).* In this case the solution minimizes the sum of the squares of the differences between the calculated and the specified doses for the optimization points.

Case 2. *Equal number of optimization points and dwell positions (determined).* With an equal number of equations and unknowns, the system has an algebraic solution.

Case 3. *Fewer optimization points than dwell positions (underdetermined).* An infinite number of solutions exist for this system, and an added criterion of minimizing the sum of the squares of the dwell times selects the solution.

A further restriction on the dwell times, minimizing the difference between successive dwell times, can avoid negative dwell times as solutions (since they would be physically impossible). A weighting factor for equal dwell-time gradients varies how important this last criterion should be considered. If the solution to the system of equations yields any negative dwell times, increasing the weighting factor will tend to level the dwell times. The overall dwell time must be positive to deliver any dose, so as the weighting factor increases, at some point negative dwell times must disappear.

In the case of large implants as, for example, perineal templates, sets of hundreds of equations (dose points and adjacent dwell times) may arise, each equation having hundreds of dwell times (see Fig.14). A perineal implant with 300 dwell positions and 200 dose points results in almost 500 equations with 300 unknown dwell times. Solving such an extensive set of equations requires a large computer memory and is very time consuming, and at a certain point it becomes prohibitive. However, the constraint on dwell times in adjacent dwell positions yields smoothly changing dwell times along each catheter. This is shown in Fig. 15, where optimized dwell times are given for a straight catheter. Such smoothly changing dwell times can be approximated by a polynomial function that describes their values along the catheter with just a few parameters, similar to a Fourier approximation.[31]

After the polynomial approximations of dwell times along the catheters, a new set of equations can be generated with the parameters as the un-

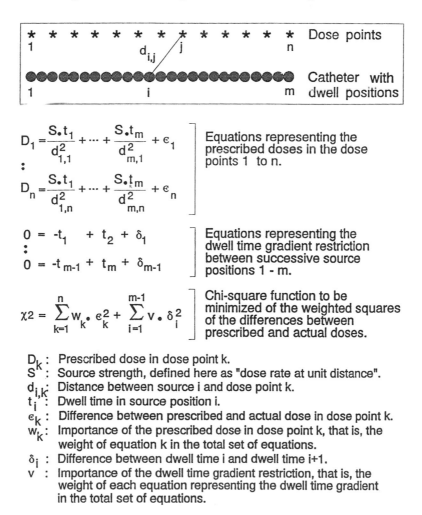

$$D_1 = \frac{S \cdot t_1}{d^2_{1,1}} + \cdots + \frac{S \cdot t_m}{d^2_{m,1}} + \epsilon_1$$

$$\vdots$$

$$D_n = \frac{S \cdot t_1}{d^2_{1,n}} + \cdots + \frac{S \cdot t_m}{d^2_{m,n}} + \epsilon_n$$

Equations representing the prescribed doses in the dose points 1 to n.

$$0 = -t_1 + t_2 + \delta_1$$
$$\vdots$$
$$0 = -t_{m-1} + t_m + \delta_{m-1}$$

Equations representing the dwell time gradient restriction between successive source positions 1 - m.

$$\chi2 = \sum_{k=1}^{n} w_k \cdot \epsilon^2_k + \sum_{i=1}^{m-1} v \cdot \delta^2_i$$

Chi-square function to be minimized of the weighted squares of the differences between prescribed and actual doses.

$D_k$ : Prescribed dose in dose point k.
$S$ : Source strength, defined here as "dose rate at unit distance".
$d_{i,k}$: Distance between source i and dose point k.
$t_i$ : Dwell time in source position i.
$\epsilon_k$ : Difference between prescribed and actual dose in dose point k.
$w_k$: Importance of the prescribed dose in dose point k, that is, the weight of equation k in the total set of equations.
$\delta_i$ : Difference between dwell time i and dwell time i+1.
$v$ : Importance of the dwell time gradient restriction, that is, the weight of each equation representing the dwell time gradient in the total set of equations.

**Fig. 14.** Optimization of dwell times to prescribed doses with dwell-time gradient restriction.

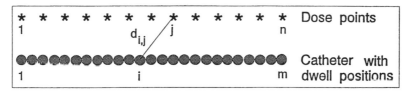

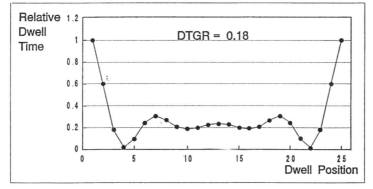

Curve of dwell time t versus distance x to first dwell position is smooth due to dwell time gradient restriction DTGR.

Approximate t(x) with polynomials P (x) to the degree p with p < m :

$$t(x) = \sum_{j=1}^{p} a_j \cdot P_j(x) \ ,$$

Suitable value for degree: $p = 2 \sqrt{m} - 1$, thus 48 dwell times in a catheter may be approximated by p = 13.

m : Number of source dwell positions.
n : Number of dose points.
p : Number of parameters.
$a_j$ : jth parameter.
$p_i^j$ : jth polynomial

**Fig. 15.** Parameterization of dwell times in $x^2$ sufficient dwell-time gradient restriction.

knowns. The coefficient matrix of this set is square, with the dimensions equal to the total number of parameters. In this way, the above mentioned perineal implant with 300 dwell positions and 200 dose points now results typically in 100 equations with 100 unknown parameters, which are easily solved. This technique of optimization with a large number of dwell positions is called *polynomial optimization.*

Although a large-volume implant can be optimized by polynomial optimization to the prescribed doses to the dose points, the resulting dose distribution may not be satisfactory. This is because it is difficult in clinical practice to place a sufficient number of dose points in and around the implant. By only placing dose points around the outside of an implant, cold spots can arise in the central portion. In that situation, because the inner dwell positions are far away from the dose points and contribute slightly to their dose, small dwell times result. The same rationale explains why placing dose points on the inside of such an implant results in inappropriately low dwell times in the outer catheters (Fig. 16).

By merging the polynomial optimization and the geometric optimization (discussed in the next section), a volume implant can be optimized to an equal dose to the dose points midway between the catheters, while suppressing a hot spot in the center of the implant. The geometric component of this combined optimization method determines which fraction of the total treatment time the source has to spend in each catheter in order to achieve dose homogeneity in the target volume. The polynomial component optimizes, within the constraint of the above-mentioned time fraction for each catheter, the dwell times to match the prescribed dose at the dose points. Thus, geometric optimization de-

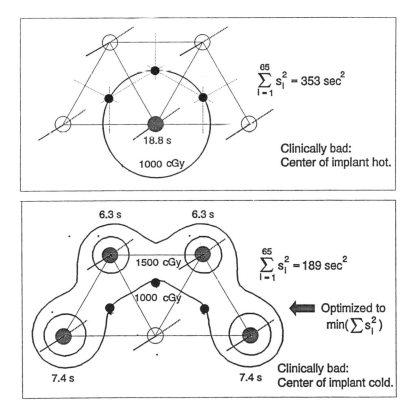

Implant of 5 catheters, each dwell positions 1 - 13, step length 0.5 cm.
Reference Air Kerma Rate is 4.0682 cGy.h$^{-1}$.m$^2$, i.e. 10 Ci $^{192}$Ir.
● : Active source dwell position
○ : Inactive source dwell position
• : Dose points, midway between catheters along 6 cm active length

**Fig. 16.** Optimization on dose points between dwell positions.

termines the time per catheter, and polynomial optimization determines the distribution of this time over the catheter to obtain the same dose to the dose points along the catheter.

The polynomial optimization without the geometric component is called optimization on distance. It is used when dose points placed along the catheters define the isodose surfaces. A typical case is an intraluminal application with only a few catheters.

The polynomial optimization with the geometric component is called optimization on volume. A typical case is the optimization of the two-plane breast implant discussed in the section on the Stepping-Source Dosimetry System earlier in this chapter.

Minimizing the square of the dwell times biologically minimizes the total imparted energy (and similarly the integral dose) the patient receives.

Rather than just solving the simultaneous equations, some investigators have looked into other methods of optimization, such as simulated annealing[32] or Newton's method.[33] As of this writing, such approaches are used only at research institutions.

### Geometric Optimization

An alternative to optimizing to specified points is optimization based solely on the configuration of the catheters. This is referred to as geometric optimization (GO). The geometric relationships among the dwell positions themselves are used to determine dwell times. To gain the full usefulness of GO, certain principles must be observed.

Geometric optimization makes use of the intersource distances to determine the relative dwell times. The basic assumption is that the dose at each dwell position is a function of the proximity of that point to each of the other dwell positions. Positions that have many neighbors will, without optimization, receive a higher dose than those with few neighbors. Thus, a function, which will decrease the dwell time of source positions with many close neighbors and increase the time of those that do not, is sought. The simplest way to do this is to calculate the sum of the inverse square distances from all the other dwell positions. This sum is a simple approximation of the dose contribution to that point from all other dwell positions. The relative time for this dwell position is set inversely proportional to this sum (Fig. 17). This works well for simple, regular implants.

In practice, however, implants are often not regular. When catheters converge strongly, this simple method results in overcompensation. Since the dwell time for a given position is dominated by its nearest neighbor, two nearby dwell positions will tend to "annihilate" one another. A constraint is needed for the maximum effect any one dwell position can have on another. If two dwell positions are very close together, they are considered to be at a certain minimum distance rather than their true distance. The user specifies this minimum distance over the range of 2.5–10 mm, but it is generally set to the effective step

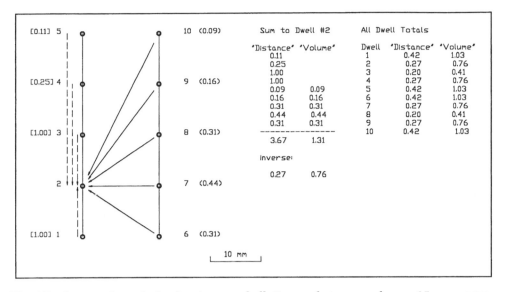

**Fig. 17.** Geometric optimization in a nutshell. Two catheters are shown, 15 mm apart, with dwell positions numbered. The numbers in parentheses are the inverse square distances to dwell #2. Relative time in dwell #2 is determined by summing the inverse square distances of all dwells (distance method) or dwells in the other catheter only (volume method), then taking the inverse of the sum. This procedure is performed once for each dwell position. The totals shown are the relative dwell times for each dwell position.

length (the distance between successive active dwell positions). It can be increased by the user in case the optimization overcompensates in an area where several catheters converge.

Another problem arises if a volume implant has a cold spot because of diverging catheters. If the distance between the catheters is much larger than the effective step size (i.e., the distance between successive dwells within a catheter), then the optimization will be dominated by the nearest neighbors, which now lie in the same catheter as the one being optimized. This leads to isodose contours that conform to the shape of individual catheters. If it is desired to "fill in" the dose between catheters, the contribution to dose from the nearby dwells in the same catheters can be excluded. The option of excluding nearby dwell positions in the same catheter goes by the designation of "volume" optimization since the target for the uniform dose covers the implanted volume. Including the same-catheter dwells so that the isodose surfaces follow the catheter at a given distance is called "distance" optimization.

Modern interstitial brachytherapy in Europe is closely associated with the PDS, in which continuous wires of Iridium-192 are placed, often with large interwire spacings. In contrast, the American experience has been based on sources consisting of nylon tubes containing short (3 mm) pieces of $^{192}$Ir wire, conventionally spaced at 1.0 cm. These are placed close together in the range of 10–15 mm between catheters. The implant consists of large numbers of point sources, spaced similarly in all three dimensions. Geometric optimization is an outgrowth of the American approach and is less effective when used with closely spaced dwell positions in widely spaced catheters (Figs.18–20). The reason for this is simply that, with very small step sizes, the optimization is dominated by nearby dwell positions in the same catheter, reducing the sensitivity to intercatheter spacing.

Geometric optimization may be used for almost all implant situations, without additional assistance from the dose-point optimization, as long as dwell positions are spaced no closer than 1.0 cm along each catheter. With smaller spacing between dwell positions, GO can be combined with the dose-point method.

When using GO for intraluminal (e.g., bronchial, biliary) implants, the radius at which the distribution is most uniform is a function of the step size. A step size of 5–10 mm results in relatively good uniformity for practical implants.

Geometrical optimization can lead to dangerously long dwell times in implants with a small number of catheters (see Fig. 21). In this case, the algorithm will attempt to producea uniform distribution midway between the catheters, with the result that the local doses near the divergent ends of the catheters are extremely high. This may be appropriate at times but requires very careful consultation between the physician and physicist. Using the distance method instead is likely to produce a more appropriate result (Fig. 22). The situation becomes especially unstable using volume optimization if one of the catheters is shortened (Fig. 23). In this case there are no nearby restraining points at the

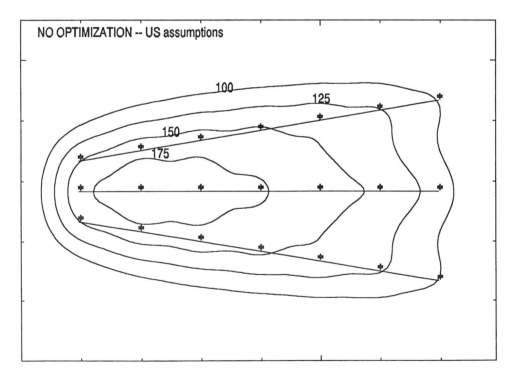

**Fig. 18.** Two-plane implant of six catheters, with deviation. Calculation is midway between planes.

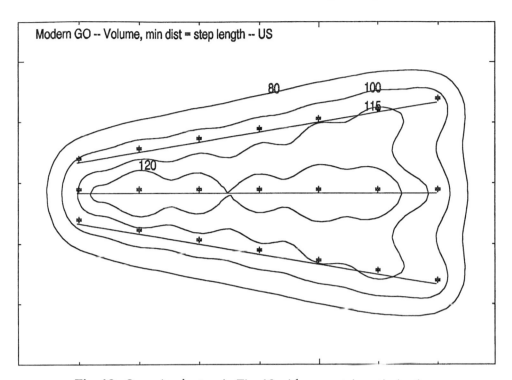

**Fig. 19.** Same implant as in Fig. 18 with geometric optimization.

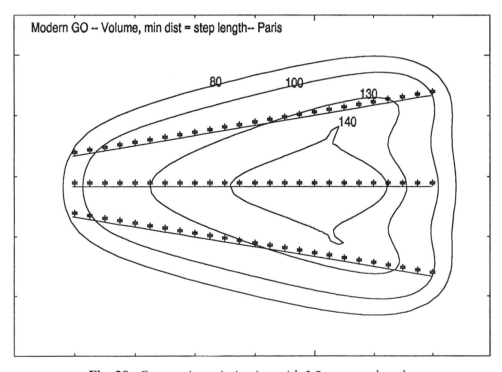

**Fig. 20.** Geometric optimization with 2.5 mm step length.

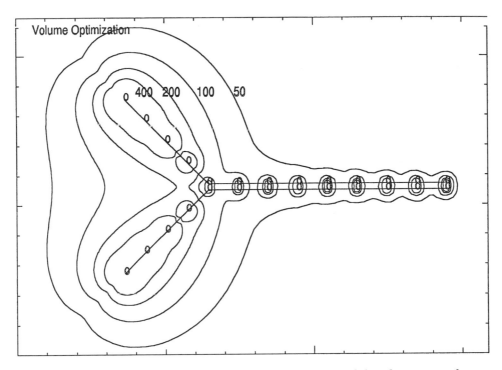

**Fig. 21.** Volume optimization on catheter implant gives equal dose between catheters. This is unlikely to be the physician's intent.

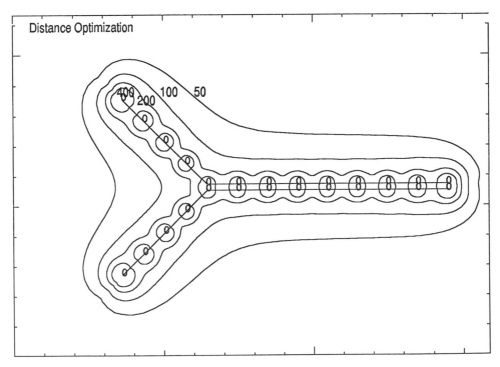

**Fig. 22.** Distance method used with the implant in Fig. 21 produces an excellent result.

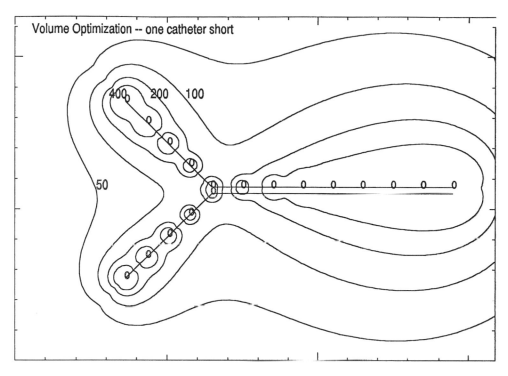

**Fig. 23.** Most dangerous situation—one catheter shorter, with volume optimization.

superior end, with the result shown. This type of inappropriate distribution usually will be obvious by the extremely large dwell times generated at one end. As always, it is important to evaluate whether the resultant distributions satisfy all prescriptive requirements prior to treatment.

## Evaluation of the Optimized Plan

### Visual Evaluation of Dose Distributions

Evaluation of a radiotherapy dose distribution is usually done by visually inspecting isodose lines in one or more planes through the target volume. Nearly all external beam treatment plans are routinely evaluated in this way. In brachytherapy, however, this approach is impeded by the following two considerations:

(1) High-dose gradients exist around the sources or dwell positions in the target volume, contrary to the low-dose gradient over the target volume in an external beam treatment plan.

(2) A straightforward definition of the RD is not possible. Although in an external beam-dose distribution the RD may be related to the dose at the isocenter or prescribed for an isodose surface encompassing the target

volume, in brachytherapy a point like the isocenter in the center of a flat dose distribution does not exist, and there is no simple relationship between the isodose surfaces surrounding the target volume and the dose distribution inside the target volume.

It has, however, become common practice to evaluate the dose distribution of a volume implant along the same lines as an external beam-dose distribution. Consequently, the aim of HDR stepping source treatment planning is to obtain as homogeneous a dose distribution in the target volume as possible, while sparing any adjacent vulnerable regions. Since the high-dose gradients around the individual dwell positions will always be there, the optimizing will aim at obtaining prescribed dose values in the volumes equidistant between the dwell positions (dots on Figs. 2 and 3). Considerable clinical experience is required to judge a treatment plan owing to the inherent inhomogeneous dose distribution in the target volume. However, volume-dose histograms are a powerful tool to obtain a figure of merit for a treatment plan. Such a figure of merit must assess the volumes of the flat dose regions between the catheters or needles throughout the target volume.[34-37]

## Distribution of Grid Points Through the Implant Volume

In order to evaluate the three-dimensional dose distribution using volume-dose histograms, the distribution must be divided into volume elements with assigned dose values. It is common practice to encompass the treatment volume with a rectangular box and to define a grid of equidistant dose points inside this box. The distance between two adjacent dose points will be called the grid dimension. Each dose point is the center of a voxel (volume element) with a volume equal to the third power of the grid dimension. Typically, the dose values must be calculated in a grid of 100,000 points in order to obtain a reasonably smooth volume-dose histogram. Due to the fact that a regular grid is applied over a more or less regular implant, there is a large redundancy of grid points (Fig. 24). Since in brachytherapy a good implant is a regular one, an ar-

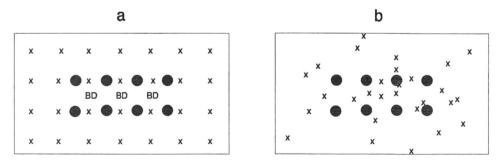

**Fig. 24.** a. Regular grid placed over a regular implant. Owing to the regularity of the grid, no grid points lie in the basal dose point regions, BD. b. Arbitrary grid placed over a regular implant. Much more information about the dose distribution is obtained with the same number of dose points as in a.

bitrary distribution of grid points is much more effective. The voxel assigned to such an arbitrary grid point then has a volume equal to the volume of the box divided by the number of grid points.[38]

The coordinates of such arbitrary grid points are generated by using random number generators. A random number generator delivers a number between 0 and 1. After scaling the random generator for the x-value to the corresponding box dimension, a random x-grid coordinate is obtained. In the same way, random y- and z-grid coordinates are obtained.

For the same histogram accuracy, the reduction in the number of grid points when they are distributed randomly instead of being equally spaced is a factor of 3 to 5 in clinical practice, depending on the regularity of the implant. A second reason for using an arbitrary grid is the fact that additional grid points only have to be added to the already existing ones; only the voxel size must be recalculated. Thus, if the amount of dose values at arbitrary grid points is not sufficient to construct a valid volume-dose histogram, the dose values at an additional set of arbitrary grid points can simply be added to the already calculated volume-dose histogram. This is not possible with a regular grid.

### Differential Volume-Dose Histogram

A differential volume-dose histogram is a graph with the dose, D, on the horizontal x-axis and the volume-dose gradient, dV/dD (the change of the volume encapsulated by the isodose surface with dose D, divided by the dose on the vertical y-axis (see Fig.25). In Fig. 26 dV/dD is visualized. If on the x-axis, a very small dose interval at dose level $D_o$ is

$$dD = D_0 - D_1, \tag{17}$$

then on the y-axis the change of volume with dose around dose level $D_o$ is

$$dV/dD = (V_0 - V_1)/(D_0 - D_1), \tag{18}$$

with $V_o$ the volume encompassed by dose $D_o$ and $V_1$ the volume by $D_1$.

Figure 25 gives the differential volume-dose histogram of an $^{192}$Ir point source in water, which delivers 1,000 cGy at 10 mm distance. Due to the inverse square law, the change of volume with dose, dV/dD, near the point source is small; at a large distance from the point source dV/dD is large. A simple calculation of dV/dD at a 10-mm and a 20-mm distance from the point source of Fig. 25 illustrates this (see Fig. 26). The point source in Fig. 26 is called "ideal" because tissue attenuation and scattering is disregarded.

The volume of a spherical isodose surface around a point source with radius r is $(4/3) \pi r^3 = 4.19 r^3$. In Fig. 26 for $r_o$ = 10 mm, $D_o$ = 1,000 cGy and $V_o = 4.19 \times 10^3$ = 4,190 mm³. Using $r_1$ = 10.1, dV/dD can be approximated by $(V_o-V_1)/(D_o-D_1)$ = −6.3 mm³/cGy. For $r_o$ = 20 mm, D = 250 cGy. If $r_1$ = 20.1 mm, then dV/dD = −202 mm³/cGy. It is common practice to disregard the negative sign in the volume-dose histograms. By doubling the distance from an

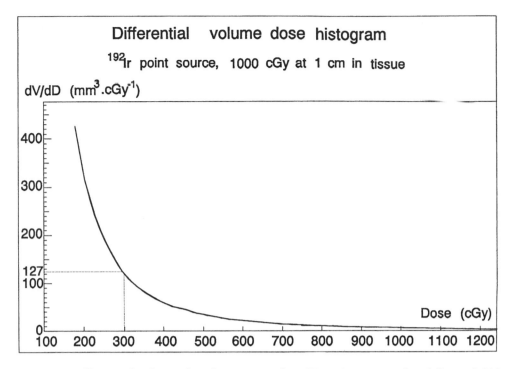

**Fig. 25.** Differential volume-dose histogram of an [192]Ir point source that delivers 1,000 cGy at 1 cm in soft tissue. The dotted line relates the 300 cGy dose with the theoretical value 127 mm³/cGy (see text).

ideal point source, dV/dD changes by a factor of 203/6.3 = 32. Because V changes with $r^3$ and D changes with $r^{-2}$, dV/dD changes with $r^5$, so

$$(dV/dD)_D = c' \cdot r^5, \qquad (19)$$

with c' a constant depending on source strength, medium etc.

Because the differential volume-dose histogram is a function of D instead of r, one gets

$$(dV/dD)_D = c \cdot D^{-5/2} \qquad (20)$$

for an ideal point source. Using $D(r) = S/r^2$, $c = -2\,\pi r \cdot S^{3/2}$ is easily derived. Thus, for an ideal point source

$$dV/dD = -2\pi \cdot S^{3/2} \cdot D^{-5/2}. \qquad (21)$$

In Figure 25 the differential volume-dose histogram is given for an [192]Ir seed in tissue for distances up to 3 cm from the seed. The corresponding histogram for a point source in air that delivers the same dose at 1 cm (but now in air) is practically the same because over the range 0–3 cm the tissue attenu-

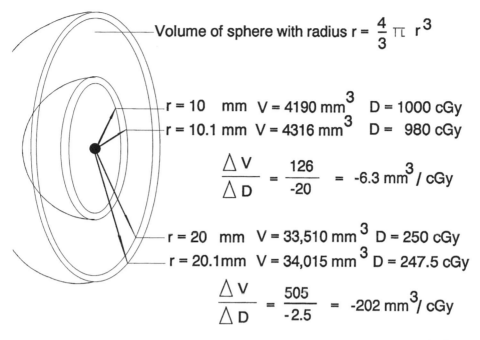

Volume of sphere with radius $r = \frac{4}{3}\pi r^3$

$r = 10$ mm $V = 4190$ mm$^3$ $D = 1000$ cGy
$r = 10.1$ mm $V = 4316$ mm$^3$ $D = 980$ cGy

$$\frac{\Delta V}{\Delta D} = \frac{126}{-20} = -6.3 \text{ mm}^3/\text{cGy}$$

$r = 20$ mm $V = 33{,}510$ mm$^3$ $D = 250$ cGy
$r = 20.1$ mm $V = 34{,}015$ mm$^3$ $D = 247.5$ cGy

$$\frac{\Delta V}{\Delta D} = \frac{505}{-2.5} = -202 \text{ mm}^3/\text{cGy}$$

**Fig. 26.** Approximation of the volume-dose gradient dV/dD around an ideal point source, which gives 1,000 cGy at 10 mm distance. dV/dD is approximated for D = 1,000 cGy, and D = 250 cGy. Tissue attenuation and scattering are disregarded.

ation and scattering influence on the histogram is hardly noticeable. So for a dose of 300 cGy one finds, using eq. (21), that

$$dV/dD = 27\pi \cdot 1000^{3/2} \cdot 300^{-5/2}$$
$$= 0.127 \text{ cm}^3/\text{cGy}$$
$$= 127 \text{ mm}^3/\text{cGy}.$$

Even when several catheters are positioned in a specific geometrical configuration, large and unavoidable dose gradients exist in the vicinity of individual dwell positions. These gradients result from the dependence of the dose on the inverse square of the distance to each one of the dwell positions. The histogram for the unoptimized breast implant of Fig. 2 is given in Fig. 27. "Unoptimized" in this context means that all sources are of equal strength, that is, all dwell times are equal. This histogram shows two peaks. The higher one at a dose of about 700 cGy is caused by the volumes around the three rows of inner dose points; the lower one at a dose of about 600 cGy is caused by the volumes around the two rows of outer dose points.

The cumulative histogram, V versus D, of the unoptimized breast implant is given in Fig. 28. This histogram directly gives, for a given dose D, the volume with doses higher than D. However, it is not suitable for evaluating the quality of the implant because of its integrating character. The two peaks visible on the differential volume-dose histogram are no longer discernible.

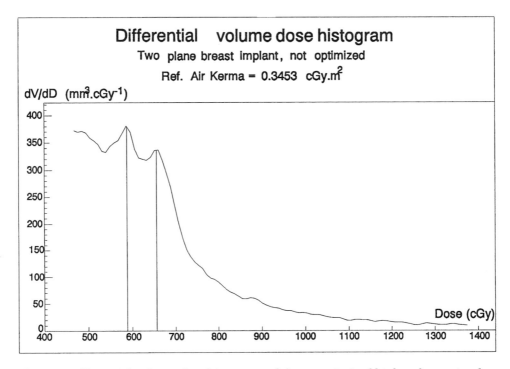

**Fig. 27.** Differential volume-dose histogram of the unoptimized biplane breast implant of Fig. 2. The peak at 660 cGy is caused by the volume around the three rows of inner basal dose points; the peak at 580 cGy is caused by the volumes around the two rows of outer basal dose points.

It is clear from these figures that, using the histograms dV/dD versus D or V versus D to evaluate the implant is of a limited value. This is caused by the influence of the inverse square law on the dose distribution. Anderson,[34] in 1986, described a histogram in which this influence was removed.

## Anderson "Natural" Volume-Dose Histogram

The previous section explained that the area under the curve dV/dD between $D_1$ and $D_2$ is the volume treated with doses between $D_1$ and $D_2$. For an ideal point source r = $(S/D)^{1/2}$, the area under the curve dV/dr between $r_1$ and $r_2$ is also the volume treated with doses between $D_1$ and $D_2$. Generally, for any function u(D), the area under the curve dV/du between $u(D_1)$ and $u(D_2)$ represents the volume treated with doses between $D_1$ and $D_2$.

Anderson[34] presented a differential volume-dose histogram, dV/du versus u, with u(D) = $-D^{-3/2}$ + const. For our purposes it suffices to set the constant term to 0. For an ideal point source, using eq. (21) and dV/du = dV/dD ·dD/du, one finds

$$dV/du = -(4/3)\pi \cdot S^{3/2}, \tag{22}$$

which is independent of dose D.

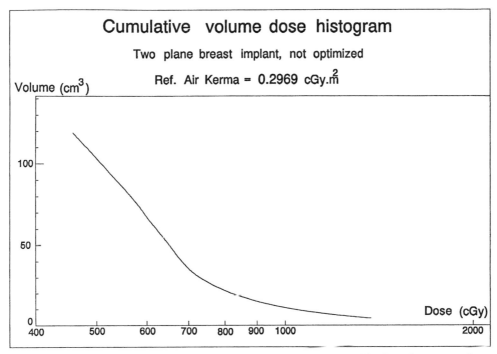

**Fig. 28.** Cumulative volume-dose histogram of the unoptimized biplane breast implant of Fig. 2. Note that the two peaks of the differential histogram of the same implant in Fig. 27 are not discernible.

It is common practice to take the absolute values of u(D) and dV/du. So, if the horizontal axis of the histogram is taken as $u(D) = D^{-3/2}$ and the vertical axis as dV/du, then an ideal point source will give a horizontal line at $(4/3)\ \pi \cdot S^{3/2}$. For the sake of simplicity, the absolute signs around dV/du are disregarded. Because u(D) decreases with increasing D, u(D) is taken in the opposite x-direction. In this way the so-called "Natural" volume-dose histogram is obtained (see Fig. 29). The solid line in this figure represents the "Natural" volume-dose histogram for a real $^{192}$Ir point source, using 100,000 arbitrarily distributed grid points. The dotted line is the theoretical value $(4/3)\ \pi \cdot S^{3/2}$ for an ideal point source, which gives the same 1,000 cGy at 1 cm in air. This value is $(4/3)\ \pi \cdot 1{,}000^{3/2}\ cm^3 \cdot cGy^{3/2} = 1{,}132.5\ mm^3 \cdot cGy^{3/2}$.

The "natural" volume-dose histogram of the unoptimized biplane breast implant of Fig. 2 is given in Fig. 30. The two peaks stand out clearly (see also Fig. 27). At a large distance from the implant, thus at a very low dose, the whole implant behaves as a point source with $dV/du = (4/3)\ \pi(nS)^{3/2}$, with S the strength of a single source (dwell position) and n the number of sources (dwell positions). For the very high doses in the small volumes around each individual dwell position, the dose is determined predominantly by the source at the position concerned, hence,

$$dV/du = (4/3)\pi \cdot nS^{3/2}. \tag{23}$$

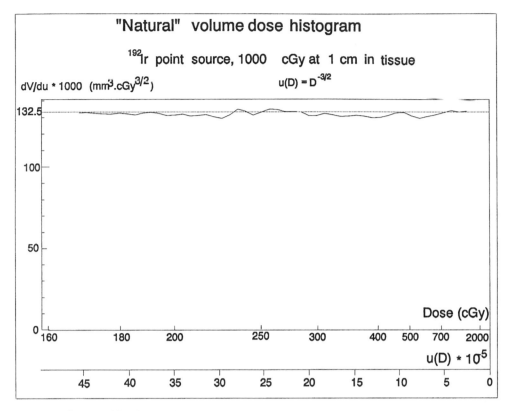

**Fig. 29.** "Natural" volume-dose histogram of an $^{192}$Ir point source that delivers 1,000 cGy at 1 cm in tissue. The " − " sign of the dV/du and u has been disregarded in the figure. ———— indicates the actual histogram. ········· indicates the theoretical value (see text).

The following dose values are defined in the "natural" histogram (see Fig. 30): the low dose (LD) is the dose with the dV/du value halfway between the peak dose value and the limit value on the low-dose side. The high dose (HD) is the dose with the dV/du value halfway between the peak dose value and the limit value on the high-dose side. The target dose (TD) is the prescribed implant dose and is defined by the radiation oncologist. The uniformity index (UI) is defined as

$$UI = \frac{V(TD - HD)}{u(TD) - u(HD)} \bigg/ \frac{V(TD)}{u(TD)} \tag{24}$$

or expressed as a function of dose:

$$UI = \frac{V(TD - HD)}{TD^{-3/2} - HD^{-3/2}} \bigg/ \frac{V(TD)}{TD^{-3/2}} \tag{25}$$

In the above equations, V(TD − HD) equals the volume between TD and HD, and V(TD) the volume with doses higher than TD. So UI is the volume

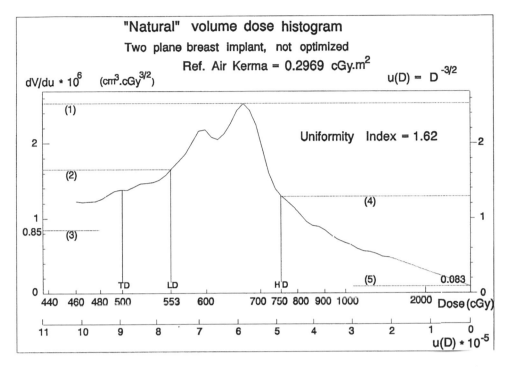

**Fig. 30.** "Natural" volume-dose histogram of the unoptimized biplane breast implant of Fig. 2. Line (1), the highest peak value, represents dV/du due to the three volumes around the basal dose points inside the implant; the lower peak value represents dV/du due to the two volumes around the outer basal dose points. Line (3) represents the theoretical limit, $(4/3) \pi (nS)^{3/2}$ of dV/du at a large distance from the implant, with n as the number of dwell positions, and $S = D(r)/r^2$, the source strength of the ideal point source. Line (2) lies midway between lines (1) and (3) and defines the so-called "Low Dose." Line (5) represents the theoretical limit, $(4/3) \pi (nS)^{3/2}$ of dV/du, for very high dose values. Line (4) lies midway between lines (1) and (5) and defines the so-called "High Dose."

between TD and HD isodose surfaces averaged over the u-interval u(TD) − u(HD), divided by the volume within the TD isodose surface averaged over the u-interval u(TD) − u(∞).

The "natural" histogram of the optimized implant of Fig. 3 is given in Fig. 31. Note the comparatively small change in the UI compared to the unoptimized implant in Fig. 30. This is caused by the different definition of TD in these implants; the unoptimized implant uses only the basal dose points in the central transversal plane, and the optimized implant uses all dose points between the catheters.

From the definition of UI follows its dependence on the target dose TD, which is similar to the RD in dosimetry systems like the Paris system. Different values of TD give quite different values of UI. So UI cannot be used to assess the quality of the implant independently of the selected TD. If such assessment is required, an implant quality index (QI) may be defined based on LD instead of TD. This index represents a Figure of Merit of the implant irre-

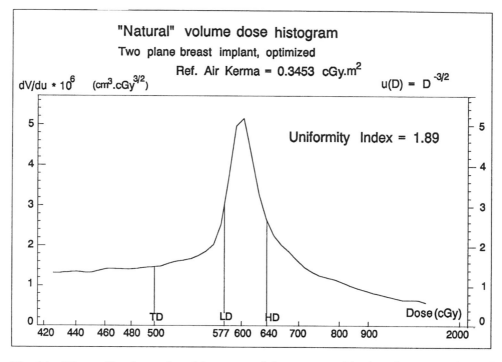

**Fig. 31.** "Natural" volume-dose histogram of the optimized biplane breast implant of Fig. 3. Note the relatively small change in the uniformity index compared to the unoptimized case (1.89 verses 1.62). This is due to the different definition of TD in the optimized and unoptimized implants. See text for further details.

spective of whether the implant covers the target volume or not. Thus, the QI is defined as

$$QI = \frac{V(LD - HD)}{u(LD) - u(HD)} \Big/ \frac{V(LD)}{u(LD)} \qquad (26)$$

or expressed as a function of dose:

$$QI = \frac{V(LD - HD)}{LD^{-3/2} - HD^{-3/2}} \Big/ \frac{V(LD)}{LD^{-3/2}} \qquad (27)$$

### Volume Gradient Ratio

In this section a Figure of Merit for brachytherapy dose distributions is defined. It is based on the difference between the differential volume-dose histogram of the implant and a point source in the center of the implant, which gives the same maximum dose on the surface of the rectangular box confining the grid points (Fig. 32) The generation of the arbitrary grid points

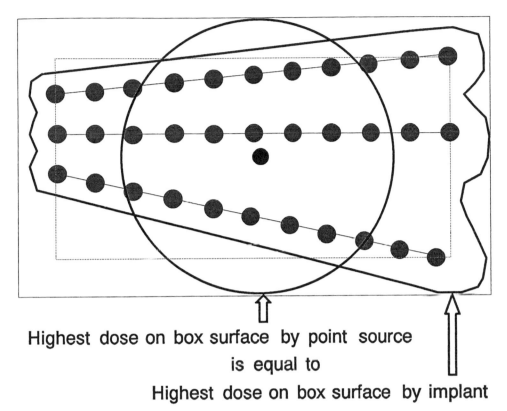

**Highest dose on box surface by point source**

**is equal to**

**Highest dose on box surface by implant**

**Fig. 32.** Definition of volume gradient ratio (VGR). The box is taken with a margin of 1 cm around the active dwell positions. The highest dose on the box surface given by the implant belongs to the lowest isodose surface still completely encompassed by the box. The virtual point source in the center of the box gives the same highest dose of the box surface as the implant. The VGR is based on the difference between the differential volum-dose histogram of the implant and the point source.

inside this box was presented in the section "Distribution of Grid Points Through the Implant Volume." The maximum dose on the box surface defines the isodose surface with the lowest dose confined completely inside the box. Any isodose surface with a dose lower than this maximum surface dose extends outside the box and cannot be presented in the volume-dose histogram. The maximum dose on the box surface, therefore, defines the minimum value on the dose axis in all volume-dose histograms based on the grid points inside the box.

In Fig. 33 the differential volume-dose histogram is given for the unoptimized biplane breast implant of Fig. 2, with an active length of 9 cm. The rectangular box defining the grid points is taken with a margin of 1 cm around the smallest box encompassing the active dwell positions. Since the active length is 9 cm, the distance between the outer needles in the lower plane is 6 cm, and the distance between the two needle planes is 1.8 cm; the grid confining box has the dimensions $11 \times 8 \times 3.8$ cm$^3$.

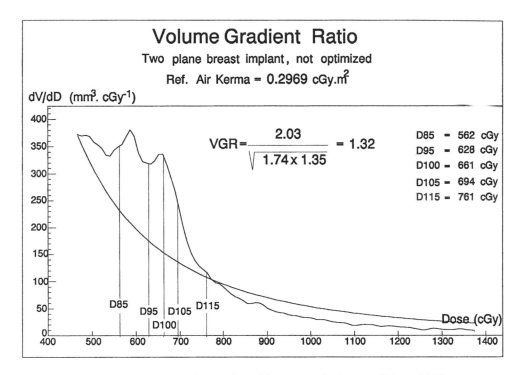

$$VR(D1\text{-}D2) = \frac{\text{area under implant histogram between D1 and D2}}{\text{area under point source histogram between D1 and D2}}$$

$$VGR = \frac{VR(D95 - D105)}{\sqrt{VR(D85 - D95) \times VR(D105 - D115)}}$$

**Fig. 33.** VGR of the unoptimized biplane implant of Fig. 2. The histogram is discussed in Fig. 27. The area under the implant histogram between doses D1 and D2 is the volume in the implant between the isodose surfaces D1 and D2, so VR is the ratio of the volume between isodose surfaces D1 and D2 of the implant and the point source.

The volume gradient ratio (VGR) is defined as follows. First the dose $D_{100}$ is defined as that dose that produces the largest difference between the histogram of the implant and the histogram of the point source (Fig. 33). Then the doses $D_{85}$, $D_{95}$, $D_{105}$ and $D_{115}$ are taken as 85, 95, 105, and 115 percent of $D_{100}$, respectively. The volume ratio $VR(D_1 - D_2)$ is defined as the ratio of the volume between the isodose surfaces $D_1$ and $D_2$ of the implant and that of the point source. The VGR is now defined as

$$VGR = \frac{VR(D_{95} - D_{105})}{\sqrt{VR(D_{85} - D_{95}) \times VR(D_{105} - D_{115})}}. \tag{28}$$

The VGR is defined by the maximum difference between the differential volume-dose histogram and the point-source histogram. Therefore, it is independent of an arbitrarily selected RD and only assesses the implant. This is conceptually similar to the PDS where the RD is defined as 85% of the mean dose at the basal dose points in the central transversal plane of the implant.

The unoptimized 9-cm-long implant of Figure 33 is used to treat a 7-cm-long target volume. The same volume is covered by a 7-cm-long implant optimized according to SSDS. The determination of VGR is given in Fig. 34.

## Execution of the Planned Treatment

As mentioned previously, the advantages of HDR include the ability to move organs to obtain a more favorable dose distribution, and once properly positioned, the equipment can be fixed rigidly in space. The correct treatment requires that the calculated planned treatment transfers from the planning computer to the treatment unit and that movement has not altered the geometry appreciably since the localization films.

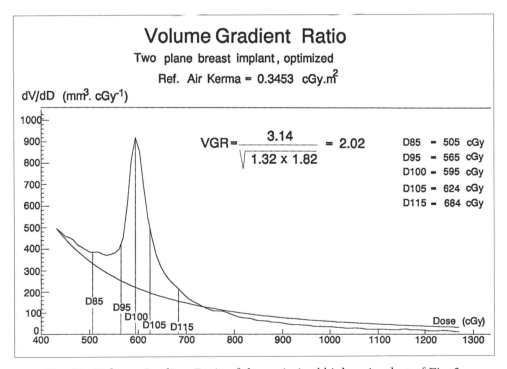

**Fig. 34.** Volume Gradient Ratio of the optimized biplane implant of Fig. 3.

## Transfer of Information from the Dosimetry Computers to the Treatment Unit

An on-board computer actually controls the progress of the source. The problem becomes how to assure the proper programming of this computer. The most direct data transfer would be using the same computer for dosimetry and treatment-unit control. At least one manufacturer currently employs that configuration. A transfer of the data via a network would also serve as a direct link, minimizing the possibility of error during transfer. A common mode of data transfer uses programmable cards or floppy disks. Although little likelihood exists for errors in the program to occur during passage from the planning computer to the treatment unit, a final pretreatment check should include a comparison between the dwell times as printed on both computer systems, not so much to look for small, occult errors as to protect from programming from the wrong patient's card. If hardware compatibility precludes data transfer between the planning and the treatment systems, manual programming based on a computer printout certainly increases the need for review of the program before treatment.

## Movement Between Localization and Execution of Treatment

In the ideal situation the procedure is performed in a dedicated room with its own localization x-ray system. Thus, once in position, with the applicator locked in position with respect to the table and the patient immobile, the treatment plan describes the delivered treatment (not counting the transit dose, as discussed above). With such a program, one team of investigators[7] found the average movement between the applicator and the patient's skeletal anatomy to be 2.6 mm. This compares to a study of LDR patients showing up to 2-cm movement over the course of an application.[39]

The patient movement in many HDR programs falls between the ideal and the LDR situation. An example is transporting a patient between localization (e.g., on a simulator) and treatment delivery (e.g., where the unit shares a room with an accelerator). Usually such a transfer takes place with the patient on a long board and the applicators fixed to the board. As of yet, no studies have compared radiographs taken for localization with some taken after treatment to look for relative movement between the sets.

# Examples of Planning by Site

## Optimization of Interstitial Implants of the Base of the Tongue

### *Introduction*

Treatment options for early and advanced primary and recurrent cancers of the base of the tongue (BOT) are classically external beam radiation therapy

(EBRT), surgery, or a combined modality treatment. As in most cancers in the head and neck, but particularly in oropharyngeal cancers, locoregional control is, even in palliative cases, extremely important when considering the overall quality of life. Although progress in reconstructive techniques has certainly made surgery a less morbid procedure than it was in the recent past, it is of value to keep in mind that especially in advanced cancers of the BOT the ultimate survival remains poor. Therefore, a treatment approach maintaining normal functions such as speech and swallowing, is to be preferred. Due to its conservation properties per se, radiation therapy (RT) should be considered seriously as the prime modality in the treatment of the BOT proper. However, normal surrounding tissues such as the cord, skin, subcutaneous tissues, mandible, temporomandibular joints, and salivary glands are dose-limiting normal tissues. Therefore, interstitial radiation therapy (IRT) as a boost dose has been suggested as a possible means of circumventing the surpassing of normal tissue tolerance. In one protocol at the Dr. Daniel den Hoed Cancer Center, Academic Hospital, Rotterdam, The Netherlands, treatment of BOT cancers consists of RT and surgery, with the neck and the primary cancer radiated by EBRT to a dose of 46 Gy; after a period of 1 or 2 weeks, the treatment is followed by a neck dissection (in case of positive neck nodes) and implantation of the BOT. For salvage treatment, if surgery is not feasible, IRT alone is sometimes considered.

Since 1991, the boost dose of IRT has been given by means of the micro-Selectron HDR. It is expected that optimization could produce better and more homogeneous dose distributions, especially in less regular implants like the volume implants of the BOT than would be possible with LDR.

A typical implant of the BOT consists of three catheters running through the BOT and, subsequently, over the dorsum of the tongue, with a number of blind-ended catheters sutured to each of them. The following sections compare the dose distribution from equal dwell times in each dwell position and that distribution resulting from so-called geometry-based optimization. Part of the goal is to restrict the active dwell positions to the part of the catheters running through the BOT and, thus, to have the parts running over the tongue surface unloaded to avoid overdosage at the tongue surface (with long-lasting severe mucositis and/or ulceration). One has to determine carefully whether or not one has an area of underdosage and, if so, how this depends on optimization.

## Description of the Implant

BOT tumors are usually implanted with three sagittal planes each consisting of one catheter (the posterior catheter), running through the BOT, caudally to the posterior margin of the primary tumor and subsequently over the surface of the tongue, with two or three blind-ended catheters sutured to it (Fig. 35). The blind-ended catheters are implanted through the tumor tissue with the proximal catheters approximately 1 cm ventrally to the anterior margin of the tumor. The proximal end of each blind-ended catheter is sutured with a button

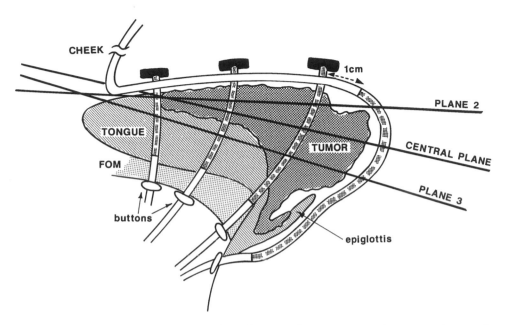

**Fig. 35.** Schematic view of BOT implant showing the posterior catheter running partly over the surface of the tongue and the blind-ended catheters sutured to it. Indicated are the position of the central plane, plane 2 at the surface of the tongue, and plane 3 running through the caudal part of the implant.

to one of the catheters running over the surface of the tongue (Fig. 35). After implantation, orthogonal radiographs, with dummy markers inserted in the catheters, are made for localization purposes. On the lateral radiograph three planes are usually indicated in which the dose distribution has to be determined (Figure 35).

After digitizing the radiographs into the treatment planning computer, the following procedure for dose planning is used. A central plane passing through the geometric center of the implant is defined, approximately perpendicular to the main direction of the blind-ended catheters (Fig. 35). In this central plane the intersections with the catheters form triangles. Following the PDS,[40] the geometric centers of these triangles are taken as basal dose points (local minima), and the average dose in these points is called the mean central dose or "the basal dose." The RD for this implant is specified at 85% of the basal dose (however, see comments in the previous section on dosimetry systems).

*Treatment Optimization*

The current comparison uses a specific patient implant that is considered representative for this type of implant. The NPS (Nucletron B.V., The Netherlands), module UPS version 11.00, has been used to calculate the dose distributions for the two situations. The line source of the LDR treatment is in this case simulated by assuming equal dwell times of a point source in each dwell position along the line. The optimized dose distribution is calculated using geometric optimization as implemented in NPS, as discussed previously.[41,42] The relative dwell weight of each dwell position is determined from the distances to other dwell positions. The dose is specified as 85% of the mean central dose. Both situations assume a source of a microSelectron HDR, having an active length of 3.5 mm and an initial reference air-kerma rate of about 4.1 cGy/h at 1 meter. Any anisotropy of this source is neglected in this study. This has been verified to be justified for volume implants of this kind. The spacing between neighboring dwell positions inside a catheter is set at 5 mm.

For the nonoptimized situation the dose distribution has been calculated for the case in which all dwell positions in all catheters are utilized with equal dwell times (Fig. 36A). It would be expected that the optimized implant could significantly reduce an overdosage at the intersection of the blind-ended catheters and the catheters running over the dorsal surface of the tongue. In order to further reduce the high-dose region occurring at the surface of the tongue, it has been suggested that an "interrupted loading" be applied to the posterior catheters. In this case only the part of the posterior catheter running through the BOT is loaded. In general this means that these catheters are only loaded at the posterior part of the implant with a separation between the active part and the posterior blind-ended catheter of about 1 cm (Fig. 36B). An underdosage at the surface of the tongue in between the catheters could occur when using a nonoptimized technique. Whether geometric optimization of this kind of implants would enable the use of an interrupted loading pattern of the posterior catheter without underdosage of the surface of the tongue has been evaluated.

The results of this evaluation use the following abbreviations for the four situations: C-NO = continuous loading, not optimized (equivalent to the general LDR treatment); C-O = continuous loading, geometrically optimized; I-NO = interrupted loading, not optimized; I-O = interrupted loading, geometrically optimized.

Isodose plots have been made in different planes passing through the implant, as indicated in Figs. 35 and 37. For further analysis volume-dose calculations have been applied. If the volumes as a function of dose are calculated as sums of discrete separate volume elements, we refer to "distributed" volume-dose analysis. If single (contiguous) volumes are determined, we use the term contiguous volume-dose analysis.[43,44] The distributed volume-dose table has been calculated using 400,000 voxels and covering a volume of 419.2 cm³. A contiguous volume-dose analysis has been applied to the above-mentioned dose distributions using voxels of 24.6 mm³ covering a volume of 440.6 cm³.

For this example 1,000 cGy has been chosen as the reference isodose in order to simplify the isodose representation.

## Results of Optimization

For this implant 11 basal dose points can be defined as shown in Fig. 37 indicated by the asterisks. Only nonobtuse triangles have been considered. The resulting relative dose contribution in each basal dose point is presented in Table 2 as a percentage of the final RD.

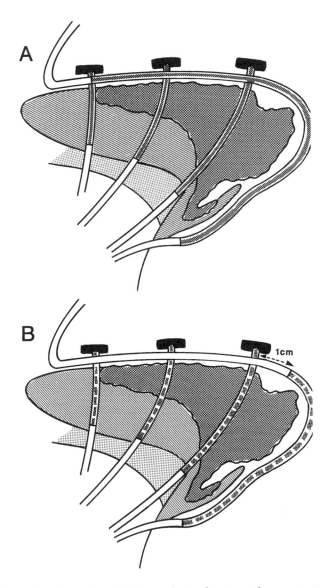

**Fig. 36.** Schematic view of a BOT implant showing the posterior catheter running partly over the surface of the tongue and the blind-ended catheters sutured to it. The shaded regions indicate the active parts of the catheters. In panel A the posterior catheter is continuously loaded. In panel B a so-called interrupted loading is applied to the posterior catheter, that is, only the part running through the BOT is loaded.

*Isodose Plots:* From all isodose plots the most relevant ones for the current investigation are presented in Figs 38 to 41. The 200%, 150%, 125%, 100%, and 80% isodose lines are shown. Figures 38 and 40 show a reduction of the overdosage at the surface of the tongue because of optimization. In the I-NO case

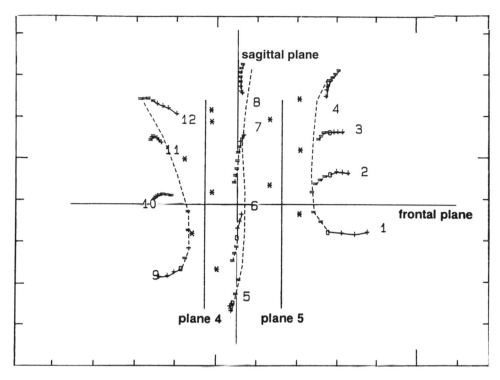

**Fig. 37.** A schematic view of the central plane with the projections of the catheters indicated. The asterisks denote the position of the basal dose points. The sagittal and frontal planes used for evaluating the dose distribution are indicated. Planes 4 and 5 represent the sagittal planes in between the sagittal source planes.

an underdosage at the surface of the tongue, which is slightly improved by optimization, is seen.

*Distributed Volume-Dose Table:* A distributed volume-dose is shown in Table 3 with the dose expressed as percentages of the reference isodose. In order to discuss the results of optimization, the ratio of the volumes due to optimized and nonoptimized cases are depicted for the continuous and interrupted loading patterns. It can be seen that in case of continuous loading, geometric optimization results in a reduction of the overdosed volume with an equal volume encompassed by the reference isodose. For the interrupted loading pattern, optimization results in an increase of the overdosed volume as well as the volume receiving at least the RD.

*Contiguous Volume-Dose Table:* The values of the largest single volume receiving at least a specified dose are presented in Table 4. For the continuous loading pattern Table 4 shows a reduction of the largest contiguous overdosed volume in combination with an equal contiguous volume receiving at least the

## Table 2

### Relative Dose Distribution in the Basal Dose Points for the C-NO, C-O, I-NO, and I-O Cases

| Basal Dose Point | Dose in Basal Dose Points (%) | | | |
|---|---|---|---|---|
| | C-NO | C-O | I-NO | I-O |
| 1 | 112 | 116 | 113 | 113 |
| 2 | 125 | 118 | 125 | 119 |
| 3 | 111 | 106 | 108 | 105 |
| 4 | 111 | 113 | 111 | 117 |
| 5 | 115 | 112 | 113 | 114 |
| 6 | 123 | 140 | 127 | 135 |
| 7 | 118 | 113 | 115 | 112 |
| 8 | 124 | 130 | 126 | 128 |
| 9 | 114 | 110 | 113 | 114 |
| 10 | 126 | 117 | 124 | 119 |
| 11 | 120 | 114 | 118 | 117 |
| range | 111–126 | 106–140 | 108–127 | 105–135 |
| 85% mean dose | 100.4 | 99.6 | 99.9 | 99.9 |
| S.D. ($\sigma_n$) | 5.5 | 9.2 | 6.5 | 7.7 |

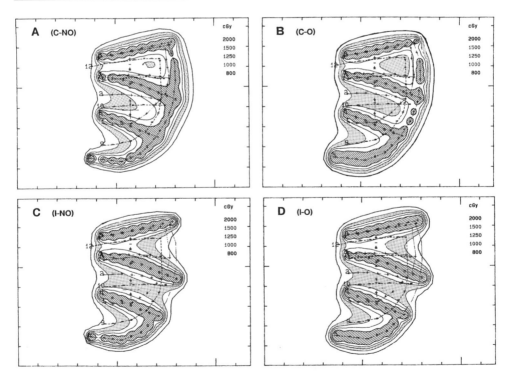

**Fig. 38.** The dose distribution in a sagittal plane running through the center of the implant. The C-NO case is presented in panel A, the C-O case in panel B, the I-NO case in panel C, and the I-O case in panel D.

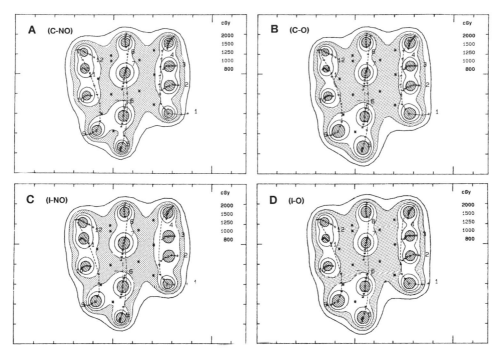

**Fig. 39.** The dose distribution in the central plane. The C-NO case is presented in panel A, the C-O case in panel B, the I-NO case in panel C, and the I-O case in panel D.

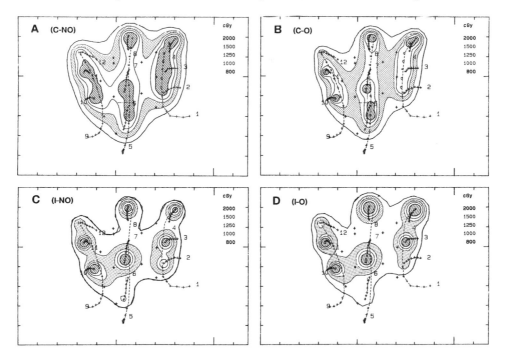

**Fig. 40.** The dose distribution in plane 2 at the surface of the tongue. The C-NO case is presented in panel A, the C-O case in panel B, the I-NO case in panel C, and the I-O case in panel D.

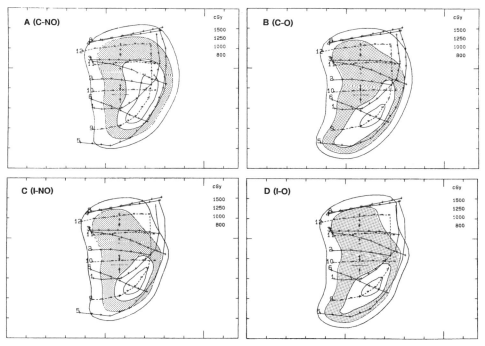

**Fig. 41.** The dose distribution in plane 4, an extra sagittal plane in between the right and central sagittal source planes. The C-NO case is presented in panel A, the C-O case in panel B, the I-NO case in panel C, and the I-O case in panel D.

RD due to optimization. In the case of an interrupted loading pattern, a slight increase is seen in the contiguous volume encompassed by the RD with a decrease of the overdosed contiguous volume.

*Natural Volume-Dose Histogram:* The natural volume-dose histograms are presented in Fig. 42 with the resulting UI shown in Table 5. The C-NO case results in a broad peak with the treatment dose situated at the low-dose side of the

## Table 3

### The Distributed Volume Dose for the C-NO, C-O, I-NO, and I-O Cases

| Dose | Volume (cm³) | | | | | |
| | C-NO | C-O | C-O/C-NO | I-NO | I-O | I-O/I-NO |
|---|---|---|---|---|---|---|
| 75% | 136.16 | 138.90 | 1.02 | 121.53 | 134.67 | 1.11 |
| 100% | 89.84 | 90.92 | 1.01 | 76.44 | 84.22 | 1.10 |
| 150% | 28.93 | 23.99 | 0.83 | 21.66 | 22.77 | 1.05 |
| 200% | 11.25 | 9.37 | 0.83 | 8.71 | 9.37 | 1.08 |
| 250% | 5.70 | 4.73 | 0.83 | 4.63 | 5.13 | 1.11 |
| 300% | 3.31 | 2.85 | 0.86 | 2.58 | 3.04 | 1.17 |

## Table 4

### The Contiguous Volume Dose For the C-NO, C-O, I-NO, and I-O Cases Showing the Largest Single Volume Receiving at Least a Specified Dose

| | *Volume (cm³) (number of volumes for a specified dose)* | | | | | |
|---|---|---|---|---|---|---|
| *Dose* | *C-NO* | *C-O* | *C-O/C-NO* | *I-NO* | *I-O* | *I-O/I-NO* |
| 50% | 223.1 (1) | 231.0 (1) | 1.04 | 206.0 (1) | 226.6 (1) | 1.10 |
| 75% | 134.0 (2) | 138.5 (1) | 1.03 | 121.0 (2) | 133.2 (2) | 1.10 |
| 100% | 87.4 (2) | 88.6 (2) | 1.01 | 74.9 (2) | 82.0 (2) | 1.09 |
| 125% | 51.5 (1) | 31.3 (2) | 0.61 | 26.8 (2) | 20.0 (3) | 0.75 |
| 150% | 19.7 (2) | 16.1 (2) | 0.82 | 7.0 (5) | 7.3 (8) | 1.04 |
| 175% | 5.8 (7) | 5.7 (7) | 0.98 | 3.3 (9) | 2.5 (9) | 0.76 |

peak almost on top of the LD. The optimized case shows a much narrower and higher peak in the histogram, indicating a significant increase in the uniformity of the dose distribution. The UI for the continuous loading pattern is respectively 1.40 for the nonoptimized situation and 1.58 for the optimized situation.

Compared to the C-NO case, both techniques using interrupted loading show narrower peaks. Again, the peak becomes narrower and higher when converting from a nonoptimized dose distribution to an optimized dose distribution. In both cases, the treatment dose level is at the high dose side of LD.

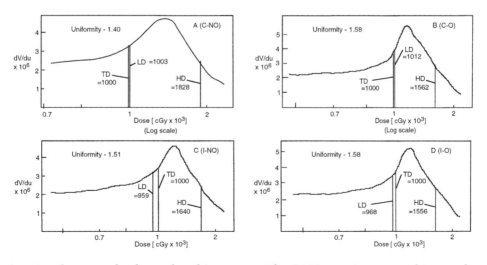

**Fig. 42.** The natural volume-dose histograms. The C-NO case is presented in panel A, the C-O case in panel B, the I-NO case in panel C, and the I-O case in panel D. The scaling of the four plots is not identical. For each case: TD = 1,000 cGy. C-NO: LD = 1,003.2 cGy, HD = 1,828.3 cGy. C-O: LD = 1,012.3 cGy, HD = 1,562.3 cGy. I-NO: LD = 959.1 cGy, HD = 1,640.0 cGy. I-O: 967.9 cGy, HD = 1,556.3 cGy.

**Table 5**

**The Dose Nonuniformity Ratios (DNR) and the Uniformity Indices (UI)
for the C-NO, C-O, I-NO, and I-O Cases**

|  | C-NO | C-O | I-NO | I-O |
|---|---|---|---|---|
| DNR | 0.32 | 0.26 | 0.28 | 0.27 |
| UI | 1.40 | 1.58 | 1.51 | 1.58 |

Interrupted loading of the posterior catheters results in UIs of 1.51 and 1.58 for the nonoptimized and optimized situation, respectively.

*Dose Nonuniformity Ratio[45]:*   The Dose Nonuniformity Ratio (DNR) resulting from the data of the distributed volume-dose table is shown in Fig. 43 as a function of the chosen reference isodose, $D_{ref}$, as a percentage of the actual reference isodose. For the C-NO case the minimum of this function is at 125% of the actual chosen reference isodose. In case of the three other situations, that is, C-O, I-NO, and C-O, the minimum of the function is at 110% for both optimized cases and 115% for the I-NO case.

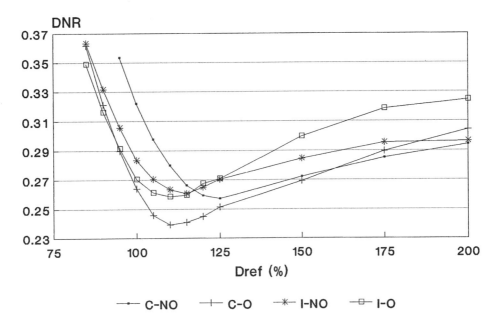

**Fig. 43.** The Dose Nonuniformity Ratio, DNR, resulting from the data of the distributed volume-dose table as a function of the chosen reference isodose, $D_{ref}$. $D_{ref}$ is represented as a percentage of the actual reference isodose, that is, 1,000 cGy. This means that in this Figure 100% is the actual chosen reference isodose. The curves are shown for the C-NO, C-O, I-NO, and I-O cases.

## Evaluation

The distributed as well as the contiguous volume-dose tables indicate for the implant with the continuous loading pattern a benefit from the optimization: the overdosed volume can be reduced with the volume enclosed by the reference isodose remaining unaffected. In the case of interrupted loading, a similar effect is only recognized from the contiguous volume-dose histogram. It shows that the overdosed volume is distributed over separate small volumes, although the total overdosed volume remains the same. Biologically, this might be of importance.

When comparing the analysis according to the natural volume-dose histogram and the dose nonuniformity curves, it follows that both methods are in agreement with each other when comparing the uniformity of the optimized and not optimized dose distributions for this volume implant. From both methods it is clear that optimization for the continuous as well as the interrupted loading pattern results in more homogeneous dose distributions than the continuous loaded, not optimized implant. When using the natural volume-dose histogram, this is expressed in a narrower and higher peak accompanied by an increase in UI. When considering the actual chosen reference isodose (100% in Fig. 43), it is seen that the lowest DNR occurs in both the C-O and I-O cases (Table 5).

In considering the implant using continuous-loaded catheters, the general conclusion drawn from this study is that optimization results in a reduction of the overdosage at the surface of the tongue, especially at the intersection of the posterior and the blind-ended catheters. Furthermore, it is clear from the volume-dose tables that there is a reduction of the overdosed volume that is accompanied with an increase in the uniformity shown by the increase in the UI and a decrease of the dose nonuniformity ratio.

In considering the implant using interrupted loading of the posterior catheters, an improvement in the dose distribution is seen due to optimization. Still, it is very difficult to draw definitive conclusions from the isodose distributions solely as to whether optimization results in a satisfactory dose distribution in this case. From the distributed volume-dose table (Table 3) it is shown that for this example the treated volume slightly decreases for the I-O case compared to the C-NO case. The contiguous volume-dose table (Table 4) shows an advantage of the interrupted loading with the overdosed volume being divided over more separate volumes than in the C-O case. Although it is shown that geometric optimization is a tool to improve the dose distribution, it should be concluded that for each implant individually one should evaluate the feasibility of using an interrupted loading pattern of the posterior catheter in combination with geometric optimization in relation to the actual implant and the clinical demand.

For such an implant the resulting dose distribution after optimization must be carefully analyzed using isodose plots in the planes mentioned in this section. If the dose distribution would be unsatisfactory, for example, a too-large indentation of the reference isodose at the surface of the tongue in one of the sagittal planes, the loading pattern of one or more of the posterior catheters should be changed and the optimization procedure restarted.

This example shows clearly the benefits of using a stepping source after-loading machine from the dose distribution point of view since it offers the opportunity to optimize the dose distribution for these rather difficult irregular volume implants.

## Optimization in Gynecologic Applications

### Cervical Carcinoma

A modest objective for treatments of the uterine cervix is to merely duplicate the distributions used for LDR applications. Success at using the same relative weightings as LDR can result in an overdose or underdose for some parts of the dose distribution. This situation comes from the differential conversion of dose to biologically effective dose with different dose levels at HDR. Since new relative weightings need to be calculated, one may as well attempt to improve the shape of the dose distribution compared with LDR applications. The construction of the LDR sources limited geometric variations to the approximately 2-cm length of the sources and limited each source term to one of four source-strength values. The flexibility of the HDR units allows for much finer specification of the resulting dose distribution. Thomadsen et al.[8] describe a technique for optimizing the treatment. For the tandem, a good distribution for treatment of the cervical volume at risk uses distance optimization with the dose specified as 100% at 18 mm lateral to the dwell position 10 mm caudal from the first position (assuming that the tip of the tandem abuts the cephalad limit of the uterine cavity and the first active dwell position falls 10 mm from the tip of the tandem) and then 20 mm lateral from the dwell position 10 mm caudal from the first point through their Points M. Points M are defined as 20 mm cephalad along the tandem from a line joining the middwell positions in the ovoids and 20 mm lateral to the tandem (see Fig. 44). Inferior to Points M the ovoids have more influence on the dose 20 mm from the tandem than the tandem itself, so optimization around the tandem stops there. The ovoid dwell times most strongly affect the dose to the vaginal mucosa in contact with the ovoid surface. Thus, optimization points for the vaginal surface should be placed at the ovoid radius lateral to the center of each ovoid. The ovoids supplied with most tandem and ovoid sets follow the LDR brachytherapy models, which evolved for use with 1.5-cm active length sources; thus, it is not surprising that the ideal spread of dwell positions covers this same 15 mm. Using a spread of dwell positions simulating 2-cm physical length projects unnecessary dose toward the bladder and rectum, while shortening the "active length" to less than 1.5 cm, undertreats the vaginal surfaces at the top and bottom of the applicator. With the stepping-source Nucletron microSelectron system, which allows the use of dwell positions separated by 2.5 mm beginning approximately 10 mm from the physical end of the applicator tip running through the center

## Comparison Pt. A and Pt. M

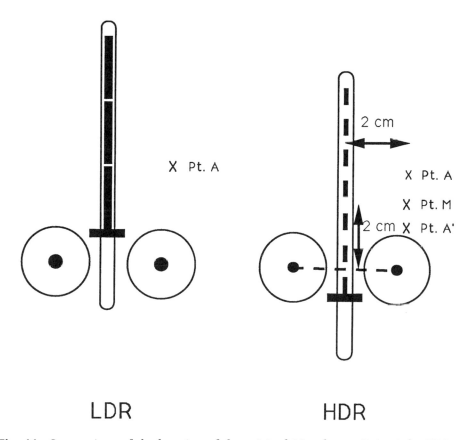

**Fig. 44.** Comparison of the location of the original Manchester Point A for LDR and HDR, the revised Point A (shown as A' on the HDR; A and A' should be approximately the same for LDR) and the Madison Point M. Notice that Point A falls too cephalad, and Point A' too caudal for the anatomical target indicated originally by Point A with LDR.

of the ovoids, using dwell position numbers 2, 4, 6, and 8 provides a good compromise between covering the ovoid surface adequately, without a significant dose to the bladder or rectum.

The biological effectiveness of the radiation delivered during an HDR fraction increases with the dose itself; that is, an 8 Gy fraction has more than twice the biological effectiveness of a 4 Gy fraction. To deliver the same relative biological dose to the vaginal mucosa in contact with the ovoid surface as with LDR (typically 145% of the dose at point A), the HDR physical dose must remain at a lower percentage to compensate for the higher dose rates at the ovoids surface compared to Point M. Table 6 presents the relative vaginal doses for a range of doses used to treat Point M. Altered anatomy or vaginal extension, just as with LDR, may require modification of the percentages. Asymme-

**Table 6**

**Dose to Ovoid Surface for Given Doses to Point M
(upper third of vagina only)**

| | Dose to point M (100%) per fraction (Gy) | Relative vaginal surface dose |
|---|---|---|
| | LDR | 145% |
| HDR | 3.7–4.9 | 140% |
| | 7.2 | 136% |
| | 8.2–10.5 | 135% |

tries between the two ovoids and the tandem can also limit how well the optimization program can succeed in achieving the desired dose distribution. Abnormalities, such as asymmetrics or unusually long or short tandems, sometimes require operator intervention into the optimization process.

In cases with vaginal extension or a narrowing of the vagina due to the course of radiation treatments, cylinders around the tandem replace the ovoids. Large volumes of the vagina cannot tolerate as high a dose as the limited portion irradiated by the ovoids. In general, treatments for involvement of two-thirds of the vagina require a decrease in the dose to the vaginal surface from 135–140% to something in the range of 100%. Treating the entire vagina limits the dose to 75–90%; however, using a differential dose along the vagina allows the application of higher doses in areas of the highest involvement. As for optimization with ovoids, the optimization points fall at the surface of the cylinders and in this case at centimeter intervals along the vaginal part of the tandem. Optimization points closer than about 0.5 cm to a junction of different radius cylinders or to where changes in dose are to occur can result in unrealistic dwell times (i.e., negative dwell times) or a poor overall match between the desired doses and the results of the optimization program owing to the necessary use of large value for the weighting for the equal dwell-time gradient (an index that tells the optimization program the importance of holding adjacent dwells to the same times—see the section on Optimization). Optimization of the uterine portion of the tandem follows the same pattern as with the tandem and ovoids, except it continues caudally below the level of Points M to 0.5 cm of the external cervical os, where the cylinders begin.

Houdek et al.[25] performed optimization for a tandem and ring applicator and found that in comparing the dose distribution to that from a conventional LDR tandem and ovoids the tandem and ring delivered a significantly lower dose to the rectum for a specified dose to Manchester Points A, by using the relative weights shown in Fig. 45.

*Inoperable Corpus Carcinoma*

Although the objective with cervical cancer is to treat the lower portion of the uterus, for corpus cancer the focus shifts toward the upper portion. LDR treatments usually used Heyman capsules to bathe the corpus in radiation. The

# Activity Distribution

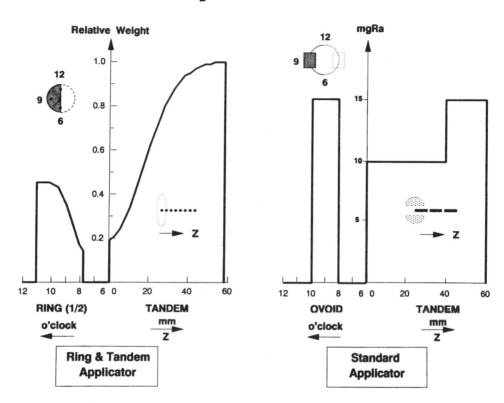

**Fig. 45.** Distribution of relative weight/activity. Left: distribution optimized for ring applicator. Right: standard activity distribution.

variable weighting available with HDR treatments allows a much larger proportion of the radiation dose to be thrown toward the tip of a tandem than with LDR sources, so that, in general, there is no need to resort to the introduction of many additional source positions. Bastin et al.[46] describe the use of tandems with corpus treatments and define two points of interest for dose specification (see Fig. 46)

Point S: defined as 1.5 cm cephalad of the tip of the tandem (usually about 2.5 cm cephalad of the first dwell position), and

Point W: defined as 2 cm caudal from the tip of the tandem and 3 cm lateral to the tandem.

Optimization entails placing optimization points at Point S, then starting at the first dwell position, placing points 3 cm laterally at 0.5-cm intervals for approximately 2 cm, and then resuming placement of lateral points about 1 cm cephalad of Points M at a distance of 2 cm at 0.5-cm intervals through Points M. Vaginal optimization follows the same procedure as for cervical carcinoma, except the vaginal dose normally is set to 89–93% but varies in cases of vaginal extension. Frequently, satisfying the optimization criteria requires the use of

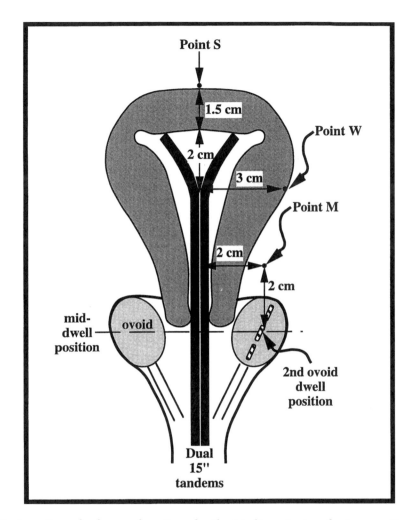

**Fig. 46.** Location of reference locations for the Madison System for inoperative cancer of the corpus. Based on Bastin et al.[46]

low values of the weighting factor for equal dwell-time gradients: the lowest value that yields non-negative dwell times probably results in the best fit.

To replace the Heyman capsules in the uterus, Bastin describes using one or two tandems, depending on the lateral diameter of the organ. If two tandems are used, they each should be 15 degrees.

## Optimization in Intraluminal Applications

Endobronchial applications comprise frequently encountered intraluminal treatments, and the same principles described here for the endobronchial treatments apply to most other intraluminal situations. As stated earlier, one advantage of the HDR stepping source configuration is that active lengths remain within the target volume compared to uniformly loaded wire (or seeds), which require extension of the source material beyond the targeted boundaries to deliver the treatment dose. Mehta et al.[47] reported on endobronchial applications with target volumes falling a 20-mm radius from the center of the applicator tube for the large-diameter bronchi and at 10 mm for small diameter bronchi. A rule of thumb developed during these treatments, and generally when using distance optimization, states that the active dwell positions begin and end inside the target volume at a distance equal to half of the target radius. Optimization points need to be placed in the four cardinal directions (to account for catheter curvature), beginning at the first dwell position and ending at the last. Usually, spacing the points 10 mm apart gives adequate spatial resolution, unless the catheter curves greatly. Additional points on the catheter at the beginning and end of the target finishes establishing the shape of the dose distribution. Often, endobronchial catheters curve greatly, giving a relatively high dose to the inside of the curve and a low dose to the outside. A decision must be made whether to deliver the specified dose to the maximum, minimum, or an average around the catheter. Unfortunately, no differential weighting can eliminate this inhomogeneity in dose.

*Acknowledgments*

The authors would like to thank Lowell Anderson, Department of Medical Physics, Memorial Sloan-Kettering Cancer Center, New York, for reviewing this chapter and N. Driver and P.C. Levendag for their work on the section on Optimization of Interstitial Implants of the Base of the Tongue.

---

# REFERENCES

1. Adams G. Errors in brachytherapy. In: Wright A, Boyer A, eds. Advances in Radiation Therapy Treatment Planning. New York: American Institute of Physics; 1983, 575-600.
2. Chassagne D, Horiot JC. Propositions pour une définition commune points de référence en curiethérapie gynéologique. J Radiol Electrol 58:371, 1977; and Chassagne D, Gerbaulet A, Dutreix A, Cosset JM. Utilization pratique dosimétrie pur ordinateur en curiethérapie gynécolgique. J Radio Electrol 58:387-393, 1977.
3. Paterson R. The Treatment of Malignant Disease by Radiotherapy, 2nd ed. Rome and London: Butler & Tanner, Ltd.; 1963, 336.
4. Pierquin B, Chassagne DJ, Chahbazian CM, et al. Brachytherapy. St. Louis: Warrem H. Green, Inc.; 1978.
5. Dutreix A, Marinello G, Wambersle A. Dosimetrie en Curietherapie. Paris, France: Masson; 1982.
6. Summarized in Meredith WJ, ed. Radium Dosage. Edinburgh and London: E. & S. Livingstone, Ltd.; 1967.
7. Stitt JA, Fowler JF, Thomadsen BR, et al. High dose-rate intracavitary brachytherapy for carcinoma of the cervix—The Madison system. I:clinical and radiobiological considerations. Int J Radiat Oncol Biol Phys 24:335-348, 1992.

8. Thomadsen BR, Shahabi S, Stitt JA, et al. High dose rate intracavitary brachytherapy for carcinoma of the cervix: The Madison system. II: procedural and physical considerations. Int J Radiat Oncol Biol Phys 24:349-357, 1992.

9. Marinello G, Valero M, Leung S, et al. Comparative dosimetry between iridium wires and seed ribbons. Int J Radiat Oncol Biol Phys 11:1733-1739, 1985.

10. van der Laarse R. Stepping source dosimetry system as an extension of the Paris system. Presented at the International Brachytherapy Working Conference; September 6-8, 1992; Baltimore, Md.

11. Edmundson GK. Geometry based optimization for stepping source implants. In: Brachytherapy HDR and LDR. Columbia, Md.: Nucletron Corp.; 1990, 184-192.

12. Quimby, EH. Dosage calculations with radioactive materials. In: Glasser O, Quimby EH, Taylor LS, et al. eds. Physical Foundations of Radiology, 3rd ed. New York: Hoeber Medical Div., Harper and Row, 1963.

13. Williamson JF, Anderson LL, Grigsby PW. American Endocurietherapy Society recommendations for specification of brachytherapy source strength. Endocurie/Hypertherm Oncol 9:1-7, 1993.

14. Meisberger LL, Keller R, Shalek RJ. The effective attenuation in water of gamma rays of gold-198, iridium-192, cesium-137, radium-226 and cobalt-60. Radiology 90:953–957, 1968.

15. van Kleffens HT, Star WM. Application of stereo x-ray photogrammetry. Int J Radiat Oncol Biol Phys 5:557-563, 1979.

16. van der Laarse R. New implementations in UPS Version 10 and its differences from UPS Version 9.11. In: Nucletron Manual. Veenendaal, The Netherlands: Nucletron; 1991.

17. Williamson JF, Perera H, Zuofeng L. Comparison of calculated and measure heterogeneity correction factors for $^{125}$I, $^{137}$Cs, and $^{192}$Ir brachytherapy sources near localized heterogeneities. Med Phys 20:209-222, 1993.

18. Williamson JF, Zuofeng L, Wong JW. One-dimensional scatter-subtraction method for brachytherapy dose calculation near bounded heterogeneities. Med Phys 20:233-244, 1993.

19. Cerra F, Rodgers JE. Dose distribution anisotropy of the Gamma Med IIi brachytherapy source. Endocurie/Hypertherm Oncol 6:71-80, 1990.

20. Kubo H, Chin RB. Angular exposure distribution measurements of a high dose rate Ir-192 source. Med Phys 18:598, 1991.

21. Baltas D, Kramer R, Loffler E. Measurements of the anisotropy of the new HDR iridium-192 source for the microSelectron-HDR. In: Mould RF, ed. International Brachytherapy. Veenendaal, The Netherlands: Nucletron International BV; 1992, 290-306.

22. Moerland MA, de Koning JHAG, Battermann JJ. The anisotropic dose distribution of a HDR iridium-192 source. In: Mould RF, ed. International Brachytherapy. Veenendaal, The Netherlands, Nucletron International BV; 1991, 286-289.

23. Houdek PV, Schwade JG, Wu X, et al. Dose determination in high dose-rate brachytherapy. Int J Radiat Oncol Biol Phys 24:795-801, 1992.

24. microSelectron; Columbia, Md.: Nucletron Corp.

25. Houdek PV, Schwade JG, Abitbol AA, et al. Optimization of high dose rate cervix brachytherapy. Part I: dose distribution. Int J Radiat Oncol Biol Phys 21:1621-1625, 1991.

26. Nath R, Meigooni AS, Meli JA. Dosimetry on transverse axes of $^{125}$I and $^{192}$Ir interstitial brachytherapy sources. Med Phys 17:1032-1040, 1990.

27. Weaver KA, Smith V, Huang D, et al. Dose parameters of $^{125}$I and $^{192}$Ir seed sources. Med Phys 16:636-643, 1989.

28. Williamson JF, Nath R. Clinical implementation of AAPM Task Group 32 recommendations on brachytherapy source strength specification. Med Phys 18:439-448, 1991.

29. Mate TP, Gottesman J, Anderson K, et al. Fractionated high dose rate $^{192}$Ir conformal prostate brachytherapy: The Seattle method. Presented at the conference on "Prostate Cancer: The Role of Interstitial Implantation"; Third Annual Symposium; June 26-27, 1992; Seattle, Wash.

30. van der Laarse R. Optimization of high dose rate brachytherapy. In: Activity—The Selectron User's Newsletter 2:14-15, 1989.

31. van der Laarse R, Edmundson GK, Luthmann RW, et al. Optimization of HDR brachytherapy dose distributions. In: Activity—The Selectron User's Newsletter 2:94-101, 1991.

32. Sloboda RS. Optimization of brachytherapy dose distributions by simulated annealing. Med Phys 19:955-964, 1992. See also Sloboda RS, Pearcey RG, Gillan SJ. Optimized low dose rate pellet configuration for intravaginal brachytherapy. Int J Radiat Oncol Biol Phys 26:499-511, 1993.

33. Holms TW. A Model for the Physical Optimization for External Beam Radiotherapy. Madison, Wisc.: University of Wisconsin; 1993. Thesis. See also Luenberger DG. Linear and Nonlinear Programming, 2nd ed., chapter 9. Reading, Mass.: Addison and Wesley; 1989, and Holms TW, Mackie TR. A comparison of three inverse treatment planning algorithims. Phys Med Biol 39:91-106, 1994.

34. Anderson LL. A "natural" volume-dose histogram for brachytherapy. Med Phys 13:899-903, 1986.

35. Chen GTY. Dose volume histograms in treatment planning. Int J Radiat Oncol Biol Phys 14:1319-1320, 1988.

36. Wu A, Ulin K, Sternick ES. A dose homogeneity index for evaluating $^{192}$Ir interstitial breast implants. Med Phys 15:104-107, 1988.

37. Loft SM, Dale RG. The incorporation of specific tissue/nuclide attenuation data into the Anderson method for producing brachytherapy volume-dose histograms. Phys Med Biol 35:1519-1531, 1990.

38. Niemierko A, Goitein M. Random sampling for evaluating treatment plans. Med Phys 17:753-762, 1990.

39. King CG, Stockstill TF, Bloomer WD, et al. Point dose variations with time in brachytherapy for cervical carcinoma. Med Phys 19:777, 1992. (Abstract)

40. Dutreix A, Marinello G, Wambersie A. Dosimétrie en Curiethérapie. Paris, France: Masson; 1982.

41. Edmundson GK. Geometry-based optimization for stepping source implants. In: Activity—The Selectron User's Newsletter 5(4):22, 1991.

42. Edmundson GK. Geometric optimisation: an American view. In: Mould RF, ed. International Brachytherapy. Veenendaal, The Netherlands: Nucletron International BV; 1992, 256–257.

43. Neblett DL, Syed AMN, Puthawala AA, et al. An interstitial implant technique evaluated by contiguous volume analysis. Endocurie/Hypertherm Oncol 1:213–221, 1985.

44. Visser AG, Levendag PC, Driver N, et al. Application of volume-dose calculations in brachytherapy: experience from "irregular" head and neck implantations. In: Mould RF, ed. Brachytherapy 2. Veenendaal, The Netherlands: Nucletron International BV; 1989, 397–403.

45. Saw CB, Suntharalingam N. Quantitative assessment of interstitial implants. Int J Radiat Oncol Biol Phys 20:135–139, 1991.

46. Bastin KT, Buchler DA, Thomadsen BR. Heyman's based model for high dose rate multi-tandem intracavitary brachytherapy. Endocurie Hypertherm Oncol 9:9-13, 1993.

47. Mehta M, Petereit D, Chosy L, et al. Sequential comparison of low dose rate and hyperfractionated high dose rate endobronchial radiation for malignant airway occlusion. Int J Radiat Oncol Biol Phys 23:133-139, 1992.

# Chapter 7

# Quality Assurance for High Dose Rate Brachytherapy

*Jeffrey F. Williamson, Gary A. Ezzell, Arthur Olch, and Bruce R. Thomadsen*

## Introduction

Despite several hundred high dose rate (HDR) remote afterloading units in active clinical use throughout the world, consensus as to the essential elements of a quality assurance (QA) program has yet to be achieved[1-4] even on such easily quantifiable issues as source-strength specification and calibration.[5] Probably in no other area of brachytherapy is such a program so essential. HDR brachytherapy is characterized by high-intensity sources with dose rates on the order of 450 Gy/h, computer optimization of implant quality resulting in differentially loaded sequences of dwell positions, a complex computer-controlled device for treatment delivery, electronic links between the treatment-planning computer and treatment-delivery device, and the delivery of large fractions (200–1,500 cGy) in a few minutes. Thus, all the elements of computer-optimized and computer-controlled delivery of a conformal dose distribution are present in HDR brachytherapy, a modality that is still in the planning stage for external-beam radiotherapy. In contrast to external-beam conformal radiotherapy, a course of HDR brachytherapy may consist of a single outpatient visit in which applicator insertion, implant imaging, treatment planning and treatment delivery must be completed in a few hours. Several serious treatment delivery errors have been reported, including positioning of the active source train outside the treatment volume,[6] mispositioning of dose prescription points,[6] and failure to detect a source that had separated from its cable and remained in the implanted catheter for 91 hours.[7]

The goal of an HDR brachytherapy QA program is no different from that in other areas of radiation oncology: to maximize the likelihood that each individual treatment is administered consistently, that it accurately realizes the radiation oncologist's clinical intent, and that it is executed with regard to safety of the patient and others who may be exposed to the source during the course of treatment. More specifically, an HDR QA program must ensure that the intended source is accurately delivered to its intended position within the correct applicator, remain there for the correct length of time, and accurately

From: Nag, S. (ed.): *High Dose Rate Brachytherapy: A Textbook*, Futura Publishing Company, Inc., Armonk, NY, © 1994.

deliver the absorbed dose required to realize the radiation oncologist's written prescription. In addition, the treatment must be administered safely so as not to exceed accepted exposure limits for members of the general public and radiation workers involved in the procedure. A comprehensive QA program addresses each of the three basic processes constituting an HDR treatment.

### Applicator Insertion Process

Applicator selection and placement in the patient is under control of the radiation oncologist and referring surgeon: its success depends on the experience and surgical skill of these physicians. Physics QA duties include documentation of the applicator system inserted, its correct operation, and the correct correlation with target volume localization information.

### Treatment-Planning Process

Treatment planning includes formulation of the prescription, radiographic examination of the implant, definition of the target volume, and computer-assisted dose-calculation and dose-optimization planning. The end result of this process is identification of the treatment-device programming parameters, that is, the "correct" dwell positions and dwell times for each catheter. "Correct parameters" means those required to accurately deliver the prescribed dose distribution, including any volume or dose constraints on irradiated normal tissue. A QA program must ensure, in general and for each treatment, that the treatment planning program functions accurately, that the system for inferring dwell-position locations from simulation radiographs performs accurately, that the target volume rendered on these films is consistent with all known tumor localization data, and that optimization endpoints used by the treatment planning program are appropriate.

### Treatment Delivery Process

This process includes entry of the programming parameters into the remote afterloader, connection of the patient to the device, and delivery of treatment. The QA program must contain procedures for validating the entered data, responding to unexpected machine malfunctions and emergencies, and documenting the delivered treatment.

## Machine Quality Assurance

A major focus of QA is to verify accurate operation of the remote afterloading device. Acceptance testing and commissioning involves comprehensive physical characterization of the device and verifying all important operating specifications. This includes establishing treatment planning and source localization procedures consistent with the method utilized by the device to control positional, temporal, and dose-delivery accuracy. Another goal is to assure patient and public safety by careful facility surveys and systematic verification of emergency response systems, error-detection capabilities, and interlock of the remote afterloading system. Well-defined QA tests to be carried out at specified quarterly, monthly, or daily intervals are designed to confirm the continuing integrity of the operating specifications of the device through time.

## Treatment Team Organization and Procedure-Specific Quality Assurance

In the authors' experience, most errors in HDR brachytherapy are the result of human errors, miscommunications, or a misunderstanding of equipment operation rather than failure of the treatment delivery and planning devices to perform properly. HDR treatment planning and delivery are complex human activities involving cooperation of physician, physicist, technologist, nurse, and dosimetrist, who must execute their functions correctly and unambiguously receive and transfer critical information from one another for overall treatment-delivery accuracy to be achieved. Development of an operational QA program requires careful definition of each participant's role, including specifying to whom variances from expected outcome are to be reported and providing training appropriate for each function. The anticipated flow of the entire procedure must be defined, and forms must be designed to clearly document critical information, including the implant drawing, catheter numbering system, intracavitary applicators utilized, and target localization data to ensure accurate communication from the physician to the physicist and treatment planner, from operating room (OR) to simulation, and from treatment planning to treatment delivery. Checks to verify accurate execution of critical staff functions, for example, identification of source positioning parameters from simulation films, must be developed. The points in the treatment planning and delivery processes at which the physicist or physician must intervene to verify correct execution as well as what is to be checked must be clearly identified. Finally, procedures must be developed for identifying and resolving variances from the expected outcome such as source fracture or other machine malfunction. Careful attention to human-factor aspects of treatment delivery is critical and all too often neglected.

Each of the four coauthors of this chapter represents an institution with clinically active HDR brachytherapy programs that has invested heavily in the development of innovative and practical QA programs. Our intent is to represent the sometimes divergent results of our collective experience, with emphasis on the process of logically developing a QA program to suit the unique needs of individual institutions.

## Quality Assurance Program Endpoints

Currently, three types of single-stepping source remote afterloading devices are available in the United States: the GammaMed 12i, the Nucletron micro-Selectron/HDR (Nucletron Corp., Columbia, Md.), and the Omnitron 2000 systems, all of which contain a single moving high-intensity $^{192}$Ir source. In addition, a programmable source-train device (Nucletron Selectron/HDR), which uses spherical $^{60}$Co sources and inactive spacers, is available. A large variety of applicator and localization systems are offered by these vendors, and clinically-active HDR brachytherapists utilize an even larger array of implantation, target-localization, and optimization techniques. Such variability in device features and clinical practice precludes development of a fixed QA protocol: from basic principles, each physicist must develop a program specifically suited to his or her individual clinical environment. Systematic development of a QA program that encompasses both device function and human factors requires that the clinical goals of the treatment program be identified, translated into physical endpoints, and assigned tolerances for acceptable performance.

For any clinical brachytherapy application, these endpoints fall into the following four general categories.[4,8]

## Safety of the Patient and the Public

This group of QA endpoints includes adequacy of the facility-shielding barriers, as well as the remote afterloader safe. The governing guidelines are spelled out in great detail by the U.S. Nuclear Regulatory Commission (NRC). Ensuring patient safety, that is, the prevention of complications due to machine failure or operator error, includes the correct functioning of relevant error recognition features, interlocks, treatment status indicators, and emergency response systems.

## Positional Accuracy

Verification of positional accuracy requires that one confirms that the correct sequence of active sources or dwell positions is delivered to the correct position in the correct applicator. "Correct position" refers specifically to the position prescribed by the attending radiation oncologist. Often, prescribed positions are defined relative to radiographic images of dummy seeds or radiographic markers that are inserted into the applicator of interest prior to simulation. For surface-dose or gynecologic intracavitary applicators, correct position may be defined as the expected position relative to the applicator surfaces. Any other definition of correct position (distance from the indexer, position on an autoradiograph) is irrelevant. Positional accuracy assessment reduces to verifying the protocol (hereafter called "simulation source localization procedure") for calculating the machine programming parameters (length, position, channel number) used to position the actual source at a desired location in the catheter defined by the radiographic marker seeds. The NRC generally demands that an accuracy criterion of ± 1 mm be met. In our experience, this may be difficult to achieve, except under laboratory conditions. A criterion of ± 2 mm, exclusive of applicator positioning errors in the patient, is achievable in most clinical applications.

An important clinical aspect of positional accuracy is definition of the target volume or area used as the basis for choosing the treatment volume: the 3-dimensional (3-D) space encompassed by the activated dwell positions. For endobronchial brachytherapy, this entails correlating bronchoscopically or computed tomography (CT)-localized tumor margins with the dummy seed positions visualized on the simulation radiographs and may require attention to applicator motion. Since this aspect of positional accuracy is highly dependent on the skill of the operating radiation oncologist and level of physicist involvement expected or tolerated, general guidelines are difficult to formulate.

## Temporal Accuracy

A treatment system achieves temporal accuracy if each source sequence or single-source "dwell position" remains at its intended position for the length of time specified by the treatment program. Tests of absolute timer accuracy are required whenever source calibration is based upon an external time standard, whereas relative tests suffice when the machine timer is used for both treatment delivery and source-strength calibration. An accuracy criterion of ± 2% seems easily achievable both by manual afterloading techniques and commercially-available remote afterloading systems. Verification of absolute temporal accuracy for a given device requires that one independently measure the time interval and that the source remains stationary at a dwell position for a range of machine timer settings. In addition, the influence of transit dose on dose delivery accuracy must be evaluated and corrected for, if necessary. Transit dose is the additional dose delivered while the source is in motion.

## Dose-Delivery Accuracy

Even with completely error-free source positioning and dwell-time delivery, many other variables must be controlled in order to assure accurate delivery of the absorbed dose in tissue. It is useful to subdivide dose-delivery accuracy into physical and clinical aspects. Physically accurate dose delivery is achieved if the predicted dose and actual dose absorbed by the medium are equal at reference points specified without positional error relative to the applicator. This category neglects the difficult problem of defining dose calculation points relative to patient anatomy. Accurate calibration of the source in terms of a well-defined physical quantity, preferably air-kerma strength, is among the most important physical dose-delivery parameters. Another factor is selection of accurate dosimetric data for calculating the single-source dose distribution. Assessment of applicator attenuation and shielding corrections is desirable to ensure that the dose distribution upon which the radiation oncologist's knowledge of clinical dose response rests is duplicated. It is difficult to assign a meaningful tolerance to this endpoint since no dosimetric data exists in the published literature either for currently available $^{192}$Ir sources or for shielding corrections. In addition, no practical and validated dose-measurement technology is available to the hospital physicist. However, a source-calibration accuracy of ± 2% relative to existing external beam air-kerma standards seems reasonable. On the basis of recent low dose rate (LDR) dosimetry experience,[9] physical dose-delivery accuracy on the order of 5% is achievable at distances of 1 to 5 cm from the source. Finally, relative to the input data supplied and the algorithm assumed, the computer-assisted dose calculations should have a numerical accuracy of at least ± 2%.

Clinical dose-delivery accuracy includes a large array of often difficult-to-solve problems. Relatively straightforward issues include the accuracy with which the dosimetrist and treatment planning computer reconstruct the relative 3-D geometry of the implant. In intracavitary brachytherapy, consistent, if not accurate, localization of bladder and rectal reference points is often important. Finally, if dwell weights are optimized to achieve dose uniformity or adequate coverage of a specified target volume, careful attention to optimization endpoints, prescription criteria, and quality of the resultant implant is required. The more difficult problems include identification of the target volume and critical organ margins relative to the implanted applicators and controlling or compensating for patient motion.

## Acceptance Testing and Commissioning of HDR Remote Afterloading Devices

The goal of acceptance testing is to confirm that a treatment device lives up to its specifications, whereas commissioning involves measurement of those physical parameters necessary to support clinical dose calculation and treatment, for example, measurement of beam characteristics for a linear accelerator. To the extent the distinction is meaningful in HDR brachytherapy, commissioning involves working intensively with the device to discover its strengths and weaknesses with respect to the principal QA endpoints, described above, and developing clinical procedures for exploiting its strengths and neutralizing its weaknesses. Acceptance and commissioning procedures are performed after installation of the device but before its clinical utilization.

## Safety of the Patient and the Public

### Radiation Safety

The NRC currently requires[11] that exposure rates in uncontrolled areas adjacent to brachytherapy sources receive less than 2 mR in any hour and 100 mR in any week (both independent of occupancy) and that no member of the general public receive more than 500 mR annually (based on estimated occupancy). These requirements are expected to change early in 1994: the hourly limit will remain the same, the weekly workload requirement will be eliminated, and the individual exposure limit will fall to 100 mR/year. For exposure of occupationally exposed workers in controlled areas, the customary interpretation of the ALARA (as low as reasonably achievable) principle generally limits whole-body personnel exposures to 500 mR annually, although both occupancy and workload factors may be used. A careful survey of primary exposure levels in all occupiable space around the HDR suite is indicated, with the source placed in air at the expected treatment position. Time can be saved by using a Geiger-Müller detector to locate the position of maximum exposure in each area, followed by quantitative measurement of exposure rate with a calibrated ion chamber survey meter. Since the HDR source is uncollimated, the adequacy of an existing teletherapy vault will depend on the thickness of its leakage and scatter barriers, not its primary beam barriers. Once the position of maximum exposure in each area has been located, it should be marked or recorded since the NRC generally requires its licensees to repeat the facility survey each time a new source is installed. The source should be placed in a scattering phantom for exposure measurements near unshielded doors protected by a maze. To verify compliance with the hourly limit, the measured instantaneous exposure rate may be weighted by the expected use or duty factor, generally 0.25. A generous estimate of the number of weekly treatments, along with some allowance for QA activities, should be used to estimate weekly and annual exposures. HDR units placed in existing $^{60}$Co teletherapy vaults, which are shielded only for scatter and leakage, may fail the more stringent Code of Federal Regulations (CFR), Part 20,[11] annual exposure limits for even modestly large workloads. This may require enhanced shielding, workload limits, or a license amendment requesting exemption from the revised Part 20. In addition to area exposure limits, the NRC usually requires that the exposure rate 1 m from the treatment head with the source in its retracted position be limited to 0.25 mR/h. The maximum exposure rate in contact with the unit casing should be noted as well. Finally, the NRC requires each source to be leak tested at 180-day intervals. For single-source $^{192}$Ir treatment units, the vendor's leak test usually suffices since the source is replaced at quarterly intervals. Since CFR Part 35[10] makes no reference to HDR brachytherapy, regulatory requirements may vary from region to region or state to state.

## Emergency Response and Error-Detection Systems

Many interlock tests and ancillary safety systems are common to all HDR remote afterloading systems. All systems should be equipped with a closed circuit television system (CCTV) for observing the patient as well as a two-way intercom system. A door interlock, which interrupts treatment and does not allow its resumption without reactivating treatment from the control console, must be provided. The room must be equipped with an independent area monitor, which indicates (both inside the room and at the operator's console) whether the source is retracted or is in treatment position. The response of the system to AC power failure should be tested. Correct response includes immediate retraction of all radioactive sources and, following restoration of power, accurate display of source position and dwell time remaining at the instant of interruption. Correct operation of visual indicators of treatment (usually a yellow light for source exposed and a green light for source fully retracted) at the console, on the treatment unit, and above the treatment room door should be verified. A flashing "High Radiation Area" sign should be located above the door. The integrity of all treatment head-to-transfer tubes and transfer tube-to-applicator connections must be checked. Any mechanical or electronic interlock systems, designed to prevent connection of applicators and treatment tubes to an incorrect treatment-head position, should be checked. The room should be properly posted, including the "High Radiation Area" sign, emergency procedures, and the NRC or agreement state notice to radiation workers. The unit should never be used without the operator's manual being present, especially for those devices that indicate machine status with numerical error codes rather than the full text of the error condition. A Geiger-Müller survey meter with a full scale of least 1,000 mR/h should be at hand for confirming source retraction prior to releasing the patient from the room. Finally, emergency equipment, needed to bring the source under control, should be present. This includes a portable safe, forceps, a wire cutter for single-stepping source machines, and any surgical instruments required to remove applicators from the patient on an emergency basis. A recently issued NRC bulletin[12] effectively requires posttreatment radiation surveys and written emergency procedures, including surgical intervention, to be followed should the source fail to retract.

## Single-Stepping Source Machines

Proper testing of many error detection, interlock, and emergency response systems requires knowledge of the specific machine design. We first consider single-stepping source machines such as the GammaMed IIi and 12i, the microSelectron/HDR (see Fig. 1), and the Omnitron 2000 devices. Each of these systems utilizes a single high-intensity $^{192}$Ir source welded to the end of a cable. Upon receiving a command to initiate treatment, the source cable advances from the internal safe of the afterloader to the first treated dwell position in the first catheter, sequentially steps through each dwell position, is retracted into the safe, and then is ejected into the next catheter to be treated. Each of these back-and-forth motions of the cable is executed by a stepper motor activated by pulses originating in the system microprocessor. All single-stepping source systems verify that the cable moves as programmed by means of an optical encoder or other device that compares angular rotation of the stepper motor shaft or cable length ejected or retracted with the number of pulses sent to the motor. This system is used to detect catheter obstruction or excessive friction during cable motion. Under various conditions, for example, source sticking upon retraction, a high-torque DC emergency motor is programmed to retract the

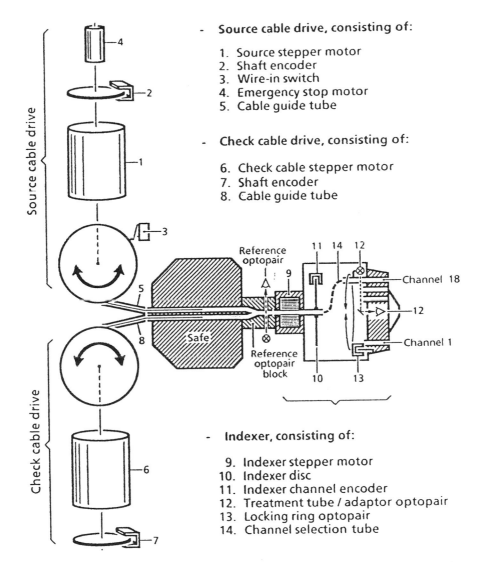

- Source cable drive, consisting of:

  1. Source stepper motor
  2. Shaft encoder
  3. Wire-in switch
  4. Emergency stop motor
  5. Cable guide tube

- Check cable drive, consisting of:

  6. Check cable stepper motor
  7. Shaft encoder
  8. Cable guide tube

- Indexer, consisting of:

  9. Indexer stepper motor
  10. Indexer disc
  11. Indexer channel encoder
  12. Treatment tube / adaptor optopair
  13. Locking ring optopair
  14. Channel selection tube

**Fig.1.** Functional diagram of a single-stepping source remote afterloading device. Courtesy of Nucletron Corporation, Columbia, Md.

source. The physicist should identify all conditions under which this system is activated, for example, contact with obstruction during ejection and failure of primary timer. The exit and return of the cable to its safe are usually confirmed by an "opti-pair," which is a paired light-sensitive detector and infrared light source that detects the cable when its tip obstructs the light path. In addition, all currently-marketed HDR devices are equipped with check cables or dummy sources that check the patency of the catheter system prior to ejection of the cable bearing the radioactive source. All single-stepping source systems are equipped with an indexer, a motor that rotates the source path within the treatment head and aligns it with the catheter to be treated. The indexer contains an array of receptacles into which source transfer or guide tubes attach. Interstitial, intracavitary, or transluminal applicators are attached to the distal ends of these transfer tubes. Correct function of each of these subsystems is checked prior to source ejection, and source motion is prevented or "interlocked" if failure is noted.

Two of the four authors of this chapter check most mechanical interlocks with a dummy source cable in place of the radioactive source assembly, allowing the physicist to safely remain in the room during simulated treatments. A principle of safety-system testing is to simulate the targeted clinical error condition as closely as possible. Such tests include: (a) activation of the emergency retraction motor by the emergency stop buttons at the control console, the room entry corridor, and on the treatment unit; (b) detection of a blocked catheter by the check cable; (c) activation of the emergency motor by blocking and restraining the active source cable with one's fingers; (d) response to unlocked indexer ring; (e) response to disconnected transfer tube and disconnected applicator; and (f) correct function of the manual crank-operated source-retraction system. Activation of the emergency retraction motor can be detected by a characteristic noise or by monitoring the voltage across its terminals.

Systematic real-life clinical testing of critical interlocks and safety systems designed to detect serious device and/or source transport errors cannot be achieved without special equipment, temporary modification of the machine, and the vendor's assistance. These catastrophic error conditions include failure of the source to retract, loss of the source tip, failure of the primary timer, and adequate emergency retraction pulling force. Consequently, such "total system" testing is currently not performed either by the vendors or clinical users. Examples of highly desirable tests in the authors' opinion include (1) measurement of the emergency motor torque, (2) response to simulated loss of source capsule, (3) simulation of timer failure, and (4) simulation of stepper motor failure. Test (4) directly checks the ability of the machine to detect discrepancies between the optical encoder output and number of transmitted motor stepper pulses. Test (2), which involves clipping off the end of a dummy source while in treatment mode, verifies that the system detects discrepancies between the cable lengths ejected and retracted, which is the principal method of detecting a lost source. Test (2) should be performed while the machine is in emergency retraction mode and in the normal operating mode. Recently, separation of a 4 Ci HDR source from its cable went undetected by the users, in part, because the machine software disabled the cable-length verification check during operation of its emergency retraction motors.[7] A different test would be needed for the GammaMed 12i device. A Geiger-Müller radiation detector, built into the base of this machine, monitors the ambient radiation level within the room to confirm source retraction.

A model for real-life testing of safety interlocks has been developed by Weinhous et al.,[13] who attempted to test every important interlock on a multiple-modality computer-controlled linear accelerator. Their approach was to simulate each targeted error condition under clinical operating conditions as closely as possible and then note whether the interlock performed its specified function. In contrast, HDR remote afterloader vendors typically test interlock logic by confronting an isolated HDR microprocessor with input signals simulating each target error condition rather than testing the entire device. Further development of more comprehensive procedures for testing individual machine responses to simulated failures and emergencies under clinically realistic operating conditions is clearly needed.

## Programmable Source-Train Machines

Systems such as the Selectron/HDR (see Fig. 2) utilize small (2.5-mm diameter) spherical $^{60}$Co sources and geometrically-identical spherical spacers that are transported from the intermediate safe to intracavitary treatment applicators by means of compressed air.[14-18] Each applicator consists of 48 fixed treatment positions, each of which can be occupied by a spacer or radioactive source, allowing any 48-pellet sequence of spacers and radioactive sources to be selected by the user. Prior to programming, the radioactive sources and spacers are segregated into separate compartments of the main safe. The Selectron "column" composes or assembles user-programmed sequences using mechanical valves to transfer individual pellets from the main safe to the appropriate compartment of the intermediate safe which, in turn, is coupled to the corresponding applicator. Opti-pairs count each pellet type leaving the main safe and arriving at each intermediate safe compartment to verify correct sequencing. The Selectron transfer tubes and applicators contain two concentric lumina that allow compressed air to flow through the inner source-transport lumen either in the proximal-to-distal direction (source-ejection mode) or distal-to-proximal direction (source-retraction mode). Throughout this chapter, "distal" and "proximal" are used to designate the directions away from and toward the afterloader. By purging the applicator with compressed air and monitoring the pressure buildup in each transfer tube, the Selectron can detect detached applicators and interrupt treatment as appropriate. Upon initiating treatment, the sequence is pneumatically transported into position within the treatment needle and held in position by a larger diameter sphere located just proximal to the pellet train. The large pellet blocks the needle aperture, preventing air flow, increasing treatment tube pressure, and signaling the Selectron microprocessor that the sequence is in treatment position.

Emergency response tests specific to the Selectron/HDR system [15] include (a) immediate retraction of the source train upon interrupting the compressed air supply, (b) preventing treatment initiation in the absence of an applicator, (c) retraction of all source trains if the applicator is removed during treatment, and (d) retraction of all source trains when the control pellet is displaced from the needle aperture. Such tests, which often require the physicist to remain in the treatment room during treatment, can be performed using a sequence of nonradioactive pellets.

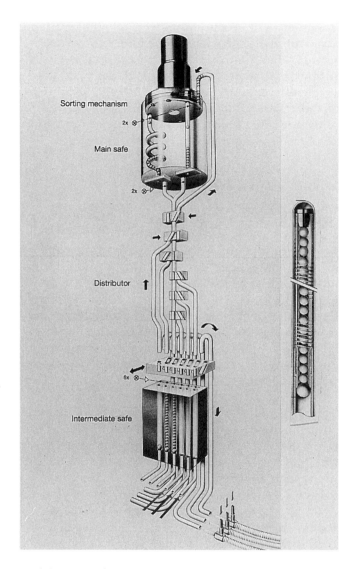

**Fig. 2.** Functional diagram of a programmable source train afterloading device, the Selectron/HDR. The inset to the right of the main figure illustrates the two concentric lumina of the applicator and the larger-diameter control pellet that defines the location of the proximal aspect of the source train. Courtesy of Nucletron Corporation.

## Positional Accuracy

For all HDR systems, verification of positional accuracy consists of two basic steps: (a) applicator-independent verification that the device accurately positions the radioactive sources or dwell positions relative to the reference position utilized by the device as its positioning criterion and (b), assuming accurate type (a) positioning, verification that the active source centers are accurately positioned at their prescribed locations in each available type of applicator system. Type (a) accuracy refers to the inherent positional accuracy of the device, for example, that a single-stepping source afterloader accurately ejects the length of source cable corresponding to its programmed length setting. Its assessment is highly dependent upon machine design. Type (b) accuracy encompasses any other condition that might cause the radioactive source to deviate from its prescribed location. Examples of type (b) positioning errors include variations in transfer-tube length, misregistration between the simulation dummy marker locations and actual source position, or source cable backlash within a large, inner diameter transfer tube resulting in a difference between the length of cable ejected and displacement of the source along the axis of the applicator system. Type (b) accuracy is dependent upon the localization procedure used, that is, the method used to infer length programming parameters from simulation radiographs or other information used to identify the prescribed location of the active dwell positions. A third source of error, type (c), can arise in individual treatments because of acute machine failure, operator programming errors, or failure to correctly execute the source localization procedure.

## Verification of Intrinsic (Type a) Positional Accuracy

Table 1 describes the mechanisms by which remote afterloader vendors active in the North American market control and verify source position. For single-stepping source devices, accurate source positioning is achieved by retracting or ejecting the appropriate length of cable as measured by a primary cable-tip or cable-end detector (usually an opti-pair). In addition, these remote afterloaders contain some type of secondary cable-motion detector for verifying the length of cable actually ejected, for example, a detector that monitors the rotation of a wheel or roller that moves with the source cable. The basic method of type (a) testing is a comparison of the radioactive source-center position with a nonradioactive marker or "source position simulator" that serves as a standard of positional accuracy. Assuming accurate agreement (± 1 mm ) is confirmed, the validated positional standard can then be used to confirm the accuracy of all clinically used combinations of applicators and transfer tubes and to assess the accuracy of source-localization protocols. Since the micro-Selectron/HDR is the most widely used machine in North America, the positional QA tests developed by the authors for this system will be discussed in detail. Adaptations of these procedures for the other systems listed in Table 1 will be discussed at the end of this section.

To specify location of the radioactive source in an applicator connected to the microSelectron/HDR, the user must specify the active dwell locations (1–48), the distance between adjacent dwell positions (2.5 or 5 mm), and the distance from the indexer face to the first (most distal) dwell position (a length between 715 and 995 mm). The device responds by ejecting the length of source cable required to place the source at the most proximal dwell position. The source then treats the remaining dwell positions, moving in the proximal-to-distal direction. The reference position, from which ejection length is reck-

**Table 1**

**Intrinsic Source-Positioning Strategies Utilized by Remote Afterloaders
Marketed in North America**

| Machine | Reference Position | Primary Detection Method | Method of Verification |
|---|---|---|---|
| Gamma Med 12i | Distal end of applicator | Always ejects 130 cm of cable from point where opti-pair detects proximal cable tip | Detects collision of check cable with applicator tip to confirm applicator-transfer tube length is within ±1 mm of 130 cm; Correct angular displacement of stepper-motor shaft |
| MicroSelectron/HDR | Distal plane of indexer head | Detection of distal cable tip by opti-pair | Correct angular displacement of stepper-motor shaft |
| Selectron/HDR | Control pellet just proximal to source position 48 | Seating of control pellet in transfer tube-applicator interface | Increase in transfer tube air pressure |
| Omnitron 2000: Normal Mode | Distal plane of indexer head | Detection of distal cable tip by opti-pair | Correct angular rotation of friction wheel in contact with wire |
| Omnitron 2000: End Seek Mode | Distal end of applicator | Detects collision of check cable with applicator tip | Cable length ejected, as measured by number of stepper-motor pulses, must be within ±1 cm of user-specified length |

oned, is defined by passage of the source tip by an opti-pair located proximal to the indexer. Since no system is provided for accurately defining the applicator end, source position is completely controlled by programming the cable length (specified as a nominal indexer-face-to-source-center distance). An adequate standard of intrinsic positional accuracy should (a) have radio-graphically visible dummy seeds over the range of programmable treatment distances, (b) allow specification of source position relative to the proximal aspect of the transfer tube rather than the applicator orifice or tip, (c) be compatible with all transfer tube-applicator combinations, and (d) have the same outer diameter and flexibility as the radioactive source cable. Restriction (b) results in a 1-m-long cable (see Fig. 3) with a reference mark on its proximal end that allows insertion depth relative to the transfer-tube indexer interface to be measured. Such an arrangement avoids any dependence on the absolute length of the transfer-tube and applicator. Restriction (d) ensures that the positional accuracy standard will duplicate the backlash characteristics of the actual source cable.

A vendor-supplied accessory, the radiographic marker (see Figs. 4 and 7) provides a clinically-relevant standard for assessing primary positional accuracy. This marker consists of a 1,050-mm-long sourcelike cable with radio-opaque markers spaced at 1-cm intervals at its distal end. It is designed so that when fully inserted into a treatment tube-applicator combination (see Fig.7a in "Verification of Clinical (Type b) Positional Accuracy"), these markers repre-

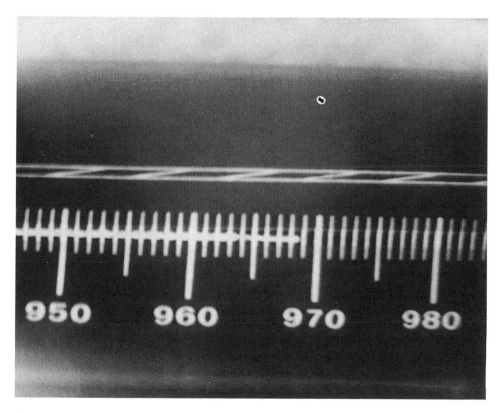

**Fig. 3.** A CCTV image of the radioactive source in the Nucletron source ruler. Type (a) positional accuracy is verified by comparing the ruler location of the radioactive source tip with the location of the radiographic marker or source position simulator seed corresponding to the programmed indexer length. It is essential to use the same transfer tube for comparing the radioactive source and radiographic marker.

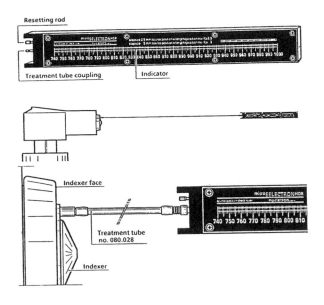

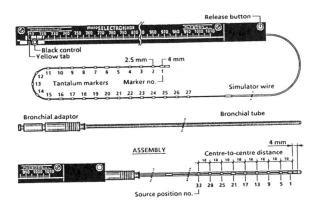

**Fig. 4.** Quality assurance accessories available for the microSelectron/HDR. The upper figure illustrates the source-position ruler, which allows the source and check cable to be viewed against a ruled scale. The lower figure illustrates the source-position simulator, which accepts the indexer mechanical interface for most types of transfer tubes. By sliding the control knob to the desired treatment length, the most distal marker simulates the position of the radioactive source center when the microSelectron is programmed to this setting. Figs. 7a (center panel) and 7b (lower panel) illustrate the use of another important QA accessory, the radiographic marker. Courtesy of Nucletron Corporation.

sent treatment lengths (relative to the HDR treatment-head reference point) of 995 mm, 985 mm, . . . , and so forth. The vendor also supplies a ruler (Fig. 4), consisting of a source guide that allows the source to be visualized against a ruled distance scale.

The most basic test consists of comparing the position of the radioactive source center with the seed positions on the radiographic marker. The following two methods[3] are in wide use.

## (1) Autoradiography Method

A transparent applicator, for example, a flexible implant tube, is securely taped to a ready-pack film and attached to a transfer tube. The radiographic marker is inserted, and a pin is used to mark several cardinal treatment lengths, for example, 995, 895, and 795 mm. Without removing the applicator from the film, the transfer tube is attached to the HDR remote afterloader and its actual source is used to expose the film at these treatment positions. The radiographic marker and autoradiographic images should correspond to within about 0.5 mm (see Fig. 5).

## (2) Closed-Circuit TV Camera Method

A CCTV camera is positioned in the treatment room so as to remotely view the source ruler when connected by means of a transfer tube to the treatment device. For a programmed treatment length of 995 mm, the ruler location of the active source tip is noted (see Fig. 3). Then, using the same treatment tube and duplicating its position and curvature, the ruler location of the 995-mm reference mark of the fully-inserted radiographic marker is noted. This ruler reading is compared to radioactive source-tip reading from which the tip-to-center-of-radioactivity distance has been subtracted.

The CCTV method is very precise (± 0.3 mm) and allows the penetration of the check cable to be measured, but it requires knowledge of the tip-to-center-of-radioactivity distance. This parameter can be obtained from the vendor's mechanical drawings of the source, a result that should be verified autoradiographically. For the CCTV positional measurement, only the location of the source tip relative to the radiographic marker is relevant, not its absolute location on the ruler. CCTV visualization of repeated source ejections can be used to measure producibility of source-tip positioning (found to be ± 0.2 mm for the microSelectron/HDR). By replacing the ruler with a closed-ended transparent catheter of known length taped to a ruler, the indexer-to-collision distances sensed by the HDR can be measured by CCTV observation. For the Nucletron device, these distances were found to be in error by as much as 7 mm and were, therefore, useless in quantitatively measuring the catheter end. In addition, it is possible to program the source center 1–3 mm beyond the catheter end, without the machine detecting a collision.[19] The radioactive source tip simply pushes up against the catheter end, compresses the source cable, and assumes a position as much as 3 mm proximal to its programmed location. To ensure that such mispositioning does not occur, the most distal dwell position must be programmed no closer than 1 mm from the catheter end. The autoradiography method is slightly less precise and flexible and is

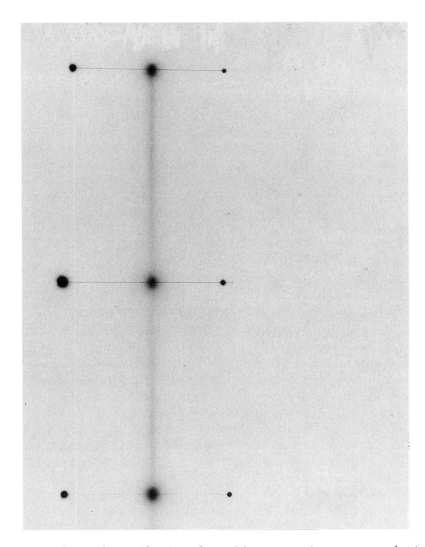

**Fig. 5.** Autoradiographic verification of type (a) accuracy. A transparent plastic applicator with an attached transfer tube was taped to a XT-L ready-packed verification film, a radiographic marker was fully inserted, and pin pricks were used to define the 995-, 895-, and 795-mm indexer locations relative to the marker. The transfer tube was then attached to the treatment unit, and the 8 Ci source was programmed to dwell at these locations for 0.3 sec. Excellent agreement was observed. The transit dose component is dramatically illustrated.

more time consuming if many measurements under varying conditions are to be made. All of the coauthors have independently found that the Nucletron device systematically mispositions the source by + 1.5–2.0 mm, that is, a programmed 995-mm length setting positions the source center at 997 mm relative to the radiographic marker. This error, according to the vendor, is due to a 0.6-mm backlash correction and a 1-mm shift of the center of radioactivity toward the source tip owing to a 1991 source-design revision.

Tests of intrinsic positional accuracy must also demonstrate that the treatment device delivers each programmed sequence to the assigned channel. This is most simply tested by exposing a multiple-channel autoradiograph, with each channel assigned a unique sequence of active dwell positions. Figure 6 illustrates an 18-channel staggered array autoradiograph, consisting of 11 dwell positions and catheter spaced at 10-mm intervals. This image demonstrates that the indexer correctly delivers each unique dwell-position sequence is to its intended channel, that positional accuracy is maintained as a function of treatment length and dwell position number, and that dwell spacing is accurately (± 0.5 mm) maintained. By building a cassette with puncture holes in its lid at known distances from the proximal ends of the cassette applicators, positional accuracy can be easily verified on a daily basis. To quantitate source position, the distance between the source image and the reference line (image-to-pin distance) is measured. The measured source position, $L_{meas}$, can be calculated by

$$L_{meas} = \text{measured image-to-pin distance}$$
$$+ \text{ pin-to-applicator-tip distance} \qquad (1)$$
$$+ \text{ treatment tube length}$$

In contrast to the microSelectron/HDR, both the GammaMed 12i and the Omnitron 2000 (in its "end seek mode") machines reference programmed source positions to the distal end of the closed applicator. The GammaMed 12i system assumes that every applicator-transfer tube assembly is exactly 130 cm long, and specifies dwell location relative to that point, while the Omnitron device allows the applicator assembly to have a variable length. By measuring the length of check cable that must be ejected to produce a collision with the catheter end, both systems are able to measure the length of the source path. The 12i system prevents treatment if the source path length deviates more than 1 mm from the expected 130 cm, whereas the Omnitron system offsets the dwell position by a user-specified length from the applicator end, regardless of source-path length. To assess intrinsic positional accuracy, both the CCTV and autoradiography tests can be used to verify that these systems offset the center of radioactivity of the actual source from the catheter end by the programmed distance. In addition, the accuracy with which these systems measure the source path length, relative to the indexer face, should be verified. A source cable, similar to the Nucletron radiographic marker, can be used to measure the transfer tube proximal tip-to-catheter end distance directly. For the GammaMed 12i, the applicator length should be varied to confirm correct operation of source path-length variance interlock.

**Verification of Clinical (Type b) Positional Accuracy**

Even though a remote afterloading device accurately ejects the programmed length of source cable relative to its designated reference point, many other factors may compromise positional accuracy within clinically implanted applicators. The transfer tube length might vary from tube to tube or depend

**Fig. 6.** An 18-channel staggered autoradiograph used to confirm the correct delivery of each unique sequence of dwell positions to the programmed channel, the correct spacing of adjacent dwell positions, and the accurate relative positioning of the most distal dwell position.

excessively on tube curvature. An inappropriate source localization procedure may lead to erroneous correlation of the prescribed treatment positions on the basis of a radiographic visualization of a dummy marker, with the programmable position parameters. Given that intrinsic positional accuracy of the device has been confirmed, Type (b) accuracy includes assessment of all transfer tube- and applicator-dependent parameters that affect source localization. The relevance of a specific parameter may depend not only on machine design, but on the design of applicators, dummy markers, and localization protocols.

Evaluation of clinical positioning accuracy consists of four basic QA tests.

(1) Verification that the radioactive source center position, for a given programmed position, is independent of the transfer tube used or type of applicator, for example, intracavitary, interstitial, or transluminal.

(2) Verification that the source position is not excessively dependent on transfer tube or applicator path curvature or loop diameter.

(3) Confirmation, either visually or radiographically, of the accuracy of each simulator-source localization protocol for each kind of transfer-tube applicator combination, using the validated radiographic marker simulating the HDR source.

(4) Verification of the assumed lengths of all transfer tubes and applicators where indicated by machine design or source localization protocol.

Tests (1) and (2) are necessitated by the phenomenon of cable backlash: a difference between the length of cable ejected or retracted and the corresponding displacement of the radioactive source along the axis of the tube constraining its path. This occurs whenever the inner tube diameter exceeds that of the source, causing the flexible cable to assume a slightly helical path. Either CCTV visualization or autoradiography can be used to check (1) and (2). The senior author's group discovered that, by varying the radius of curvature of the old-style (pre-1992) Nucletron transfer tubes, source position variations as large as 4 mm could be observed. The improved guide tubes currently marketed by this vendor show variations of only 0.5 mm. Backlash is a potential problem for all machines, regardless of the direction of cable motion during treatment or whether the device references source position to a detector in the treatment head or by collision with the applicator tip. Transfer tube length, when required, can be easily measured using a validated radiographic marker as illustrated by the central figure of Fig.7b. The transfer tube is connected to a closed-ended applicator of known length $L_a$. Then, as illustrated by Fig. 7b, the radiographic marker is inserted so that the marker tip is in contact with the applicator end, and the offset, $O_r$, measured. Let $L_t$ denote the transfer tube length (the distance from indexer face to applicator orifice when coupled to tube) and $L_{RM}$ the indexer-to-radiographic marker tip distance (usually 999 mm for Nucletron markers). $L_{RM}$ is the programmed distance setting corresponding to the radiographic marker tip when fully inserted into a treatment tube ($O_r = 0$). These parameters are related by the equation, $L_t + L_a = L_{RM} - O_r$. Then the transfer tube length $L_t$ is given by

$$L_t = L_{RM} - (O_r + L_a) \tag{2}$$

Tests (3) and (4) are highly dependent on applicator design and the localization technique used as well as on machine design. We will review the source localization problems specific to the microSelectron/HDR in some detail and only briefly comment on the QA of other machine designs. Two simulation source-localization procedures (Fig. 7) are in common use with the microSelectron/HDR: the applicator orifice method and applicator distal tip method.

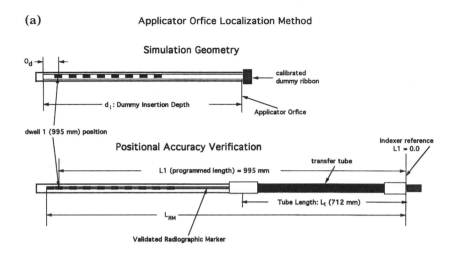

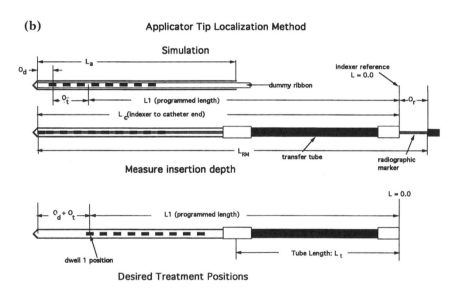

**Fig. 7.** Illustration of two simulation-source localization schemes used in conjunction with the microSelectron/HDR or other machines that internally reference source location within the treatment head. (a) Dummy simulation marker referenced to the proximal orifice of the implanted applicator and (b) Dummy marker referenced to the closed distal end of the applicator. To validate method 7a, the simulation dummy seed locations (upper panel 7a) are compared to those of a radiographic marker (lower panel 7a) when fully inserted into a transfer tube attached to the applicator. The applicator tip method (b) directly references the applicator end to the afterloader indexer by sounding each catheter-transfer tube combination (center panel of 7b) with a 1-m validated radiographic marker.

The applicator orifice method (upper panel, Fig. 7a) is used whenever the dummy ribbon (or "simulation marker" in Nucletron jargon) is referenced to the proximal aspect or orifice of the implanted applicator or when the applicator does not have a well-defined end, for example, when the interstitial loop technique is used. The dummy ribbons (upper panel, Fig. 7a) marketed by Nucletron for both interstitial and intracavitary applicators are based upon this localization concept. The maximum insertion depth, $d_i$, of each dummy marker relative to the applicator orifice is constrained by a small cap on its proximal end. The seed markers, usually spaced at 1-cm intervals, are designed to correspond to cardinal source positions of 995 mm, 985 mm, and so forth, when the marker is fully inserted. Positional accuracy tests must identify the relationship between source position, as specified by the machine relative to its indexer, and the location of the dummy seeds, specified relative to the proximal aspect of the applicator. The lower panel of Fig. 7a illustrates the basic measurement: a transfer tube is attached to the applicator, a type-(a) validated radiographic marker is fully inserted into the tube, and the radiographic marker seed positions are compared to those of the dummy ribbon. For flexible, transparent interstitial applicators, direct visual comparison can be used, whereas for intracavitary or other opaque applicators, transmission radiographs of the two-marker geometries must be obtained. Figure 8 illustrates such radiographs of a Fletcher-Suit shielded colpostat, loaded with a dummy marker (left) and a radiographic marker with the appropriate transfer tube attached (right). The senior author has observed deviations as large as 3 mm for this test. For intracavitary applicators, these images can be used to (a) assess correct positioning of the dwell-position sequence along the applicator axis, (b) to choose treatment dwell positions that are symmetrically placed between anterior and posterior colpostat surfaces, and (c) to verify thickness, location, and shape of any internal shielding.[4] Alternatively, superposition of an autoradiograph of the radioactive source and a transmission radiograph with the dummy ribbon in place can be used. However, this technique is limited to those applicators that permit close proximity of the active dwell positions with the film plane.

Examination of Fig. 7a shows that dummy-ribbon insertion depth ($d_i$), indexer distance setting (L1) to dummy position 1, transfer tube length ($L_t$), and dummy tip-to-position distance ($O_d$) are related as follows:

$$L1 = L_t + (d_i - O_d) \tag{3}$$

Equation (3) demonstrates that if the transfer tube length is incorrect or shrinks or expands through time, the applicator orifice method will yield incorrect distance settings. To preserve the accuracy of this localization technique, the constancy of transfer tube length must be periodically verified. Alternatively, the basic test, illustrated by Fig. 7a, can be repeated for each transfer tube. The senior author found that the old-style Nucletron interstitial applicator transfer tubes varied in length by as much as 4 mm, indicating that these conditions cannot simply be assumed.

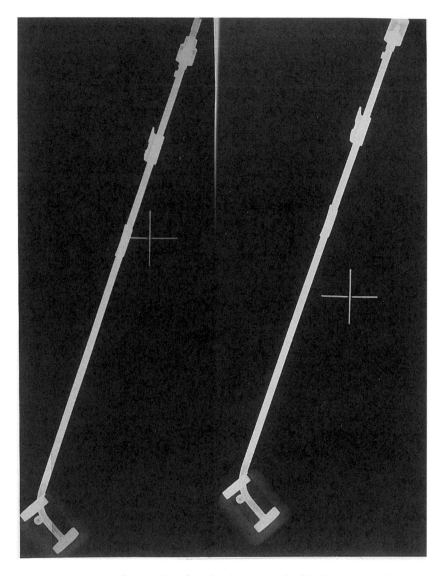

**Fig. 8.** Transmission radiographs of a Fletcher-Suit shielded colpostat, loaded with a simulation marker (right) without a transfer tube and with a radiographic marker (left) with the appropriate transfer tube attached.

Equation (3) can be used directly to calculate HDR distance settings for those users who opt to use conventional manual afterloading dummy ribbons for simulation rather than purchasing the very expensive calibrated dummies from the vendor. At simulation, conventional dummy ribbons are inserted into the applicators prior to imaging. Then, each dummy ribbon is carefully withdrawn, and its insertion depth, $d_i$, measured and recorded on a form similar to that shown in Fig. 15 (see "Quality Assurance During Treatment Planning . . .". Equation (3) can then be used to calculate the programmed indexer distance to the most distal dummy seed center. In contrast to the calibrated dummy ribbon case, the transfer tube length, $L_t$, must be explicitly known.

The other common source-localization technique, the applicator-tip localization method (see Fig. 7b), uses the end of the closed tip of each applicator to localize the dummy marker relative to the indexer face frame of reference. The method works as follows: (a) simulation markers are fully inserted into each implanted catheter and simulation radiographs obtained as usual, (b) the appropriate transfer tubes are attached to the applicators, and (c) each transfer tube-applicator assembly is "sounded" using a validated radiographic marker, measuring its offset, $O_r$, from full insertion as illustrated by the center panel of Fig. 7b. Step (c) relates the applicator-tip reference point to the indexer face reference position L = 0.0. The indexer-to-catheter end distance, $L_c$, is given by

$$L_c = L_{RM} - O_r \qquad (4)$$

The patient radiographs then are examined, the treatment volume identified, and the offset, $O_t$, between the most distal dummy seed and treated dwell position centers recorded. The dwell 1 programmed treatment distance is given by

$$L1 = L_c - (O_t + O_d) \qquad (5)$$

where $O_d$ is the distance from the dummy ribbon tip to its most distal seed center. This system has the advantage of automatically correcting for transfer tube-to-transfer tube length variations as well as shrinkage or expansion through time. The length of each transfer tube-applicator combination must be less than $L_{RM}$, and the user must be able to accurately match the radiographic image of each dummy ribbon with the corresponding catheter number. Validation of this method consists of the following steps: (a) Using eq. (5) and Fig. 7b to calculate the indexer distance to several of the dummy seed centers; (b) programming the HDR or mechanical source simulator with these treatment lengths; and (c) verifying that the radioactive source is located at the same position (within ± 1 mm) in the catheter as the corresponding dummy seed centers. Coincidence of radioactive source center and dummy seed can be confirmed by visual comparison of the source-position simulator with the dummy seed, by comparing autoradiography, or by CCTV viewing of the radioactive source.

Extension of the positional accuracy validation principles, described above, to other remote afterloading devices is straightforward. The Omnitron 2000 device, in its default localization mode, uses the applicator tip reference method. The system is supplied with sounding accessories, similar to those illustrated by Fig. 7b, that are applicable to all applicator types. The GammaMed 12i remote afterloader requires that the transfer tube-applicator distance always be 130 cm. Commissioning of a 12i unit must include measurement of all transfer tube lengths, $L_t$, and development of a sounding measurement that can be used to verify the correct length ($130 - L_t$) of each purchased applicator before placing it in clinical service. Since type (a) accuracy testing of "end seek" positioning mode machines such as the Omnitron 2000 or GammaMed 12i has already established that the device accurately positions the source with respect to the distal end of the applicator, type (b) testing is less complex than for the microSelectron/HDR. Opaque applicators, for example, vaginal colpostats, should be radiographed with a validated radiographic marker in contact with the applicator end to confirm that the selected dwell positions are correctly positioned with respect to the applicator surfaces and axis of symmetry.

## Temporal Accuracy

Verification of temporal accuracy consists of independently measuring the length of time the radioactive source remains at the specified dwell position and comparing this time interval with the programmed time setting. Potentially, three quantities must be evaluated: (1) absolute timer accuracy, (2) timer linearity and reproducibility, and (3) end or transit dose effects. If measured dwell time is inferred from the dosimeter readings, for example, an ion chamber, end effect manifests itself by deviation from linearity at small dwell times. This phenomenon is due to an extra dose deposited at the measurement point arising from the finite velocity of the source cable as it moves from position to position and to and from the shielded safe. This dose component is known as the "transit dose." At minimum, HDR commissioning must include verification of timer linearity and reproducibility and verifying that transit dose effects are sufficiently small that they can be ignored in clinical treatment planning. Whether absolute timer accuracy must be quantitatively verified depends upon the time standard assumed by the source-calibration technique. If integrated calibration readings, corrected for source transit, are obtained under HDR timer control and converted to ionization current without reference to an external time standard, then absolute timer accuracy is not relevant. If the HDR timer is inaccurate by $+10\%$, that is , if a programmed dwell time of 60 sec really yields a 54-sec exposure, this error will be canceled by a compensating $-10\%$ error in source-strength calibration. Then, only relative dwell-time measurements are needed to establish timer linearity and precision. On the other hand, if source strength is measured by integrating against an independent time standard, then the absolute accuracy of the HDR timer must be verified. This is the case if a re-entrant chamber[20] is used with an air-kerma strength/ionization current ($cGy \cdot cm^2 \cdot h^{-1} \cdot A^{-1}$) calibration factor obtained from an Accredited Dosimetry and Calibration Laboratory (ADCL).

### Timer Accuracy and Linearity

In the clinical environment, ion chamber measurements are generally used to assess timer accuracy and linearity. The experimental setup, used at the Mallinckrodt Institute of Radiology, but typical of that used by all the authors, is illustrated by Fig. 9. It consists of a 0.6-cm³ thimble chamber positioned parallel to and about 1.5 cm from an interstitial needle, both fixed within a machined lucite phantom. Since this device doubles as a daily output check phantom, it is permanently mounted on the wall near the remote afterloader to facilitate quick setup. The relative timer accuracy/linearity check consists of measuring integrated charge $Q_1$, $Q_2$, $Q_3$, and so forth, under control of the HDR timer for several programmed timer settings $t_1$, $t_2$, $t_3$, and so forth (typically 0.1 to 180 sec) for a single dwell position opposite the center of the ion collection volume. $Q_i$ is plotted against $t_i$ and fit to a linear function: $Q_{meas} = a \cdot t_{set} + \Delta Q$. The deviation of individual measurements from the line is an in-

## Measurement of Remote-Afterloader Dwell Time Accuracy

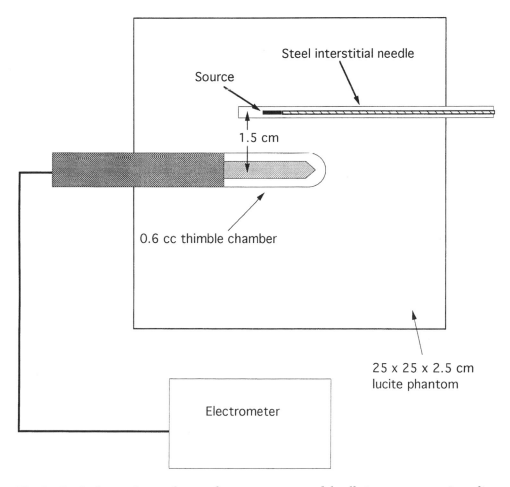

**Fig. 9.** Typical experimental setup for measurement of dwell-time accuracy, timer linearity, and end effect using ion chamber measurements. A relatively small (1–2 cm) source-to-detector distance should be chosen, both to obtain an adequate ionization current and ensure that the measured transit dose (which is distance dependent) is representative of that encountered in clinical practice.

dication of timer nonlinearity while $\Delta Q$ is proportional to transit dose. The ratio $\Delta Q/a \cdot t_{set}$ indicates the relative values of stationary and the transit dose at the point of measurement. Since the transit dose is highly distance dependent (its importance relative to stationary dose increases with increasing distance), care must be taken in extrapolating this ratio to other treatment distances and geometries.

The timer measurement technique, described above, yields only a relative measure of stationary dwell time. Meigooni et al.[21] have modified the ionometric technique to support absolute measurement of dwell time. The experimental setup is as illustrated by Fig. 9. The source is programmed to dwell for an extended period (999 sec) opposite the chamber. While the source is in this stationary position, a stopwatch is used to measure the time interval, t, required to increase the integrated charge from $Q_1$ to $Q_2$. Then, $I_{sta} = (Q_2-Q_1)/t$ is the stationary ionization current or charge integrated per second of stationary dwell time. $I_{sta}$ excludes the effects of source transit, is defined in terms of an independent time standard, and serves as a temporal calibration factor for the experimental setup. Then, as for the relative dwell time measurement, several integrated readings, $Q_{meas,i}$, are obtained under control of the remote afterloader timer for corresponding programmed timer settings, $t_{set,i}$. Unlike $I_{sta}$, each integrated charge, $Q_{meas}$, includes the transit as well as stationary dose. The corresponding measured "effective" dwell time, $t_{meas}$, given by $Q_{meas}/I_{sta}$. $t_{meas}$ is the sum of the actual stationary time and additional dwell time needed to give a dose equal to the transit dose. Timer linearity and end effect are quantified by fitting $t_{meas}$ to a linear function of $t_{set}$ (see Fig. 10).

$$t_{meas} = \alpha \cdot t_{set} + \Delta t_{tr} \qquad (6)$$

The deviation of the slope, $\alpha$, from unity is a measure of absolute HDR timer accuracy while $\Delta t_{tr}$ is an effective increase in dwell time due to source motion during ejection and retraction. In our experience, $\Delta t_{tr}$ varies from 0.06 to 0.15 sec at 1.5 cm while $\alpha$ ranges from 0.997 to 1.008, indicating that the Nucletron timer accuracy is better than 1%. For dwell times greater than 1 sec, the timer was linear within 1%, as indicated by the deviation of measured from calculated dwell times. For this nonclinical geometry, neglecting transit dose (end effect) produces errors of less than 2% for dwell times > 5 sec. The estimated precision of the measurement is 0.5% and can be improved by using a larger volume chamber at a larger treatment distance.

## Evaluation of Transit Dose

Clinical treatment planning for single stepping-source machines generally neglects the transit dose, that is, the dose delivered to tissue while the source is in motion and assumes that clinically-significant dose delivery occurs only while the source is stationary. In fact, the source moves with a finite velocity, depositing an additional dose within the target volume and an unprescribed

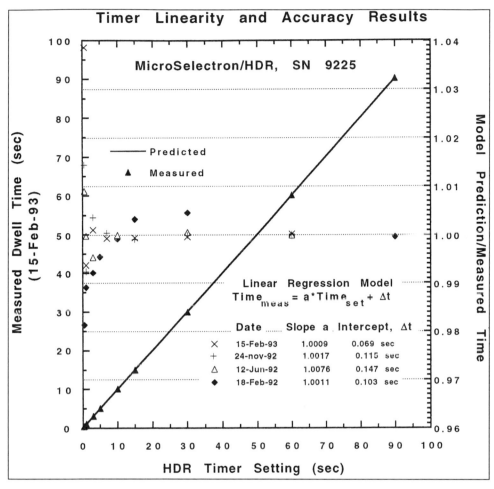

**Fig. 10.** Results of four quarterly ionometric timer-accuracy and linearity measurements performed on the HDR remote afterloader at the Mallinckrodt Institute of Radiology. The left scale shows the measured effective dwell times (closed triangles) and the linear regression fit (solid lines) for the most recent quarter. The right scale shows the ratio of times predicted by the linear model to the measured times for all four quarters (various symbols), which serves as an indication of linearity.

dose along the source trajectory proximal to the target volume. General treatment of the problem requires measurement of the source velocity, v, under various conditions. Then, the validity of the stationary source dosimetric approximation can he evaluated and appropriate corrections implemented if necessary. Simply measuring the transit dose in a fixed geometry is not adequate since this information cannot he directly extrapolated to other treatment geometries. Several approaches have been developed to evaluate source speed. Meigooni et al.[21] used a video camera to measure both dwell time and source transfer velocity and found transfer velocities ranging from 35 to 53 cm/sec over transport distances of 5 cm to 40 cm for a microSelectron/HDR. Houdek et al.[22] used an oscilloscope to count microSelectron/HDR stepper motor pulses as a measure of source speed. This elegant study found source transfer velocity to be highly dependent on source displacement: velocity ranged from 23 cm/sec for a 0.25-cm displacement to 50 cm/sec for a 99.5-cm displacement. Bastin et al.[23] used thermoluminescent dosimetry (TLD) to measure transit dose directly and found a value of 0.31 cGy/(Curie-fraction) 5 mm from a microSelectron HDR endobronchial catheter. However, these procedures are time consuming, require special equipment and expertise, and are probably not suitable for large-scale clinical use. Source speeds of 4–15 cm/sec have been reported for the Atomic Energy of Canada, Ltd. (AECL) Brachytron[24], and the original Omnitron remote afterloader was designed to transport its source at 13 cm/sec (now much faster according to the vendor). At these velocities, the transit dose could easily exceed 5% of the prescribed dose in some treatment geometries. That transit dose is negligible for any remote afterloader should not be assumed. This is especially true for those devices (includes all but the microSelectron/HDR) whose potential for transit effects have not been reported in the peer-reviewed literature.

We describe a simple method developed at the Mallinckrodt Institute of Radiology[21] for inferring source velocity from ionization measurements, which is suitable for routine use in clinical acceptance testing of remote afterloaders. The basic geometry of the ionization method of source speed measurement is illustrated by Fig. 11. A single catheter, supported by a jig in air, is programmed to deliver dwell time $t_1$ to two active dwell positions (n = 2 in Fig. 11), $P_1$ and $P_2$, separated by a distance $2 \cdot s$ (set to 20 cm). A 100 cm³ spherical ion chamber is placed at distance d (15 cm) from the source path midway between $P_1$ and $P_2$. The distances s and d are selected so as to make the stationary and transit integrated charge components approximately equal, to ensure that the measured ionization current is large relative to background leakage and to ensure that the gradient correction factor[25] does not vary with source position within the catheter. The procedure is as follows.

(1) Determine the stationary ionization current, $I_{1,2}$, defined as the measured charge due to 1 second of stationary dwelling by $P_1$ and $P_2$. Measure the integrated charge, $Q_{1,2}(t_1)$, arising from dwell times $t_1$ at dwell positions $P_1$ and $P_2$ and repeat the measurement for a second dwell time $t_2 > t_1$, yielding charge $Q_{1,2}(t_2)$. $I_{1,2}$ is given by

$$I_{1,2} = \frac{Q_{1,2}(t_2) - Q_{1,2}(t_1)}{t_2 - t_1} \tag{7}$$

By repeating this measurement with only the proximal dwell position, $P_2$ activated, the stationary ionization current, $I_2$, can be measured.

(2) Determine the transit charge, $Q_{tr}(1 \leftrightarrow 2)$, arising from two passes (ejection and retraction) of the source between positions $P_1$ and $P_2$. This requires knowledge of any internal correction the remote afterloader makes for finite source velocity. According to Nucletron, if N dwell positions spaced at inter-

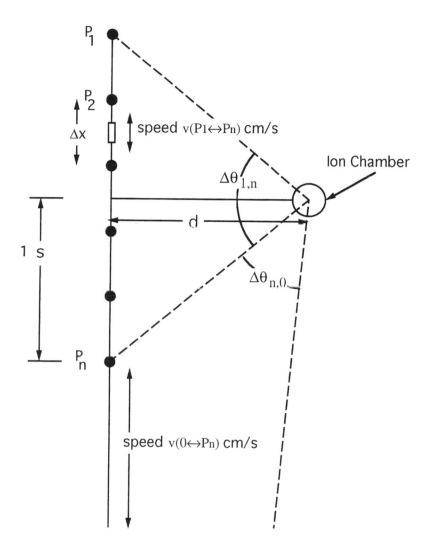

**Fig. 11.** Basic geometry for measurement of HDR source speed using a large volume ion chamber. A single catheter is suspended in air at distance d (15 cm) from a 100-cm³ spherical ion chamber midway between dwell positions $P_1$ and $P_n$. These positions are separated by 20 cm. For the basic measurement, only the two extreme active dwell positions, $P_1$ and $P_n = P_2$, are used. The distances s and d are chosen so as make the transit and stationary doses of the same order of magnitude and to avoid gradient effects.

vals of $\Delta x$ are programmed to deliver dwell times $T_1, \ldots, T_N$ at positions $P_1$, $P_2, \ldots P_{N-1}$ and $P_N$, the dwell times actually administered by the microSelectron/HDR are

$$T_1 - \min\left[0.1, \frac{\Delta x}{v}\right], \ldots, T_{N-1} - \min\left[0.1, \frac{\Delta x}{v}\right], \ldots, T_N. \qquad (8)$$

That is, if the dwell positions are relatively close together, the clock for a given dwell position actually starts the instant the source leaves the previous position. For widely separated positions, a maximum of 0.1 sec is deducted from the programmed dwell time. The transit charges, $Q_{tr}(1 \leftrightarrow 2)$ and $Q_{tr}(0 \leftrightarrow P_2)$, corresponding to source transits between $P_1$ and $P_2$ and between the indexer and $P_2$, respectively, are given by

$$Q_{tr}(P_1 \leftrightarrow P_2) = Q_{1,2}(t_2) - t_2 \cdot I_{1,2} \cdot C_{1,2}(t_2) - t_2 \cdot I_2 \cdot C_2(t_2)$$

$$Q_{tr}(0 \leftrightarrow P_2) = Q_2(t_2) - t_2 \cdot I_2 \cdot C_2(t_2) \qquad (9)$$

The factors $C_{1,2}(t)$ and $C_2(t)$ are ratios of the total administered dwell time to the total programmed dwell time for the two- and one-dwell measurement geometries, respectively. Since the microSelectron does not correct a solitary dwell position for source transit, $C_2(t) = 1.0$. For the two-dwell geometry, $C_{1,2}(t) = \frac{2 \cdot t - 0.1}{2 \cdot t}$ since $2 \cdot s/v > 0.1$ sec.

(3) Calculate the average velocities, $v(P_1 \leftrightarrow P_2)$ and $v(0 \leftrightarrow P_2)$. This calculation assumes that both stationary dwell current and transit charges are proportional to the product of dwell time and an inverse square-law factor

$$I_{1,2} \propto 2 \cdot (d^2 + s^2)^{-1}$$

$$Q_{tr}(P_1 \leftrightarrow P_2) \propto \left(\frac{4 \cdot s}{v(P_1 \leftrightarrow P_2)}\right) \cdot \left(\frac{\Delta\theta_{1,2}}{2 \cdot s \cdot d}\right) \qquad (10)$$

The second part of eq. (10) assumes that the source activity is uniformly spread over a line source of active length 2s for a duration of 4s/v (two passes). $\Delta\theta_{1,2}$ is the angle in radians subtended by the active length 2s, and the second bracketed term is the result of integrating $1/r^2$ over this line.[26] Solving these equations for velocity yields

$$v(P_1 \leftrightarrow P_2) = \frac{2 \cdot (d^2 + s^2) \cdot \tan^{-1}(s/d)}{d} \cdot \frac{I_{1,2}}{Q_{tr}(P_1 \leftrightarrow P_2)}$$

$$v(0 \leftrightarrow P_2) = \frac{4 \cdot (d^2 + s^2) \cdot \tan^{-1}\left(\frac{L}{2 \cdot d}\right)}{Q_{tr}(P_1 \leftrightarrow P_2) \cdot d} \cdot \frac{I_2}{Q_{tr}(0 \leftrightarrow P_2)} \qquad (11)$$

where L = 99.5 cm − $P_2$.

To and from the safe to position $P_2$, the above measurements yielded a speed of 55 cm/sec. Between two widely spaced dwell positions, a velocity of 40 cm/sec was found. When Eqs. (7) and (9)–(11) were generalized to accommodate multiple dwell positions uniformly spaced at 0.5, 1.0, and 2.0 cm intervals, average velocities ranging from 45 to 57 cm/sec were found. That consistent results were obtained for all dwell spacings, for which the internally applied correction factors C(t) were large, lends warrant to the vendor's description of this algorithm. Unlike the measurements of Houdek et al.[22] the ionization technique yields an average of the dwell-to-dwell displacement velocity and the velocity of source retraction. For clinical dose calculations, it seems reasonable to use a single average value of 52 cm/sec for the Mallinckrodt microSelectron/HDR. Using a video camera to record the motion of an HDR source, the velocity measured by the ionization method was confirmed within 5%.

Equipped with an accurate measure of source speed, v, it is simple to make worst-case estimates of clinical transit doses using dosimetric approximations. For example, to find the transit dose per fraction, $D_{tr}(d)$, in the central transverse plane at distance d from a single catheter consisting of N dwell positions spaced at intervals of $\Delta X$, the line source approximation can be used.

$$D_{tr}(d) = S_K \cdot \left(\frac{10^4 \text{ cm}^2/\text{m}^2}{3600 \text{ s/h}}\right) \cdot \overline{(\mu_{en}/\rho)}_{air}^{wat} \cdot \left(\frac{\Delta\theta}{L \cdot d}\right) \cdot \left(\frac{L}{v}\right) \qquad (12)$$

where $S_K$ is the air-kerma strength (in units of $cGy \cdot m^2 \cdot h^{-1}$), L is the equivalent active length ($N \cdot \Delta X$), $\Delta\theta$ is the angle (in radians) subtended by the active length at the point of interest, and $\overline{(\mu_{en}/\rho)}_{air}^{wat}$ is the ratio of mass energy absorption coefficients, used to convert air kerma into water kerma. Equation (12) neglects the transit dose contributed to the treatment volume by source motion proximal to the N-th active dwell position and includes transit dose due only to source retraction since the microSelectron corrects for dwell position-to-position source motion (eq. 8). Outside the target volume, the equation is identical, except that the last term is replaced by $2 \cdot (99.5 - L)/v$ since the source makes two passes (ejection and retraction) through this tissue for which the microSelectron makes no correction. Assuming d = 1 cm, L = 10 cm, and $S_K$ = 4.08 $cGy \cdot m^2 \cdot h^{-1}$, $D_{tr}$ is less than 1.0 cGy. On the surface of an interstitial catheter (d = 0.1 cm) proximal to the treated length, $D_{tr}$, becomes 15 cGy/ fraction assuming L = 50 cm. This compares favorably with the estimate of Bastin et al.[23] of 10 cGy. The transit dose to a large volume implant (4 × 4 array × 16 dwell positions at 0.5 cm intervals and 1.2 cm needle spacing) can be estimated by using Paterson-Parker calculations. Transit time over 8 cm of catheter adds 0.15 sec of dwell time per catheter, which is equivalent to 1.7 $cGy \cdot cm^2$ of integrated reference air kerma (IRAK),[27] resulting in a total excess IRAK of 28 $cGy \cdot cm^2$ or 3.9 mgRaEq−h to the entire implant. Based on the Manchester volume implant tables, this results in 4 cGy/fraction of extra dose to the implant, which is 1% or less relative to the prescribed dose (typically 300–1,000 cGy/fraction). Just proximal to the implanted volume, the transit dose will be approximately twofold larger. We conclude that for source velocities on the order of 50 cm/sec, the stationary-source treatment planning approximation is accurate within 2% within or near the implanted volume.

Radiation oncologists should be aware that transit doses to catheter surfaces can be as high as 15 cGy/source insertion.

# Dose Delivery Accuracy

Given that an HDR treatment unit accurately positions its source at the prescribed location and remains at the location for exactly the specified dwell time does not assure that the prescribed dose distribution is accurately administered to the patient. Additional QA tests to assure physically accurate dose delivery include (a) accurate experimental implementation of an appropriate source calibration technique, (b) selection of physically accurate dosimetric data to calculate the single-source dose distribution that is consistent with the source-strength specification quantity selected, (c) an accurate knowledge of applicator attenuation and shielding corrections, and (d) numerically accurate and artifact-free performance of the HDR computerized treatment planning system. Additional requirements for clinically accurate dose delivery include (a) accurate performance of the dosimetrist and digitizing tablet in entering the 2-dimensional (2-D) projections of the implant dwell locations into the treatment planning system, (b) accurate positioning of the catheters with respect to the target volume. (c) accurate correlation of the imaged dwell locations with respect to imaging studies and other clinical data defining the location and extent of the target volume, and (d) specification of prescription and optimization endpoints, for example, dose points, consistently with respect to the location of the implant relative to the target volume.

## Source Calibration

Since source calibration is covered in detail in Chapter 5, only its integration into the overall HDR QA program will be addressed in this chapter. First, an appropriate dosimetric quantity for specifying HDR source strength must be selected. As recommended by the American Association of Physicists in Medicine (AAPM)[28] and the American Endocurietherapy Society (AES),[27] the authors recommend the quantity air-kerma strength, $S_K$, for this purpose, rather than quantities such as equivalent mass of radium and apparent activity. Currently, the National Institute of Standards and Technology (NIST) maintains no air-kerma strength standard directly applicable to HDR [192]Ir sources, and vendor-supplied calibration certificates are based upon a variety of homemade standards, whose precision and traceability to NIST standards are often obscure. Thus, each HDR hospital physicist should establish an institutional secondary standard, with clear traceability to the NIST external-beam air-kerma standards, and use his or her own measured values of air-kerma strength as the basis of dose calculation. The de facto community standard of practice in this regard has become the interpolative secondary standard method of Goetsch et al.[29]

Institutional secondary standards, based upon air-kerma rate measurements with calibration external beam chambers are subject to many potential errors, such as inaccurate measurement of source-to-detector distance, malfunction of calibration equipment, absence of appropriate buildup cap, absence of chamber bias voltage, or errors in data analysis or computation.[5] Use of calibrated re-entrant ion chambers,[20] although less time consuming and simpler, are subject to similar pitfalls. A carefully developed, well-documented form-based calibration protocol can greatly reduce the likelihood of omissions or calculation errors by providing a checklist that requires documentation of critical positive actions where possible. For example, having a line in a checklist to document that chamber bias is turned on is good, but recording the measured bias is better. An example of such a system is illustrated by Fig. 12. Another mechanism for reducing errors is to require a second physicist to review the calibration report. New HDR users should conduct two or three independent calibrations of the same source, at least one of which is performed by a different physicist, to ensure that the procedure is bug-free and to get a feeling for precision of the measurement.

One of the most effective protections against errors in primary calibration is to establish a spot-check system using independent instrumentation, that is, a different electrometer, ion chamber, and cable. Permanently mounting a treatment needle or catheter in a plastic phantom equipped with a machined cavity for an ion chamber or diode allows a signal, proportional to source strength, to be measured quickly but reproducibly. This system must be calibrated against the institutional secondary standard during commissioning or whenever source construction changes.

Finally, following calibration, the source strength stored in the treatment planning system and treatment unit itself must be updated. All inventories, source decay charts, and other source-strength dependent manual calculation aids must be updated as well.

## Selection and Verification of Dosimetry Data

Selection and validation of dosimetric data for HDR [192]Ir sources and associated applicators are hampered by two factors: (1) an almost complete absence of peer-reviewed publications containing clinically-useful dosimetry data, and (2) lack of accurate two- or three-dimensional brachytherapy dose-measurement systems, similar to external-beam scanning water phantoms, that are sufficiently foolproof and efficient for widespread use in the clinical environment. Despite several hundred HDR remote afterloaders using high-intensity [192]Ir sources in active use across the world, the authors could find only two peer-reviewed publications in the literature[30-31] that describe clinically-useful dosimetry data based on now-obsolete HDR source designs. No published transverse-axis or 2-D dose distributions for the current generation of sources are available.

Meli et al.[31] and Cerra et al.[30] used small ion chambers to measure the transverse-axis dose distribution for a GammaMed IIi source consisting of a 5.5 mm

3. Source Leak Test: Date_____    Performed by_____
                    Test Result_____    Acceptable: YES or NO

**D. Operational Performance**

Positional Accuracy                           Max Error    Satisfactory   Unsatisfactory

1. Check source extension against source simulator   ____       ▢         ▢
2. Dummy source penetrates 4mm beyond most
   distal dwell normal type position         ____       ▢         ▢
3. 18 Channel autoradiograph: 0.5 cm spacing     ____       ▢         ▢

Timer Accuracy: Spot Check Phantom:

    Model and SN of Ion Chamber :_____    Electrometer:_____

    _____ cm between source and chamber center in constancy phantom

    Current measurement. Readings:_____    Stopwatch time:_____

    Measured Current:_____ Amperes

| Timer setting $t_{set}$ (sec) | Ionization Reading (Q) | Measured Time, $t_{meas}$ | Predicted time $a \cdot t_{set} + b$ | % Diff. meas/set | pred/set |
|---|---|---|---|---|---|
| ____ | ____ | ____ | ____ | ____ | ____ |
| ____ | ____ | ____ | ____ | ____ | ____ |
| ____ | ____ | ____ | ____ | ____ | ____ |
| ____ | ____ | ____ | ____ | ____ | ____ |
| ____ | ____ | ____ | ____ | ____ | ____ |
| ____ | ____ | ____ | ____ | ____ | ____ |
| ____ | ____ | ____ | ____ | ____ | ____ |

    Timer Accuracy (attach curve-fitting results) a:_____    Transit error b:_____ sec
    Minimum Dwell Setting giving < 2% error ignoring transit time:_____ sec
    Satisfactory ▢    Unsatisfactory ▢

**E. Independent Calibration Check (use timer accuray instrumentation)**
    Bias:_____ V  T =_____ °C  P =_____ mm Hg  $C_{T,P}$ =_____
    Reading-to-$S_K$ conversion, $C_K$ =_____    Reading/time_____

$$S_K = \frac{}{(RDNG)} \times \frac{}{(C_{T,P})} \times \frac{}{(C_K)} = \text{_____} \ cGy \cdot cm^2 \cdot h^{-1}$$

    $\dfrac{S_K \text{ in-air}}{S_K \text{ spot check}} = \text{_____}$   Satisfactory ▢       Unsatisfactory ▢

    Source Strength updated: Nucletron RTP ▢  Microselectron/HDR ▢  Quarterly Inventory ▢

**F. Comments**

_____

_____

_____

Measurements by:_____ Date_____ Reviewed by:_____

ROC 09/91

---

**HDR Ir-192 Open-Air Calibration**

HDR SN _____    Institution _____

Measurement Date _____    Source SN _____    Vendor Calibration _____ on _____date

(A) In-Air Calibration

    (1) Ion Chamber: Model: _____    SN: _____    Volume: _____ cm$^3$

        Ir-192 Air-kerma calibration factor ($N_{K,Ir}$): _____ cGy/C   Radius/length _____ / _____

    (2) Electrometer: Model: _____    SN: _____    Scale Used: _____ Calibration Factor($C_{el}$): _____ C/Rdg

        T = ____ °C  P = ____ mm Hg  $C_{T,P}$ = _____  Leakage = ____ A

$$\dot{K}_{air} \ (cGy/h) = \frac{RDG(C)}{Time(s)} \times C_{T,P} \times C_{el} \times N_{K,Ir} \times P_{grad}* \times 3600$$

    (3) Readings

| Chamber Position | Source-to-Chamber Distance (cm) | Integrated Reading (C) | Integration Time (s) | $P_{grad}*$ | Average $\dot{K}_{air}$ (cGy/h) |
|---|---|---|---|---|---|
| ____ | ____ | ____ | ____ | ____ | ____ |
| ____ | ____ | ____ | ____ | ____ | ____ |
| ____ | ____ | ____ | ____ | ____ | ____ |
| ____ | ____ | ____ | ____ | ____ | ____ |
| ____ | ____ | ____ | ____ | ____ | ____ |
| ____ | ____ | ____ | ____ | ____ | ____ |
| ____ | ____ | ____ | ____ | ____ | ____ |
| ____ | ____ | ____ | ____ | ____ | ____ |

*See Kondo and Randolf, Radiation Research 13:37-60, 1960.

**Fig. 12.** Example of a form-based HDR calibration protocol developed at the Mallinckrodt Institute of Radiology. The top panel documents (a) verification of positional accuracy, (b) verification of timer accuracy and linearity, (c) verification of primary calibration using a spot-check phantom with independent instrumentation, and (d) verification that source strength in the treatment-planning system and the HDR device have been updated. The bottom panel is used for quarterly source calibration (using the method of Goetsch et al.[29]).

long by 0.5 mm [192]Ir pellet encapsulated in a 8.5 mm $\times$ 1.1 mm stainless-steel capsule. In addition, Cerra used small diode detectors to measure angular anisotropy profiles at distances of 2 to 20 cm from the source center. Both authors concluded that the classic Meisberger et al.[32] polynomials accurately characterized the water-to-air media exposure-rate ratios on the transverse axis. Assuming an f-factor for water of 0.96, this suggests that the dose-rate constant, $\Lambda_0$ defined as the dose rate (cGy/h) in water at a distance of 1 cm on the transverse axis per unit air-kerma stength (cGy·cm$^2$·h$^{-1}$), has a value of 1.12 cm$^{-2}$. Cerra's angular profiles demonstrated a moderate level of dose anisotropy, resulting in longitudinal-axis dose rates, relative to the corresponding transverse-axis values, ranging from 60% at 3 cm to 80% at 10 cm. Unrefereed symposium proceedings[33-34] suggest that self-absorption in the 3.5-mm long active core of the current microSelectron/HDR reduces dose along its longitudinal axis by 20% to 45% at distances of 3 to 7 cm. However, none of these papers completely characterizes the dose distribution: none report absolute dose-rate measurements, and the 2-D measurments were made at inappropriately large distances, often with detectors (film and diode) known to have poor energy response. There is no evidence that the Sievert line source model accurately describes [192]Ir relative dose distributions,[35] rendering this avenue of extrapolation to current source designs suspect. Finally, almost nothing has been published documenting the dose distributions about the many shielded colpostats and rectal/vaginal cylinders available for HDR brachytherapy. Reasonably accurate 1-dimensional (1-D) computational models exist for shielded [137]Cs applicators: none of these has been validated for [192]Ir applicator dosimetry.[35] In view of the increased emphasis HDR therapy places on physical optimization of the dose distribution, accurate dose measurements and dose-calculation algorithms are urgently needed.

Until HDR dose measurements become available, clinical dosimetry for HDR sources based on air-kerma strength calibrations should utilize the transverse-axis absolute dose-rate distributions derived from conventional LDR [192]Ir seeds. Williamson et al.[9,36] has recently reviewed and critically compared measured data, derived from TLD and diode dosimetry,[36-38] and theoretical data, derived from 3-D Monte Carlo photon-transport simulations. These data sets were in close agreement with one another and the Meisberger data: reported values of $\Lambda_0$ varied from 1.10 to 1.12 cm$^2$. The dosimetric quantity, $\Lambda_0$, is the dose rate in medium 1 cm from the source on its transverse axis per unit air-kerma strength.[38-39] When measurement of applicator shielding corrections is clinically required, high atomic number detectors, such as diodes and radiographic film, should be avoided. For example, Williamson et al.[36] have shown that the response (silicon diode reading/unit dose to water) varies by as much as 75% over the 1–10-cm distance range from an LDR [192]Ir seed. Currently, the method of choice for dose measurement about intermediate-energy brachytherapy sources is TLD dosimetry in machined solid water phantoms.[37-38] Alternatively, for those with the expertise and the computer software and hardware resources, Monte Carlo photon-transport simulation has been shown to be a practical and accurate alternative to direct measurement.[9,36]

**Quality Assurance of Computer Treatment Planning Systems**

Relatively little has been written on QA of clinical treatment planning systems in general, next to nothing for brachytherapy treatment planning, and absolutely nothing for HDR treatment planning. Williamson[4] has sketched out some tests for conventional brachytherapy: however, HDR software is generally equipped with more complex and advanced features such as catheter-trajectory reconstruction algorithms, dwell-weight optimization algorithms, and dose-volume histogram-based figures of merit for ranking implant quality. Such software packages are so complex that it is impossible to test the response of the program to all possible sequences of user input. All one can hope to do is verify its major computational and graphic display functions in relatively simple testing situations. Many subtle input-history dependent bugs will reveal themselves only in the course of intensive clinical use. Prevention of software-related treatment errors requires careful scrutiny of each clinical treatment plan. Williamson's[4] list of computer planning software tests, expanded to accommodate specialized HDR funtions, is reproduced in Table 2. Working through the tests described in Table 2 not only tests the software, it familiarizes the physicist with the details of system operation and pitfalls likely to be encountered during patient planning. Planning a complex or unfamiliar type of implant can be a stressful experience since one is under pressure to complete it as quickly as possible: the clinical setting is clearly not the time to gain familiarity with and to test unfamiliar program options.

# Periodic Quality Assurance

The purpose of periodic QA of an HDR treatment unit is to ensure the integrity of its basic physical and functional specifications through time. In contrast to commissioning, periodic testing need not directly measure fundamental parameters such as source strength or source transit speed, but merely verify that they have not changed since last measured. Thus, periodic tests should be simple, comprehensive, and nonspecific and can often be relative rather than absolute. A good test is one that validates several parameters simultaneously: acceptable test outcome should imply all that all parameters are within acceptable range while test failure may not identify the offending parameter. The frequency of testing of any given system component depends on the likelihood of failure or change of that component and the severity of the effect expected from such a failure. Since an HDR unit is designed to identify hundreds of possible error conditions, and many other unchecked error conditions potentially exist, exhaustive verification of machine function obviously is not feasible. Specified testing intervals as well as specific test frequency vary significantly among the chapter coauthors: annual, quarterly, monthly, and daily QA protocols are all represented. In no other area of HDR physics is practice so variable. Three of

## Table 2
## HDR Brachytherapy RTP Quality Assurance

| Function | Benchmark Data | Frequency |
|---|---|---|
| Verify input parameters of all precalculated single-source arrays | Published recommendations; source vendor's mechanical drawings | Initially, annually |
| Verify point calculations for all source files | Published dose-rate tables; manual calculations or output of independent RTP | Initially, annually; new software version or source identity |
| Accuracy of single-source isodoses | Point source output | Initially; new software version |
| Accuracy of multiple-source isodoses | Point source data for symmetric source arrays | Initially; new software version |
| Accuracy of plan rotation matrix | Constancy of point doses, source positions, and isodoses under repeated orthogonal rotations for symmetric source arrays | Initially; new software version |
| Consistency of printed plan documentation | Assumed input parameters | Every clinical use |
| Accuracy of digitizer and coordinate reconstruction | Radiograph phantom with known catheter geometry | Initially; new software version |
| Accuracy of electronic downloading of treatment parameters to HDR unit | Comparison of treatment unit and planning-system printed output | Initially; new software version |
| Dose-volume histogram | Use isotropic point source or segment of line source allowing analytic calculation of DVH | Initially; new software version |
| Optimization software | Run series of test cases based on idealized implant geometries of various sizes; develop a sense of what optimization does to an implant compared to uniform loading before trying it on patients | Initially; Spot check when software changes by duplicating old cases |

*(continued)*

the four institutions organize QA into quarterly, monthly, and daily intervals, while one performs tests at annual, quarterly, and daily intervals.

### Daily Quality Assurance

A morning preparation routine forms the foundation for the QA program and should be designed to comprehensively, if nonspecifically, assess most QA endpoints. Such tests should be completed before beginning applicator insertion in the first patient, so that any machine malfunctions are identified before subjecting the patient to any risk-bearing medical procedure such as anesthesia. Generally, most facilities assume that the daily QA protocol need be performed only on days when patients are treated and then only before treating the first patient when multiple patients are to be treated the same day. Table 3 lists the core tests performed by the authors' institutions and attempts to describe the considerable institution-to-institution variation. Some of the listed tests are performed at monthly or quarterly intervals by some institutions.

Most of the tests are straightforward and require only observation of correct operation. Some tests require some special equipment. At the University of Wisconsin, Madison, a jig that constrains a flexible catheter into a 3-cm diameter loop is used to confirm that the afterloader correctly detects curvatures too sharp for the source cable to negotiate. At least one manufacturer discourages frequent testing of their device's obstruction detection system, fearing that repeated collision of the check cable with the catheter end could damage the cable.

Several groups have developed clever devices for simultaneously testing many basic parameters. At Mallinckrodt, a simple check phantom (see Fig. 9) containing an ion chamber near an interstitial needle is used to test accuracy of the timer, source calibration, expected value of source strength obtained by the operator from the source inventory and positional accuracy within ± 3 mm (obviously not a good substitute for the required ± 1-mm positioning accuracy test). A 60-second integrated reading is obtained at a specific dwell position and multiplied by a factor previously derived by intercomparison against the in-air calibration apparatus, yielding an estimate of air-kerma strength. In order that a 1.5-mm error in position yields a 5% change in the reading, the catheter must lie 6.5 mm or less from the chamber. DeWerd et al.(personal communication, 1993) have developed a source collimator (see Fig. 13) that allows a re-entrant chamber to accurately verify source position as well as timer accuracy and source strength. Such simple daily output checks, using integrated ionization from either a well chamber or thimble chamber placed at a fixed distance, are highly recommended: a single reading can confirm the reproducibility or accuracy of source strength, dwell time, and transit time. Although nearby walls and furniture induce unwanted signals in such detectors, spurious scatter causes no problems for consistency checks, as long as such scattering centers remain the same day to day. Mounting the test jig on a wall or in a corner adds convenience for the daily checks.

## Table 3
### Daily Core Quality Assurance Tests for an HDR Remote Afterloading Facility

| Test Endpoint | Test Methodology |
|---|---|
| Verify critical data in treatment unit and planning computer | Date, time, and source strength |
| Verify treatment status indicator lights and critical source-control functions | Source ejected/retracted lights function on treatment unit, console, and above door. Pressing "interrupt" button causes source retraction. Count down of timer to zero terminates treatment. |
| Door interlock function | Opening door interrupts treatment (open door prevents treatment activation from console) and closing door does not resume treatment without reset action from console. |
| Missing applicator interlock functions | Machine prevents source ejection when applicator is not connected to programmed channel or indexer ring is not locked. Audible and visual error condition indicators work. |
| Area radiation monitor functions correctly | Area monitor visual indicator flashes when source is ejected and, when powered only by battery backup power, flashes when test source is held against detector. |
| Audio and visual communication systems correctly function | Visual and aural contact with treatment room occupants verified. |
| Verify response to power failure | Interruption of AC power during source ejection results in immediate retraction. Upon restoring power, programmed treatment parameters and dwell time remaining are correctly recalled. |
| Source positioning accurate to within 1 mm | Many possible tests: repeat primary type (a) accuracy test for a single catheter; deviation of reading from ion chamber placed near a programmed dwell position; obtain a multiple-channel autoradiograph of every active dwell position used in the patient treatment and compare programmed position to that calculated by equation (1); visually check, using CCTV, that relative position of the source tip within the check ruler reproduces from day to day. |

*(continued)*

**Table 3**

**(*continued*)**

| Test Endpoint | Test Methodology |
|---|---|
| Timer accuracy | Many possible tests:<br>use stopwatch to time duration of "source ejected" light;<br>perform a spot check of radiation output for a timed interval using jig similar to that of Fig. 9<br>compare times of source arrival and departure from a dwell position on the printed treatment documentation with a stopwatch. |
| Emergency equipment and essential accessories present | Area correctly posted including emergency instructions; emergency equipment present including forceps, emergency safe, surgical supplies, etc.; operator's manual present; portable survey meter present and functioning. |
| Miscellaneous tests performed by some authors and not others | Operation of emergency retraction motor; for Selection/HDR, response to interruption of compressed air; check source retracts when excessive friction/applicator obstruction is encountered; verify applicator/transfer tube length when required by simulator localization procedure or product reliability; verify correct function of dedicated fluoroscopy/imaging system if present. |

## Monthly, Quarterly, and Annual Quality Assurance Procedures

Among the authors of this chapter, there are two basic aproaches to periodic QA. Three of the four institutions represented here developed monthly and quarterly QA protocols, the latter coinciding with the quarterly source change for $^{192}$Ir-based treatment units. The monthly protocol, modeled after the NRC-mandated $^{60}$Co teletherapy monthly calibration check, is sometimes required by NRC license reviewers. Table 4 lists the core tests. The fourth institution performs periodic testing at daily, quarterly, and annual intervals. Their daily QA protocol is structured so as to include all critical monthly tests including a source-strength spot check using a tertiary standard. In addition to regulatory compliance, a goal of monthly QA is to verify critical treatment parameters, such as source output, in analogy to external beam radiotherapy. Clearly, such a monthly calibration check should be performed if a reasonably rigorous output and timer checks are not being performed on a daily basis. A second purpose of monthly QA is to perform a relative check on those para-

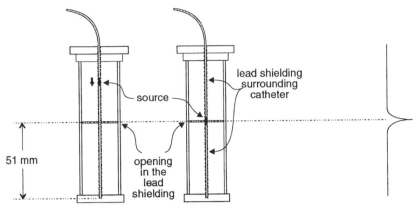

**Step 1** - Insert catheter to bottom of insert (nominally position zero).
**Step 2** - Position source on either side of the opening.
**Step 3** - Move source past opening to obtain measurements.

**Step 4** - Calculate (1) Source positioning, (2) Timer consistency, (3) Source calibration consistency.

**Fig. 13.** Cutaway view of a re-entrant chamber modified to accurately verify positional accuracy. A disk-shaped 4-mm thick tungsten-alloy shield, through which the source passes, is used to detect the passage of the source. The minimum of the ionization versus indexer-distance curve accurately defines the HDR distance setting, corresponding to alignment of the radioactive source center with the shield center. (Reproduced with permission by Standard Imaging, Middleton, Wisconsin).

meters the physicist believes could change through time. For example, many localization procedures assume a known, or at least unchanging, transfer tube length, necessitating the extensive positional accuracy tests listed in Table 4. The quarterly QA protocol should include absolute measurement of parameters that are potentially influenced by source replacement. Clearly, this includes source strength and rigorous assessment of type (a) positional accuracy since all HDR treatment devices allow some internal adjustment of this parameter. Treatment constancy checks and timer accuracy tests may be performed either at quarterly or monthly intervals, depending on the historical track record of these components. Table 5 lists the tests typically included in the quarterly protocol.

Only one of the four coauthors has developed a formal annual QA protocol. This procedure (see Table 6) should include review of the secondary dosimetry system from which the primary quarterly calibration is derived. For free-air calibration setups, this should include an intercomparison with the departmental substandard using external beam exposures as a relative or absolute reference. For those physicists using re-entrant chambers calibrated by an ADCL, annual intercomparison of this calibration against the free-air calibration procedure described by Goetsch et al.[29] is recommended. In addition, other fundamental parameters, such as transit dose, should be discussed. Finally, other infrequently checked assumptions, for example, treatment planning system accuracy, shielded colpostat integrity, source-tip-to-center-of-radioactivity distance and training compliance, should be checked. The length of all transfer tubes should be verified at this time.

**Table 4**

**Monthly Core Quality Assurance Tests for an HDR Remote Afterloading Facility Adapted from University of Wisconsin-Madison Protocol**

| Test Endpoint | Test Methodology |
| --- | --- |
| Verify source strength calibration | Use either secondary or tertiary calibration setup. |
| Inspect and confirm correct operation of all applicators and transfer tubes and source localization dummies | Examine all dummies for kinks or bends that may shorten their axial displacement through applicator assembly. Check integrity of all transfer tube-applicator interfaces. |
| Radioactive source center positioned within 1 mm of expected position defined by simulation marker used for each applicator type | UW-Madison tests: superposed auto-radiograph/transmission radiograph for each applicator and radiographic marker type. Endobronchial catheter with adapter and 1-m radiographic marker; Interstitial applicator with HDR-simulation marker fully inserted; Intrauterine tandem applicator loaded with Nucletron simulation marker (as illustrated by Fig. 7b). For treatment units (e.g., Gamma Med 12i), which require fixed-length treatment tubes and permanent applicators, all lengths should be checked. |
| Verify interlock function for all daily QA tests | Power-failure, emergency retraction motor, and applicator obstruction tests should be performed if not included in daily protocol. |
| All daily tests of treatment status indicators, audio-visual communications, area monitor function, and emergency equipment readiness | Area monitor indicator flashes when source is ejected and, when powered only by battery backup power, flashes when weak test source is held against detector. |
| Audio and visual communication systems correctly function | See Table 3. |
| Verify response to power failure | Interruption of AC power during source ejection results in immediate retraction. Upon restoring power, programmed treatment parameters and dwell time remaining are correctly recalled. |

**Table 5**

**Quarterly Core Quality Assurance Tests for an HDR Remote Afterloading Facility Adapted from Mallinckrodt Institute of Radiology Protocol**

| *Test Endpoint* | *Test Methodology* |
| --- | --- |
| Personnel safety (generally NRC mandated) | Head survey with source retracted: < 0.25 mR/h at 1 m; Facility survey: within 10 CFR, Part 20 limits. Use calibrated ion chamber survey meter; All required postings and emergency procedures in place |
| Patient safety | All treatment status indicators including treatment fault correctly function; Area monitor and audio/visual communications functioning; Important interlocks function: obstructed applicator, missing applicator, door and indexer ring |
| Inspect and confirm correct operation of all applicators and transfer tubes and source localization dummies | Examine all dummies for kinks or bends that may shorten their axial displacement through applicator assembly. Check integrity of all transfer tube-applicator interfaces. |
| Type (a) positional accuracy | Use CCTV to confirm that the radioactive source center agrees with the radiographic marker and source position simulator within .05 mm. Confirm check cable operation. |
| Type (b) positional accuracy: Radioactive source center positioned within 1 mm of expected position defined by simulation marker used for each applicator type for which source localization simulation procedure is not self-correcting for transfer tube shrinkage or expansion. | Obtain 18-channel staggered autoradiograph: verify that dwell-position spacing, assignment of dwell sequence to programmed channel, and relative indexer length to dwell 1 are correct within 1 mm. Also confirm that documented autoradiograph transfer-tube and pin-to-needle orifice lengths used for daily position check are correct. For all transfer tubes, which are assumed to be of fixed length (e.g., Nucletron GYN tubes 1-3), obtain transmission radiograph for each tube attached to a GYN applicator with 1-m radiographic marker fully inserted. Verify that 995 marker position has not changed, i.e., transfer tube length unchanged. |

*(continued)*

**Table 5**

**(*continued*)**

| Test Endpoint | Test Methodology |
|---|---|
| Source calibration | Use secondary apparatus (Goetsch-Attix free-air calibration technique or calibrated re-entrant chamber technique) to obtain air-kerma strength of new source. |
| Verify source calibration | Verify that measured air-kerma strength is within 10% of vendor value; Use tertiary daily output checking system to confirm primary calibration within 5%. Different electrometer and ion chamber must be used. |

## Personnel Requirements

As of this writing, the NRC specifies minimum credentials and training only for the radiation oncology physician. To prescribe any type of brachytherapy, the physician must satisfy 10 CFR 35.940, which requires either board certification or, alternatively, training consisting of 200 hours of classroom and laboratory instruction in radiation physics, radiation protection, mathematics of radioactivity, and radiation biology, 500 hours of supervised work experience maintaining a brachytherapy source program, and 3 years of clinical experience under the supervision of an NRC authorized user. Partly in response to an HDR source loss that went undetected by the users,[7] the NRC is currently revising HDR QA and personnel qualifications and is expected to define minimum credentials for brachytherapy physicists.

A successful program requires a well-qualified and integrated treatment delivery team with substantially more expertise than that listed above. Figure 14 shows one proposed model organization for gynecologic applications. This model team consists of the following specialists.

*Radiation Oncologist* —A board-certified radiation oncologist with special expertise in brachytherapy, preferably HDR brachytherapy, is required. To perform HDR gynecologic brachytherapy, the physician should have extensive training and experience with at least one established and documented LDR system. Since HDR gynecologic brachytherapy remains a somewhat experimental, continuously evolving technique, this experience should include following patients and quantifying clinical outcomes. This, in turn, requires appropriate biometry resources. Before beginning an HDR practice on patients, time should be spent visiting facilities with ongoing programs.

*Brachytherapy Physicist* —A board-certified, radiation-oncology physicist with expertise in brachytherapy is required. Just as with the radiation oncologist, the physicist should train at a facility already performing HDR treat-

**Table 6**

**Additional Annual Quality Assurance Tests for an HDR Remote Afterloading Facility Adapted from Mallinckrodt Institute of Radiology Protocol**

| Test Endpoint | Test Methodology |
| --- | --- |
| Review calibration of secondary source strength measurement apparatus | Intercompare chamber and electrometer used for free-air calibration against departmental substandard using a Co-60 beam. Obtain new calibration from ADCL if calibration is more than two years old.<br>If a well chamber is used for quarterly calibration, perform Goetsch-Attix free-air calibration to verify its calibration factor. Verify well-chamber response as function of axial source position. |
| Type (a) accuracy: verify that source tip-to-center of radioactivity is correct if CCTV method is used quarterly | Intercompare CCTV course tip vs. radiographic marker measurement to autoradiographic method. |
| Transit dose | Measure source speed using the excess ionization method. |
| Constancy of transfer tube length | Measure the lengths of all transfer tubes using a transparent applicator of known length. |
| Simulation marker-source localization procedure accuracy: interstitial brachytherapy | Using transparent applicator taped to ruler, confirm that each dummy-source position agrees with validated radiographic marker when used according to source localization protocol. |
| Simulation marker accuracy and applicator integrity: intracavitary brachytherapy | Obtain orthogonal radiographs of every colpostat and cylinder loaded with corresponding simulation marker. Check for symmetric source positioning, integrity of internal shielding, and other structures.<br>For one applicator of each type, compare lateral radiographs of the applicator loaded with simulation dummy and applicator-transfer tube assembly loaded with a validated radiographic marker. |
| Additional interlock tests | Have radioactive source removed and replaced by dummy cable.<br>Check in-room emergency DC motor retraction buttons and hand crank.<br>Check that emergency motors are activated when source cable (not check cable) is restrained during retraction, encounters obstruction during ejection, or is displaced during stationary dwelling.<br>During stationary dwelling, cut off cable tip to verify correct detection of source capsule loss following retraction not yet implemented. |

(continued)

**Table 6**

**(*continued*)**

| Test Endpoint | Test Methodology |
|---|---|
| Treatment-planning-system checks | Accuracy of digitizer and plotter;<br>Accuracy of single-source dose file: compare point-dose calculations against published dosimetry data;<br>Run standard plan to verify correct overall system performance;<br>Check accuracy of treatment planning-treatment unit communication |
| Verify absolute timer accuracy and linearity. Confirm that transit dose is unchanged. | Use daily output check apparatus and procedure in "Timer Accuracy and Linearity" |
| Miscellaneous | Update source strength in treatment planning computer initialization file, treatment unit and quarterly inventory.<br>Have a second physicist independently review the quarterly report<br>Check that treatment unit corrects decay source strengths and corrects dwell times for decay<br>Review accuracy of all standard treatment configurations stored in treatment unit<br>Review quality assurance manual and update if necessary<br>Review compliance with personnel training requirements |

ments before beginning his or her own program. Vendor-supplied training for both the treatment unit and treatment planning system should be obtained.

*Dosimetrist* —An individual with a good background in brachytherapy treatment planning is required. Formal qualifications include certification as a radiation therapy technologist or an undergraduate degree in physics or radiological sciences. This individual should have vendor-supplied training on operation of both the treatment unit and treatment planning system.

*Treatment-Unit Operator* —This individual must have vendor-supplied training on the HDR unit and must spend extensive time practicing with the unit before treating patients. A physicist, dosimetrist, technologist, or nurse may be designated to deliver the treatment, although some states may require HDR operators to be licensed radiation therapy technologists. The operator must not feel hesitant to enter the room and follow the emergency procedures should the source fail to retract into its shielded position.

Physicians, department heads, and administrators must realize that development and maintenance of a safe and effective HDR program requires a significant time commitment on the part of the physicist and must provide adequate staffing and equipment resources.

## HDR FLOW DIAGRAM

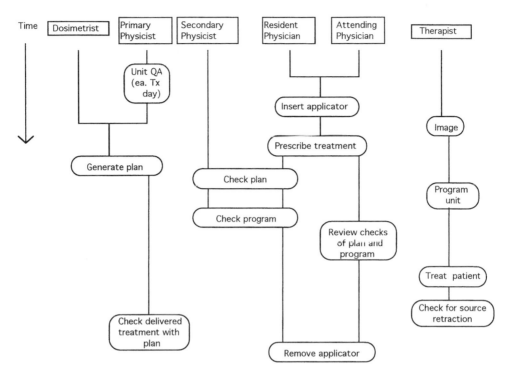

**Fig. 14.** Diagram illustrating the HDR procedure flow and assignment of tasks to treatment-delivery team personnel as practiced at the University of Wisconsin-Madison.

## Quality Assurance During Treatment Planning and Treatment Delivery

Most HDR treatment errors are caused by human errors or misjudgments made during treatment planning and execution, rather than to failure or malfunction of the equipment. In the authors' experience, it is generally the physicist's role to define the organization and responsibilites of the treatment delivery team members and to provide for their training. The time interval surrounding the HDR treatment is often extremely hectic since the time interval of the applicator remains in the unanesthetized patient must be minimized, creating an unforgiving environment in which errors and miscommunications can easily occur. Three basic principles should be followed: (1) carefully define the procedure flow and duties of each team member, (2) develop a good system of documentation and check-off forms to ensure good communication and QA compliance, and (3) isolate the vulnerable points where error is likely and institute redundant checks.

Figure 14 illustrates HDR procedure flow, task assignment, and redundant checks made at the University of Wisconsin, Madison. In this model, the primary physicist works with the dosimetrist, and a secondary physicist is utilized to review the treatment plan, HDR programming, and associated documentation prior to initiating treatment. The primary physicist catches and corrects a significant number of errors before optimization and dose calculation and directs the computer optimization process when its complexity exceeds the dosimetrist's capabilities or the ability of treatment planning system to adequately document the treatment plan (e.g. positioning of dose points) Similarly, use of the resident physician provides a redundant observer during the applicator insertion phase. This particular model requires a large staffing commitment and may not be feasible in smaller facilities. To avoid compromising patient safety, such facilities could practice simpler computer optimization procedures (allowing the dosimetrist to plan independently) or develop an alternative approach to independently checking critical decision points in the process. The other three authors generally utilize only a single physicist in HDR treatment, distributing many critical primary physicist tasks to the brachytherapy technologist and dosimetrist.

Good documentation is essential to a well-organized HDR facility. Figure 15 illustrates a prescription form used at one of the author's institutions. Each facility should design such a form that meets its needs. However, any prescription form should provide for a clearly-defined prescription, including the fraction size, dose-prescription location relative to the active dwell positions, the time interval between fractions, and authorized user signature along with signature blocks for the physicist and physician to document their pretreatment review of the plan. Space for a diagram of the implant, showing dwell locations relative to anatomy, should be available as well as a description of the applicator. Finally, the form should contain a daily treatment record showing the date of each treatment, the dose delivered, and the cumulative dose administered so far in the treatment course to prevent erroneous delivery of additional fractions. Preferably, this summary information should be contained on a single page valid for the entire treatment course, with separate sections or pages for each fraction. Additional essential documentation includes clear descriptions of all dwell-time calculations, a diagram indicating which dwell positions are activated and the indexer distance to the first dwell position, and forms documenting source-position localization. Figure 16 illustrates one system for documenting active dwell positions: it contains check-off blocks documenting that the treatment plan, treatment-specific autoradiograph, simulator films and treatment-unit programming parameters have all been intercompared to assure positional accuracy. Figure 17 illustrates a form that both defines and documents in checkable form the applicator localization measurements and treatment length calculations. The AES brachytherapy dose specification recommendations[39] contain many useful suggestions for documenting target volume location and shape, prescription criteria, and applicator characteristics that are applicahle to HDR brachytherapy.

Another extremely useful type of form is the QA checklist, an example of which is illustrated by Fig. 18. All critical QA checks and redundant observations are listed on the form. It serves to remind all treatment delivery person-

**. Barnes Radiation Oncology Center
Mallinckrodt Institute of Radiology**

## HIGH DOSE-RATE BRACHYTHERAPY    CAUTION

Name: _____    Birthdate: _____

Primary Site: _____    Ref. Physicians: _____

Stage: _____    Histopathology: _____

Date: _____    Radiotherapists: _____

R    L

**Prescription**

No. Fractions _____ Total Dose _____ cGy

Dose/Fraction: _____ Time Interval between

Fractions _____

Dose delivered to _____

_____

Signed: _____ M.D. Date: _____

Modifications: _____

_____

Applicator: _____

_____

| Date | | | | | | |
|---|---|---|---|---|---|---|
| Fraction No. | 1 | 2 | 3 | 4 | 5 | 6 |
| No. of catheters | | | | | | |
| Applicators | | | | | | |
| Dose this Fraction (cGy) | | | | | | |
| Total Dose (cGy) | | | | | | |
| Source Strength (cGy·m²/hr) | | | | | | |
| Integrated Reference Air-kerma (cGy m²) | | | | | | |
| Mg-hrs | | | | | | |
| Total Dwell Time(s) | | | | | | |
| Treatment Reviewed and authorized by: (Physician) | | | | | | |
| Planned by: | | | | | | |
| Physics Review:    (Physicist) | | | | | | |
| Delivered by:   (Technologist) | | | | | | |
| Post-treatment physician review and date | | | | | | |

2751-31 rev. 2/93

**Fig. 15.** The prescription form used at the Mallinckrodt Institute of Radiology illustrating the essential components of this document. A summary of the entire treatment course and its current status, an implant diagram, a clearly defined prescription, and treatment plan review signature blocks.

nel of essential checks, provides a simple and easily auditable record for demonstrating compliance, and is a useful tool for training newcomers in system operation.

HDR Localization Verification

Patient Name: _____  ROC No.: _____  Date: _____  Fraction No. _____

Step Length: _____  Matches Treatment Plan ☐  HDR Tape ☐  Auto Radiograph ☐  Nominal Catheter Length _____

| Channel | Check Active Dwell Positions |
|---|---|
| 1 | 1 _ _ 5 _ _ 9 _ _ 13 _ _ 17 _ _ 21 _ _ 25 _ _ 29 _ _ 33 _ _ 37 _ _ 41 _ _ 45 _ _ _ |
| 2 | 1 _ _ 5 _ _ 9 _ _ 13 _ _ 17 _ _ 21 _ _ 25 _ _ 29 _ _ 33 _ _ 37 _ _ 41 _ _ 45 _ _ _ |
| 3 | 1 _ _ 5 _ _ 9 _ _ 13 _ _ 17 _ _ 21 _ _ 25 _ _ 29 _ _ 33 _ _ 37 _ _ 41 _ _ 45 _ _ _ |
| 4 | 1 _ _ 5 _ _ 9 _ _ 13 _ _ 17 _ _ 21 _ _ 25 _ _ 29 _ _ 33 _ _ 37 _ _ 41 _ _ 45 _ _ _ |
| 5 | 1 _ _ 5 _ _ 9 _ _ 13 _ _ 17 _ _ 21 _ _ 25 _ _ 29 _ _ 33 _ _ 37 _ _ 41 _ _ 45 _ _ _ |
| 6 | 1 _ _ 5 _ _ 9 _ _ 13 _ _ 17 _ _ 21 _ _ 25 _ _ 29 _ _ 33 _ _ 37 _ _ 41 _ _ 45 _ _ _ |
| 7 | 1 _ _ 5 _ _ 9 _ _ 13 _ _ 17 _ _ 21 _ _ 25 _ _ 29 _ _ 33 _ _ 37 _ _ 41 _ _ 45 _ _ _ |
| 8 | 1 _ _ 5 _ _ 9 _ _ 13 _ _ 17 _ _ 21 _ _ 25 _ _ 29 _ _ 33 _ _ 37 _ _ 41 _ _ 45 _ _ _ |
| 9 | 1 _ _ 5 _ _ 9 _ _ 13 _ _ 17 _ _ 21 _ _ 25 _ _ 29 _ _ 33 _ _ 37 _ _ 41 _ _ 45 _ _ _ |
| 10 | 1 _ _ 5 _ _ 9 _ _ 13 _ _ 17 _ _ 21 _ _ 25 _ _ 29 _ _ 33 _ _ 37 _ _ 41 _ _ 45 _ _ _ |
| 11 | 1 _ _ 5 _ _ 9 _ _ 13 _ _ 17 _ _ 21 _ _ 25 _ _ 29 _ _ 33 _ _ 37 _ _ 41 _ _ 45 _ _ _ |
| 12 | 1 _ _ 5 _ _ 9 _ _ 13 _ _ 17 _ _ 21 _ _ 25 _ _ 29 _ _ 33 _ _ 37 _ _ 41 _ _ 45 _ _ _ |
| 13 | 1 _ _ 5 _ _ 9 _ _ 13 _ _ 17 _ _ 21 _ _ 25 _ _ 29 _ _ 33 _ _ 37 _ _ 41 _ _ 45 _ _ _ |
| 14 | 1 _ _ 5 _ _ 9 _ _ 13 _ _ 17 _ _ 21 _ _ 25 _ _ 29 _ _ 33 _ _ 37 _ _ 41 _ _ 45 _ _ _ |
| 15 | 1 _ _ 5 _ _ 9 _ _ 13 _ _ 17 _ _ 21 _ _ 25 _ _ 29 _ _ 33 _ _ 37 _ _ 41 _ _ 45 _ _ _ |
| 16 | 1 _ _ 5 _ _ 9 _ _ 13 _ _ 17 _ _ 21 _ _ 25 _ _ 29 _ _ 33 _ _ 37 _ _ 41 _ _ 45 _ _ _ |
| 17 | 1 _ _ 5 _ _ 9 _ _ 13 _ _ 17 _ _ 21 _ _ 25 _ _ 29 _ _ 33 _ _ 37 _ _ 41 _ _ 45 _ _ _ |
| 18 | 1 _ _ 5 _ _ 9 _ _ 13 _ _ 17 _ _ 21 _ _ 25 _ _ 29 _ _ 33 _ _ 37 _ _ 41 _ _ 45 _ _ _ |

Page 2 - HDR Localization Verification    Patient Name: _____  ROC No.: _____
Date: _____  Fraction No.: _____

| Channel | Insertion Depth[1] | Offset[2] | Treatment Length[3] | Active Length[4] | Length, Off-Set, Active Positions Checked Against: | | | |
|---|---|---|---|---|---|---|---|---|
| | | | | | HDR Tape | Treatment Plan | Simulation | Auto Radiograph |
| 1 | | | | | ☐ | ☐ | ☐ | ☐ |
| 2 | | | | | ☐ | ☐ | ☐ | ☐ |
| 3 | | | | | ☐ | ☐ | ☐ | ☐ |
| 4 | | | | | ☐ | ☐ | ☐ | ☐ |
| 5 | | | | | ☐ | ☐ | ☐ | ☐ |
| 6 | | | | | ☐ | ☐ | ☐ | ☐ |
| 7 | | | | | ☐ | ☐ | ☐ | ☐ |
| 8 | | | | | ☐ | ☐ | ☐ | ☐ |
| 9 | | | | | ☐ | ☐ | ☐ | ☐ |
| 10 | | | | | ☐ | ☐ | ☐ | ☐ |
| 11 | | | | | ☐ | ☐ | ☐ | ☐ |
| 12 | | | | | ☐ | ☐ | ☐ | ☐ |
| 13 | | | | | ☐ | ☐ | ☐ | ☐ |
| 14 | | | | | ☐ | ☐ | ☐ | ☐ |
| 15 | | | | | ☐ | ☐ | ☐ | ☐ |
| 16 | | | | | ☐ | ☐ | ☐ | ☐ |
| 17 | | | | | ☐ | ☐ | ☐ | ☐ |
| 18 | | | | | ☐ | ☐ | ☐ | ☐ |

[1] Faceplate to ☐ end of catheter  ☐ Dwell 1
[2] Insertion-depth reference to first dwell position
[3] Programmed distance: Faceplate to Dwell 1
[4] Distance: Proximal-to-distalmost active dwell position

Calculated by: _____  Checked by: _____

**Fig. 16.** Active dwell-position localization form developed at the Mallinckrodt Institute of Radiology illustrating active dwell positions and treatment distances for each catheter. After the physician indicates the target region on the simulator films, the physicist identifies the dwell positions from the film and fills in the form. This work is checked by the dosimetrist before beginning the treatment plan. The form contains check-off blocks documenting catheter-by-catheter intercomparison of the treatment plan, autoradiograph, simulator films, and treatment-unit programming parameters.

**BARNES RADIATION ONCOLOGY CENTER**
**MicroSelectron HDR Interstitial Implant Localization Form**

Patient Name: ______________ Date: ______________

$O_d$ = dummy offset = ribbon end-to-distal seed center
$O_t$ = Dwell 1 offset = distal dummy seed center-to-first dwell position
$O_r$ = Marker offset = marker cap to proximal end of treatment tube
Radiographic marker No. _____ Length _____ ($L_{RM}$)
Constraints

$L_c = (L_{RM}) - O_r$ $L_1 = L_c - (O_d + O_t)$

Note: $L_c - L_1 \geq 2$ mm Catheter length $\leq 283$ mm

$L_1$ - (no. dwells - 1) x step length $\geq 715$ mm

$L_1 \leq 995$ mm

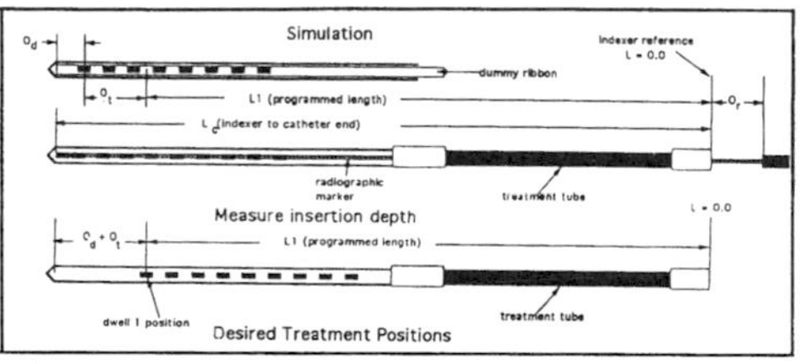


| | | SIMULATION | | | TREATMENT | | | | |
|---|---|---|---|---|---|---|---|---|---|
| Channel Number | Catheter Number | Dummy Offset $O_d$ | Marker Offset $O_r$ | Dummy Identity | Dwell 1 Offset | First/Last Treated Positions | Number of Dwell Positions | Applicator Length $L_c$ | Programmed Dwell 1 Length, $L_1$ |
| 1 | | | | | | | | | |
| 2 | | | | | | | | | |
| 3 | | | | | | | | | |
| 4 | | | | | | | | | |
| 5 | | | | | | | | | |
| 6 | | | | | | | | | |
| 7 | | | | | | | | | |
| 8 | | | | | | | | | |
| 9 | | | | | | | | | |
| 10 | | | | | | | | | |
| 11 | | | | | | | | | |
| 12 | | | | | | | | | |
| 13 | | | | | | | | | |
| 14 | | | | | | | | | |
| 15 | | | | | | | | | |
| 16 | | | | | | | | | |
| 17 | | | | | | | | | |
| 18 | | | | | | | | | |

Catheter length: _______ Step Length: _________ Calculated By: ______________ Checked By: ______________

2751-9 NEW 12/92

**Fig. 17.** The form developed at the Mallinckrodt Institute of Radiology for documenting the applicator tip localization method for interstitial implants using flexiguides or closed-end flexible implant tubes. This form is filled out in the simulator room as each catheter-transfer tube assembly is sounded by the dosimetrist or brachytherapy technologist, and the calculations are reviewed by the physicist.

# Treatment Specific Quality Assurance

In the following sections, examples of QA checks and pitfalls for each phase of treatment delivery will be described. Implementation of such measures by a specific facility will necessarily be very individualized, taking into account procedure complexity and frequency, staff available, and skill level of available personnel.

## Applicator Preparation

Upon scheduling a procedure, the appropriate applicator kit should be assembled, reviewed for correct operation and completeness, and sent for sterilization. It is useful to make a list of required kit components for each procedure type so that appropriate localization dummies. adapters, and so forth, are not forgotten. If single-use applicators are used, they should be checked for correct and error-free operation on the HDR and sounded if the localization procedure

Mallinckrodt Institute of Radiology
High Dose-Rate Brachytherapy Checklist

Patient Name: _____    Date: _____    ROC Number: _____

Fraction No.: _____ of _____

|  | Completed | Comment |
|---|---|---|
| 1. Daily QA completed | _____ | _____ |
| 2. Prescription completed and signed by authorized physician | _____ | _____ |
| 3. Correct source strength stored in HDR | _____ | _____ |

4. Simulation

| | | |
|---|---|---|
| (a) For interstitial treatments, insertion depths measured and verified | _____ | _____ |
| (b) Treatment volume marked by physician | _____ | _____ |
| (c) For ISI, localization form filled out and checked | _____ | _____ |
| (d) For non-optimized plans, manual calculation completed by physicist and checked | _____ | _____ |

5. Computer Treatment Plan

| | | |
|---|---|---|
| (a) Reviewed and accepted by physician | _____ | _____ |
| (b) HDR console programmed and stored by dosimetrist or physicist | _____ | _____ |
| (c) Autoradiograph exposed and program reloaded | _____ | _____ |

6. Final Plan Review

| | | |
|---|---|---|
| (a) Treatment plan, autoradiograph, prescription, source localization form, simulation films and HDR printout checked by physicist and signed | _____ | _____ |
| (b) Treatment plan, documentation reviewed and treatment record by physician | _____ | _____ |
| (c) HDR printout checked against treatment plan and prescription by Technologist | _____ | _____ |

7. Treatment

| | | |
|---|---|---|
| (a) Patient identified by two methods | _____ | _____ |
| (b) Signed consent form present | _____ | _____ |
| (c) Emergency equipment present | _____ | _____ |
| (d) Emergency responses reviewed for this patient | _____ | _____ |
| (e) Physician, physicist and technologist are present | _____ | _____ |
| (f) Check matching of HDR channel and applicator nos. | _____ | _____ |
| (g) Tubes free of obstructions and imperfections | _____ | _____ |
| (h) Treat patient. | _____ | _____ |
| (i) Survey patient | _____ | _____ |
| (j) Physician has initialed and dated treatment record post treatment | _____ | _____ |

Instrument: _____    Reading above background: _____    Physicist's Signature _____

Form #155
MIR - ROC 1/92

**Fig. 18.** A QA checkoff list developed at the Mallinckrodt Institute of Radiology defining step-by-step essential QA duties. It is useful for teaching newcomers the treatment-delivery process and for documenting for NRC license compliance. Developing such a form forces one to think through and define the treatment-delivery flow.

requires them to have a fixed length. Until the procedure frequency builds up to the level that OR support personnel become "trained," any specific equipment required, for example, a fluoroscopic examination table, a particular bronchoscope, topical anesthetic, and so forth, should be ordered in advance.

## Applicator Insertion

Insertion of intracavitary, interstitial or transluminal applicators is the responsibility of the radiation oncologist: the level of physics team involvement in the operative procedure depends on procedure complexity, physician familiarity with the equipment, and the receptivity of physician-to-physicist participation in this aspect of treatment delivery. In general, it is recommended that a member of the physics team, a technologist or dosimetrist for routine procedures or a physicist for complex or unfamiliar ones, attend the operative procedure. The essential operating room responsibilities of the physics team are to (a) ensure that the appropriate applicators and accessories are present, handed to the physician in the proper order, and installed in a fashion compatible with the mechanical and geometric requirements of the afterloading device, (b) ensure that tumor localization data (direct visualization, fluoroscopy, bronchoscopy, etc.) available only in the operating room are properly recorded and correlated with dwell position settings for later use in defining the treatment volume, and (c) document on the prescription form the applicators used and their location. In the experience of the senior author, physics attendance (usually a technologist) has prevented numerous errors, such as cutting catheters too short for attachment to the transfer tubes, leaving the solid plastic inserts inside flexible implant catheters used to form 180° loops, placing mini-ovoid caps with their 4-mm-thick rather than 8-mm-thick sides directed laterally, and preventing insertion of LDR-compatible rather than HDR-compatible gynecologic applicators. Especially in a teaching hospital in which senior residents or junior staff with varying levels of brachytherapy experience must take charge of a procedure, providing an experienced technical support person has proven to be an essential QA measure.

**Implant Localization and Simulation**

During radiographic examination of the implant in preparation for treatment planning, several key steps are taken that influence positional accuracy of the treatment. For multiple-catheter transluminal implants or interstitial implants, each applicator should be labeled externally with the corresponding channel number and a correctly labeled sketch of the implant drawn on the prescription form. Generally, each applicator is loaded with a radiographically distinct or recognizable sequences of dummy seeds. The identity of each simulation marker should be carefully recorded on the implant diagram to facilitate matching of corresponding dwell positions and catheters on orthogonal or variable-angle films. Finally, the localization procedure may require each catheter or catheter-transfer tube combination to be sounded, the results of which must be correctly recorded on the localization form (Fig. 17). Incorrect execution of these steps may result in delivering the wrong sequence of dwell positions and times to a catheter. We strongly recommend that two persons work together to gather the localization information; one to perform the labeling and measurement functions and a second to record the information and check the accuracy of the first. Finally, an experienced treatment planner should approve the films as adequate for implant reconstruction before the patient leaves the table.

Radiographic visualization of plastic intracavitary applicators, for example, vaginal cylinders, can be achieved by inserting small radio opaque seeds or spacers near the surface of such applicators.[40] Such marking systems not only improve anatomical localization of applicator surfaces, but support radiographic verification of colpostat and vaginal cylinder diameters as well.

### Treatment Prescription

Following simulation, the physician then reviews the films along with other pertinent localization data and (a) defines the target volume or dwell positions to be activated, (b) defines where the prescribed dose is to be delivered or specified, and (c) defines the prescribed dose and fractionation scheme and completes and signs the prescription. Unless procedure frequency is high enough to allow this procedure to be unambiguously routinized, this activity should involve consultation between the physician and the physicist. The physicist's role is to confirm that all relevant tumor-imaging studies and localization data are correctly correlated with the simulation marker images, to aid the physician in articulating clinical intent in terms of quantitative endpoints, and to develop a clear strategy for optimizing the implant, for example, does the volume outlined on the films indicate the dwell positions to be activated or a target surface with the dwell positions to be selected so as to achieve a desired balance between dose uniformity and target volume coverage? Generally, an experienced physicist should be able to recommend a combination of prescription criterion and a margin of implanted volume about the target surface necessary to achieve this goal without lengthy computer planning.

The final step in the prescription phase of treatment delivery is to describe the dwell positions to be activated in terms of the treatment planning system and treatment-delivery unit input parameters, such as dwell position numbers and treatment lengths. For intracavitary and transluminal treatments, such localization calculations are straightforward. However, for interstitial implants, where the distal surface of the target volume may not follow the surface defined by the distal catheter tips, this process may require matching the localization film images of each catheter with the corresponding channel number, an often time-consuming activity. In this case, one person, for example, the dosimetrist, should perform the matching and a second person, for example, the physicist, should verify the catheter image-channel number correspondence and localization calculations (see Fig. 17).

### Treatment Planning

Treatment planning begins with a consultation between the dosimetrist and physicist regarding the location of active dwell positions and dose prescription points, the choice of optimization algorithm, and the selection of optimization endpoints, that is, "dose points," if any, to use Nucletron jargon. We recommend that the actual treatment planning be performed by a second individual independently of the reviewing physicist. When physicist and dosimetrist work too closely together, mistakes tend to be made together, compromising the physicist's ability to review the plan with unbiased expectations and to detect errors. In the single-physicist model of treatment delivery, such independence may be difficult to achieve, especially if the dosimetrist is not highly experienced or skilled and requires constant physicist supervision and coaching. In addition, there are several key operations, such as correct placement of dose points, that are nearly impossible to verify unless the physicist watches the planning process. If the involvement of the primary physicist in treatment planning is extensive, as it will be until the staff acquires sufficient experience, the two-physicist University of Wisconsin model (Fig. 14) should be seriously considered. As experience grows, the senior author has found that he can check the progress of planning at agreed-upon intervention points and feel sufficiently independent to avoid calling in a colleague in most instances. This has been achieved by developing a well-defined optimization and dose-prescription protocol, which greatly limits the options available to the dosimetrist. For example, only geometric optimization[41] can be applied to interstitial implants (eliminating the need for dose-point placement), and the dose is always prescribed as a fixed fraction (0.75–0.90) of the central minimum dose defined by placing applicator points in the central transverse plane of the implant at a specified point in the program flow. The prospective HDR user is warned: the current DOS-based treatment-planning program distributed by Nucletron, although functionally powerful, is not well documented, does not have a clear, easily understandable user interface, and sometimes unpredictably transfers control from one module to another. Use of this system by inexperienced or inattentive personnel can give rise to serious dose-delivery errors.

## Pretreatment Physicist Review of the HDR Treatment Plan

An important function of the physicist charged with reviewing the treatment-planning process is to ensure that the physician's clinical intent has been communicated accurately to the planners, and that the resulting plan is consistent with that intent. For example, it may not be clear whether a volume marked by the physician on the localization films describes the treatment volume or the target volume to be enclosed by the prescription isodose or whether the prescription distance is specified relative to the applicator center or its surface. It may seem self-evident that clear communication between physician, physicist, and planner is necessary, but over time expectations and assumptions can become implicit and unstated and, therefore, lead to misunderstanding in the event of staff changes, and so forth. An effective physics review encompasses much more than verification of computer plan accuracy: it includes assessment of clinical appropriateness and consistency of the final treatment program with target localization data, simulation films, treatment prescription, and computer treatment plan.

The specific review of each plan should begin with verification of input data, including whether

(1) source strength matches the decayed value;

(2) correct customizing file is used;

(3) magnification factors, source-film distances, and so forth, were correct;

(4) the source-position reconstruction algorithm used was consistent with the simulation film geometry. Since some systems do not completely document the relevant parameters, for example, films correctly oriented on a digitizer, the three orthogonal dimensions of the volume formed by the peripheral catheters indicated on the graphic plan output should be compared directly with the localization radiographs. The dimensions of the prescription isodose line should match both the written prescription and the radiographically-defined implant dimensions;

(5) correct units were used for all quantities;

(6) machine variables, such as step length, were correct;

(7) optimization scheme and prescription criterion chosen are consistent with implant geometry and clinical intent;

(8) dose per fraction matches the treatment prescription;

(9) distances between reference points on the plan match those measured on the films;

(10) distance from the treatment unit to the first programmed dwell location is correct for each channel;

(11) dwell times and locations programmed in the treatment unit match those on the plan;

(12) program card, stored standards, or the equivalent, used for subsequent treatment match the parameters of the first treatment.

Especially with respect to positional parameters (dwell positions active, spacing, indexer lengths etc.), the simulation radiographs, graphical plan representation, localization form and treatment-unit printout should all be intercompared. At one institution, each programmed treatment is autoradiographed immediately upon completion of computer planning and is available for physicist review, along with the other documentation.

Finally, the plan should be checked for "reasonableness" using an appropriate figure of merit. Just as mgRaEq-h/dose ratio is a useful parameter for judging LDR implants using radium substitutes, the (source strength · dwell time)/dose ratio should fall within the range expected for the given implant geometry. Quantitative verification of computer-generated dwell time calculations is reviewed in "Manual Verification of HDR Computer Calculations."

Prior to initiating treatment, the attending physician should review the treatment plan, treatment unit programming, and associated documentation. At minimum, the physicist's signature documenting plan review, the fraction size, the dose prescription site, the consistency of dose distribution size and location with target volume coverage should be reviewed, along with any other factors influencing clinical appropriateness. Satisfactory physician and physicist review should be documented by signature on the prescription form or QA checkoff list.

## Patient Setup and Treatment

While the physician and physicist are reviewing the treatment documentation, the technologist can move the patient into the HDR room and proceed with positioning and connection of the applicators to the indexer. The technologist should verify that all emergency equipment is present, that the survey meter is present and in good operating order, and that informed consent forms are properly signed and filed in the chart. In addition, the U.S. NRC Quality Management Program[42] requires that the patient be identified by two means, for example, by comparing the patient's appearance with a photograph or asking the patient's name or social security number and comparing this response with the chart. A second individual, for example, the physicist, should check that transfer tubes are free of kinks and that the applicator-channel number correspondence agrees with the source localization documentation.

At this point, all treatment documentation should be fully reviewed and available to the technologist, including the written prescription, a table of dwell times and position settings, and the treatment plan. Prior to initiating treatment, the operator should check that (a) a signed prescription is available, (b) that physicist and physician have signed-off on plan review, (c) that the fraction size listed on the computer plan and the prescription agree, (d) that the treatment to be given is consistent with the prescribed cumulative dose and fractionation schedule, and (e) that dwell times, length settings, and step sizes programmed into the treatment unit agree with the computer plan listing or table prepared by the physicist. For complex treatments one individual should read the dwell times on the HDR printout, while comparing these values to the treatment plan. Since manual keyboard entry of the treatment parameters describing a complex implant may require several hundred keystrokes, the liklihood of data entry error is high. Meticulous checking of such manually-entered data is essential: whenever possible, prestored standard configurations or direct entry from the treatment planning computer via the programming card should be used.

The authors recommend that both the physician and primary physicist attend the treatment and be prepared to detect emergency conditions and implement the appropriate responses. As of May 20, 1993, the NRC requires that both an authorized user (a radiation oncologist authorized to prescribe brachytherapy) and a qualified physicist be physically present at all HDR treatments.[12] If warranted by the patient's medical condition, a nurse and proper monitoring equipment should be present. Emergency procedures should be reviewed by the team, including how and under what conditions applicators are to be removed and who does what. Upon initiating treatment, the physicist should observe the treatment console and should be aware of which catheter is involved should an alarm condition interrupt treatment. *Whenever treatment is interrupted, it is essential to check the area monitor to confirm that the source has heen retracted.*

### Posttreatment Quality Assurance

After treatment is completed and the area monitor indicates no exposure in the room, the room and patient should be surveyed with a hand-held detector to confirm that the source is fully retracted into its shielded storage position. A hand-held Geiger-Müller detector that is able to detect a radiation field in excess of 1 mR/hr is suitable. As a final check on treatment accuracy, the administered dwell times listed on the treatment unit printout should be compared to the originally programmed time. All QA checklists and documentation should be reviewed for completeness and filed away in the chart along with the treatment history printed out by the HDR unit. The room and HDR key should be secured as specified by the user's license.

## Manual Verification of HDR Computer Calculations

Stepping-source remote afterloading technology allows the treatment time at each active dwell position to be independently programmed. Mathematically elegant and clinically appealing optimization algorithms are widely available, which vary the relative dwell times (or weights) of each activated dwell position so as to maximize dose uniformity, target coverage, or other dosimetric constraints chosen by the user. The result is often a highly nonuniform distribution of dwell times. When such algorithms are applied to conventional implant geometries, dose homogeneity is often improved, and the length of the implanted volume needed to adequately cover the target volume may be reduced. Such flexibility creates a number of quality assurance problems, many of which have been discussed elsewhere in this chapter. An important issue is how to verify the accuracy of optimized calculations with practical manual calculation techniques. "Practical" in this context requires that the assessment take only a few minutes. In addition, the calculation check must have a high probability of detecting significant errors. A minimum goal is suggested by the NRC misadministration rule for brachytherapy, which defines the actionable threshold at 20%. Clearly, more precise methods are preferable, but the 20% value may be taken as a minimum.

A standard technique is to evaluate some characteristic parameter of the plan and compare it to an expected value. For example, at distances sufficiently far from the implant the dose is determined primarily by the source strength and total treatment time and is insensitive to local dwell time variations. One physics group (John Hicks, Ph.D., personal communication, 1993) calculates the dose at points ± 10 cm from the approximate center of the implant in the direction most orthogonal to the treatment applicators. The mean dose, divided by the current source activity and total treatment time, is then compared to expectation values, which depend on the type of implant geometry. Table 7 lists representative numbers. Readers are cautioned that the specific values depend on many variables, such as the quantity used to specify source strength, single-source dosimetry data selected, and the optimization scheme applied. At such long distances, the specific form of the tissue attenuation and scatter factor (radial dose factor) used by the planning computer needs to be considered since some expressions may extrapolate poorly.

This method can detect errors in source strength input, unauthorized changes in physical dose factors, or calculation "bugs," which affect dose globally. Its insensitivity to local dose variations means that it is not capable of detecting some errors that determine the dose at clinically relevant distances. For example, consider a situation in which the planner intended to place active dwell positions at 1.0-cm intervals but inadvertently specified 0.5-cm spacing. If the number of dwell positions were not doubled, then the implant would be smaller than desired. The "dose at a distance" method would not detect such an error.

The next logical step is to develop expectation values based on doses at typical prescription distances, which are sensitive to implant geometry. The group at the University of Wisconsin has developed dose indices for a variety of implant types: endobronchial, gynecologic (tandem and ovoids, ovoids only, vaginal cylinder), and volume implants. For example, Thomadsen et al.[43] describe two indices for tandem and ovoid treatments based on the ratio of dose at the primary prescription point to the dwell time in one particular position in the tandem and the total dwell time.

Table 7 also describes the University of Wisconsin method of verifying total treatment time for volume implants (Bruce Thomadsen, Ph.D., personal communication, 1993). This table was derived from the original Manchester volume implant table,[44] by applying corrections for modern units and factors (1.065; see [26]), for the ratio of stated to minimum dose (1.11) and conversion from mgRaEq-h to Ci-s. When applied to geometrically-optimized (distance option) volume implants, the table has an accuracy of better than 8% when the reference dose (RD) is defined to be 90–95% of the central minimum dose.

Kubo and Chin[45] have reported simple mathematical formulas for checking single catheter treatments when the dose is prescribed at distances of 7.5 mm or 10 mm from the catheter center. For example, for a 10-mm dose description, the total treatment time was found to be

$$T = 0.01 \cdot \frac{D}{S} \cdot (2.67 \cdot L + 78.6) \tag{13}$$

where      T is the total treatment time in seconds.
                    D is the prescribed dose in cGy.
                    S is the source activity in Ci, and
                    L is the total treatment length in millimeters.

Again, the numerical values in the formula depend on the specifics of the dose calculation data and the optimization algorithm assumed. A different for-

## Table 7

## Manual Dose Verification Methods for Optimized Implants

*Expected Values of Dose Index 10 cm from Implant in its Central Transverse Plane*

*(J. Hicks, Ph.D., personal communication)*

$$\text{Dose Index} = \frac{100 * \text{Average of doses at } +10 \text{ cm and } -10 \text{ cm [cGy]}}{\text{Activity [Ci]} * \text{Total time [s]}}$$

| Implant Type | Expected range of dose index |
|---|---|
| Pulmonary | 1.05—1.20 (lower if highly elongated, higher if curved) |
| Vaginal Cylinder | 1.10—1.20 (i.e., short single catheter) |
| Long Esophagus | 0.95—1.10 (i.e., long single catheter) |

*Expected Total Treatment Time for Volume Implants*

*(B. Thomadsen, Ph. D., personal communication)*

$$\text{Total time} = \frac{\text{Reference dose [Gy]} * R_v * \text{Elongation Factor}}{\text{Activity [Ci]}}$$

| Volume (cm³) | $R_v$ [Ci s/Gy] | Length/Diameter | Elongation Factor |
|---|---|---|---|
| 50 | 314.0 | 1.5 | 1.03 |
| 60 | 354.7 | 2.0 | 1.06 |
| 80 | 429.2 | 2.5 | 1.10 |
| 100 | 498.4 | 3.0 | 1.15 |
| 140 | 623.9 | | |
| 180 | 737.1 | Note: Reference dose chosen to be 90–95% | |
| 220 | 842.9 | of central minimum dose for geometri- | |
| 260 | 942.6 | cally optimized volume implants | |
| 300 | 1036.8 | | |
| 340 | 1127.0 | | |
| 380 | 1212.5 | | |

Note: Choose prescribed dose so as to limit that significant hot spots to 110%

*Expected Values of Dose Index for Geometrically Optimized Planar Implants[46]*

$$\text{Dose index I} = \frac{\text{Dose at distance H from plane [cGy]} \cdot \text{Area [cm}^2\text{]}}{\text{Activity [Ci]} \cdot \text{Total time [s]}}$$

Equivalent Length $E = 2(L \cdot W)/(L + W)$ [cm] where L, W are the length and width of implanted and area $A = L \cdot W$

$$I = A + B \cdot E + C \cdot E^2 \text{ where A, B, and C depend on H.}$$

| H [cm] | A | B | C |
|---|---|---|---|
| 1.5 | 0.4025 | 0.9228 | −0.01707 |
| 2.0 | −0.2582 | 0.8356 | −0.01481 |
| 2.5 | −0.6189 | 0.7514 | −0.01261 |
| 3.0 | −0.8216 | 0.6732 | −0.01057 |

Note: For curved implant surface, increase I by 10%; for implants with deviated catheters and significant cold spots, decrease I by 5%.

mulation has been used at Wayne State University,[46] where a simple dwell time pattern for single catheter implants was developed using film dosimetry instead of a mathematical optimization scheme. Their relationship between the same parameters is given by

$$\frac{D}{S \cdot T} = \frac{23.09}{L} + 0.0537 \tag{14}$$

Equation (14) assumes anisotropy corrections, active lengths of 50 to 230 mm, a 5-mm separation between adjacent dwell positions and the following pattern of relative dwell weights: (1.5, 1.4, 1.3, 1.2, 1.1, 1.0, . . . . , 1.0, 1.1, 1.2, 1.3. 1.4, 1.5).

Optimized square and rectangular single-plane implants have also been systematically analyzed, and dose indices developed in support of dose calcu lation verification.[46] The dose index I is defined as follows:

$$I = \frac{D \cdot A}{S \cdot T} \tag{15}$$

where    D is the dose in cGy at a reference distance H from the plane of
the implant.
A is the area of the implant in cm², 
S is the source activity in Ci, and
T is the total dwell time in seconds.

The expected value of I is a simple quadratic function of the length, E, of the equivalent square implanted area, which, in turn, is calculated from the familiar area/perimeter rule. Table 7 gives the quadratic coefficients A, B, and C for several different reference distances H, assuming intercatheter spacings of 1–1.5 cm and geometric optimization (reference E). For idealized implants, ranging in area from 3.0 × 3.5 cm² to 25.5 × 22.5 cm², Table 7 predicted the index, I, to within 5%. The index I was calculated for a series of clinical implants, most of which were used to treat the tumor bed following surgical excision of extremity sarcomas. Despite significant deviation from ideal planar geometry following closure of the operative wound, the observed index agreed with the predicted value within 10% for all cases.

In practice, applying these methods requires that the implant dimensions be determined independently from the localization films and the activity be taken from a precalculated table. If these parameters are taken directly from the computer output, errors in the computation may go unnoticed.

## Conclusions

HDR brachytherapy utilizes complex treatment delivery devices to position radioactive sources within the patient, a process that is easily verifiable by direct observation in manual afterloading brachytherapy. In addition, HDR brachytherapy is largely an outpatient treatment modality, with the result that applicator insertion, simulation, treatment planning, and treatment delivery are compressed into a relatively short time interval. Finally, only a few minutes of irradiation time may be needed to give a large dose fraction to the target volume. Despite many opportunities for error and despite pressure to perform efficiently in an often high-stress environment, HDR brachytherapy is a highly precise and safe method of radiation dose delivery. Achieving a high standard of accuracy and patient safety requires a well-trained and organized team, consisting of a physician, a physicist, a dosimetrist, and a technologist. Comprehensive acceptance testing of the treatment unit and its accessories along development of a formal QA system for assuring performance integrity in the future is also essential. The foundation of this organizational structure is an effective operational QA program.

*Acknowledgments*

The authors would like to thank the following vendor representatives for the information supplied regarding their equipment operation and QA procedures: Bart Adriance (Omnitron), Uli Bormann (GammaMed), Steven Teague (Nucletron), and Dr. Ann Wright (Omnitron).

---

## REFERENCES

1. Ezzell GA. Acceptance testing and quality assurance for high dose rate remote afterloading systems. In: Martinez AA, Orton CG, and Mould RF, eds.: Brachytherapy HDR and LDR. Columbia, Md.: Nucletron Corporation; 1990, 138-159.
2. Flynn A. Quality assurance checks on a microSelectron-HDR. Selectron Brachytherapy Journal 4(4):112-115, 1990.
3. Glasgow GP, Bourland JD, Grigsby PW, et al. Remote afterloading technology. Report of the American Association of Physicists in Medicine Task Group No. 41. New York, N.Y.: American Institute of Physics, 1993.
4. Williamson JF. Practical quality assurance in low-dose rate brachytherapy. In: Proceedings of American College of Medical Physics: Symposium on Quality Assurance in Radiotherapy Physics. Madison, Wisc.: Medical Physics Publishing Company; 1991, 139-182.
5. Ezzell GA. Calibration intercomparison of an $^{192}$Ir source used for high dose rate remote afterloading. Selectron Brachytherapy Journal 3:13-14, 1989.
6. Thomadsen BR, Shahabi S, Buchler DA, et al. Anatomy of two high dose-rate misadministrations. Med Phys (abstract) 18:645, 1991.
7. U.S. Nuclear Regulatory Commission. Loss of an iridium-192 source and therapy misadministration at Indiana regional cancer center, Indiana, Pennsylvania on November 16, 1992. Report NUREG-1480, 1993; Washington, D.C. Nuclear Regulatory Commission.
8. Jones CH. Quality assurance in brachytherapy. Med Phys World 6:4-11, 1990.
9. Williamson JF. Comparison of measured and calculated dose rates in water near I-125 and Ir-192 seeds. Med Phys 18:776-786, 1991.

10. U.S. Nuclear Regulatory Commission. Title 10, Chapter 1, Code of Federal Regulations-Energy, Part 35, Medical Use of By-product Material. Washington, D.C.: Government Printing Office, 1987.

11. U.S. Nuclear Regulatory Commission. Title 10, Chapter 1, Code of Federal Regulations-Energy, Part 20, Standards for Protection Against Radiation. Washington, D.C.: Government Printing Office, 1988.

12. U.S. Nuclear Regulatory Commission. Release of patients after brachytherapy treatment with remote afterloading devices. NRC Bulletin 93-01, 20 April 1993. Washington, D.C.: U.S. Nuclear Regulatory Commission.

13. Weinhous MS, Purdy JA, Granda CO. Testing of a medical 1 Linear accelerator's computer-control system. Med Phys 17:95-102, 1990.

14. van't Hooft E. The selectron, brachytherapy 1984. In: Shearer DR, ed.: Recent Advances in Brachytherapy. New York, NY: American Institute of Physics; 1981, 167-177.

15. Mesina CF, Ezzell GA, Campbell JM, et al. Acceptance testing for the Selectron high dose rate remote afterloading cobalt-60 unit. Endocurie Hypertherm Oncol 4:253-256, 1988.

16. Chenery SGA, Pla M, Podgorsak EB. Physical characteristics of the Selectron high dose rate intracavitary afterloader. Br J Radiol 58:735-740, 1985.

17. Dean EM, Lambert GD, Dawes PJDK. Gynecological treatment using the Selectron remote afterloading system. Br J Radiol 61:1053-1057, 1988.

18. van't Hooft F. The Selectron LDR. philosophy and design. In: Brachytherapy 1984; Proceedings from the 3rd International SELECTRON Users Meeting. Innsbruck, Austria, 1984, 52-58.

19. Evens MDC, Arsenault CJ, Cygler J, et al. Quality assurance for variable-length catheters with an afterloading brachythcrapy device. Med Phys 20: 251-254, 1993.

20. Goetsch SJ, Attix FH, DeWerd LA, et al. A new re-entrant ionization chamber for the calibration of iridium-192 high dose rate sources. Int J Radiat Oncol Biol Phys 24:167-170, 1992.

21. Meigooni AS, Williamson JF, Slessinger ED. Practical quality assurance tests for positional and temporal accuracy of HDR remote afterloaders. Presented at the 15th Annual Meeting of the American Endocurietherapy Society. Beaver Creek, Colo.: Dec. 9-12, 1992. Endocurie Hypertherm Oncol 9:46, 1993.

22. Houdek PV, Schwade JG, Wu X, et al. Dose determination in high dose-rate brachytherapy. Int J Radiat Oncol Biol Phys 24:795-801, 1992.

23. Bastin KT, Podgorsak MS, Thomadsen BR. The transit dose component of high dose-rate brachytherapy: direct measurements and clinical implications. Int J Radiat Oncol Biol Phys 26:695-702, 1993.

24. Seay DG, Hilbert JW, Moeller J, et al. Therapy using a new remote-controlled high-intensity afterloading device. Radiology 105:709-711, 1972.

25. Kondo S, Randolph ML. Effect of finite size of ionization chambers on measurements of small photon sources. Radiat Res 13:37-60, 1960.

26. Shalek RJ, Stovall M. Dosimetry in implant therapy. In: Attix FH, Tochilin E, eds. Radiation Dosimetry, III. New York, NY: Academic Press; 1969, 743-808.

27. Williamson JF, Anderson LL, Grigsby PW, et al. American Endocurietherapy Society recommendations for specification of brachytherapy source strength. Endocurie Hypertherm Oncol 9:1-7, 1993.

28. Nath R, Anderson L, Jones D, et al. Specification of brachytherapy source strength. A Report by Task Group 32 of the American Association of Physicists in Medicine. New York, NY: American Institute of Physics; 1987.

29. Goetsch SJ, Attix FH, Pearson DW, et al. Calibration of [192]Ir high-dose-rate afterloading systems. Med Phys 18:462-467, 1991.

30. Cerra F, Rodgers JE. Dose distribution anisotropy of the Gamma Med IIi brachytherapy source. Endocurie Hypertherm Oncol 6:71-80, 1990.
31. Meli JA, Meigooni AS, Nath R. On the choice of phantom material for the dosimetry of $^{192}$Ir sources. Int J Radiat Oncol Biol Phys 14:587-594, 1988.
32. Meisberger LL, Keller RJ, Shalek RJ. The effective attenuation in water of the gamma rays of gold-198, iridium-192, cesium-137, radium-226, and cobalt-60. Radiology 90:953-957, 1968.
33. Moerland MA, de Konig JH, Battermann JJ. The anisotropic dose distribution of an HDR iridium-192 source. In: International Brachytherapy: Programme and Abstracts, 7th International Brachytherapy Working Conference, Baltimore, Md., 6–8 September 1992. Veenedaal, The Netherlands: Nucletron International B.V.; 1992, 286-289.
34. Baltus D, Kramer R, Löffler E. Measurements of anisotropy of the new HDR iridium-192 source for the microSelectron/HDR. In: International Brachytherapy: Programme and Abstracts, 7th International Brachytherapy Working Conference, Baltimore, Md., 6–8 September 1992. Veenedaal, The Netherlands: Nucletron International B.V.; 1992, 290-306.
35. Williamson JF. Recent developments in basic brachytherapy physics. In: Smith AR, ed. Radiation Therapy Physics. Berlin, Germany: Springer-Verlag; 1994, in press.
36. Williamson JF, Perera H, Li Z, et al. Comparison of calculated and measured heterogeneity correction factors for $^{125}$I, $^{137}$Cs, and $^{192}$Ir brachytherapy sources near localized heterogeneities. Med Phys 20:209-222, 1993.
37. Nath R, Meigooni AS, Meli JA. Dosimetry on the transverse axes of $^{125}$I and $^{192}$Ir interstitial brachytherapy sources. Med Phys 17:1032-1040, 1990.
38. Weaver KA, Smith V, Huang D, et al. Dose parameters of $^{125}$I and $^{192}$Ir seed sources. Med Phys 16:636-643, 1989.
39. Anderson LL, Nath R, Olch AJ, et al. American endocurietherapy recommendations for dose specification in brachytherapy. Endocurie Hypertherm Oncol 7:1-12, 1991.
40. Podgorsak MB, Paliwal BR, Thomadsen BR, et al. Radiographic visualization of vaginal cylinders in gynecologic high dose-rate brachytherapy. Int J Radiat Oncol Biol Phys 25:252-527, 1993.
41. Edmundson GK. Geometry-based optimization for stepping source implants. In: Martinez AA, Orton CG, Mould RF, eds. Brachytherapy HDR and LDR. Columbia, Md.: Nucletron Corporation; 1990, 184-192.
42. U.S. Nuclear Regulatory Commission. Quality management program and misadministrations. Federal Register 56 (143): 34104-34122, Thursday, 25 July, 1991.
43. Thomadsen BR, Shahabi S, Stitt JA, et al. High dose rate intracavitary brachytherapy for carcinoma of the cervix: the Madison system: II. Procedural and physical considerations. Int J Radiat Oncol Biol Phys 24:349-357, 1992.
44. Parker HM. A dosage system for interstitial radium therapy. Part II: physical aspects. Br J Radiol 11:313-339, 1938.
45. Kubo H, Chin RB. Simple mathematical formulas for quick-checking of single-catheter high dose rate brachytherapy treatment plans. Endocurie Hypertherm Oncol 8:165-169, 1992.
46. Ezzell GA. Quality assurance of treatment plans for optimized high dose rate brachytherapy. Med Phys 20:880, 1993. (abstract).

# Part II

# Clinical Body Sites

# Chapter 8

# High Dose Rate Brachytherapy in the Treatment of Malignant Gliomas

*Delia M. Garcia, Lucia Zamorano, and Fritz Mundinger*

## Introduction

Approximately 15,000 new cases of primary malignant brain tumors are diagnosed in the United States each year, accounting for 1.5% of all malignancies. The overall incidence varies with race, sex, and age, but most cases are diagnosed in patients aged 50–80 years, with a small but significant peak occurring at 5–10 years of age.

Malignant gliomas such as anaplastic astrocytoma (AA), glioblastoma multiforme (GBM), and anaplastic oligodendroglioma (OLG) are infiltrating tumors that produce neurological damage by local invasion and by producing pressure with displacement of the normal brain. The central nervous system has no lymphatics, and hematogenous spread is rare. The inability to control the tumor locally is the major reason that patients with malignant gliomas die prematurely. After surgery and postoperative irradiation, 90% of local tumor recurrences are located within a 2-cm margin of the primary site.[1-4]

The role of external irradiation in the treatment of malignant gliomas remains undisputed. Randomized trials by the Brain Tumor Study Group (BTSG)[5,6] demonstrate the ability of external beam irradiation to increase median survival in patients with GBM and AA as compared to surgery and chemotherapy controls. Likewise, there is a dose response with statistically significant improvement in median survival for patients receiving 6,000 cGy as compared to 5,000 cGy.[7] Unfortunately, external-beam doses greater than 6,000 cGy may result in necrosis and other irreversible effects including leukoencephalopathy.[8] For this reason, interstitial brachytherapy has appeal since local therapy may allow higher doses to be delivered directly to the tumor and thereby confine radiation necrosis to the tumor with relative sparing of the surrounding normal brain.

In 1914 Frazier performed the first radioactive seed implant for a brain tumor.[9] Since the development of the Leksell stereotactic frame in the mid 1950s, implanting isotopes into brain tumors has become more accurate.[10]

---

From: Nag, S. (ed.): *High Dose Rate Brachytherapy: A Textbook*, Futura Publishing Company, Inc., Armonk, NY, © 1994.

Fritz Mundinger is a pioneer in the stereotactic implantation of radioactive sources for inoperable brain tumors. Since the early 1950s, Mundinger has advanced the development of interstitial brachytherapy techniques and has published numerous articles on his work.[11-25] In 1963, Mundinger's group developed a remote afterloading device, GammaMed (Isotopen-Technik, Haan/ Reinland I, Germany), to deliver high-dose irradiation utilizing high-activity iridium-192.[21]

Improved imaging techniques such as computed tomographic (CT) scanning, which became widely available in 1974, and more recently, magnetic resonance imaging (MRI) has also improved the feasibility of interstitial implantation. Although various isotopes have been used, [192]Iridium ([192]Ir) and [125]Iodine ([125]I) are the best radioactive materials for interstitial brachytherapy, not only because of their favorable physical characteristics but also because of their radiation safety advantages. Permanent implants with [125]I have been used,[26] but removable implants with [192]Ir or [125]I are more popular. With removable implants, one has the advantage of greater control of the radiation dose since source placement can be rearranged for better dose distribution and the time of the implant can be controlled. Removable [125]I is used in BTSG protocol 8701, a phase III study in which patients are randomized postoperatively to receive brachytherapy (6,000 cGy), plus conventional treatment (external irradiation and chemotherapy) versus conventional treatment alone. When high dose rate (HDR) remote afterloading is used, additional advantages of temporary implants include the lack of exposure to anyone but the patient and dose optimization by programming the high-intensity [192]Ir source in preplanned positions within the catheters to achieve the desired dose distribution.

Currently, few centers use HDR techniques for the management of brain tumors. However, as technology continues to evolve, we expect increasing numbers of treatment centers to become proficient at treating malignant gliomas with HDR afterloading techniques. In this chapter, two approaches are described: one in which multiple catheters are used to deliver an interstitial "boost" following external irradiation, and one in which a single catheter centrally placed within the tumor is used to deliver interstitial HDR irradiation as primary therapy.

## Brachytherapy: The Multiple Catheter Technique (D. Garcia and D. Welsh)

The technique developed in St. Louis, Missouri, uses multiple nylon catheters through which HDR treatment is administered using a spatially programmed, remote afterloading [192]Ir source (Nucletron microSelectron HDR unit). This treatment also uses moderate-temperature interstitial hyperthermia as a physical radiosensitizer. The implant and treatment are performed 2 weeks after completion of external-beam irradiation of 46 Gy in 23 fractions.

### Implantation

The catheters are implanted percutaneously in the CT suite, using interactive CT scanning and surgery.[27-30] After induction of general anesthesia, the

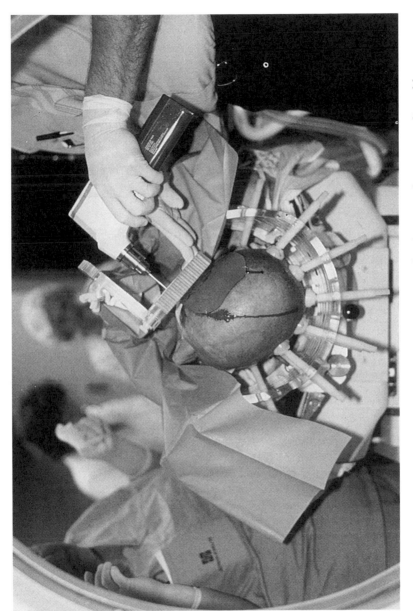

**Fig. 1.** CT-mounted stereotactic frame for interstitial catheter implantation. Adjustable pads support the patient's head and eliminate the need for skull perforation. Sterilized acrylic template attached to the headframe guides the drill and catheters and maintains the desired intercatheter spacing.

scalp is shaved, and the patient's head is secured in the stabilization frame (Cook Stereotaxic Guide, Cook Inc., Bloomington, Indiana) with the tumor uppermost. The scalp is then prepared with an antibacterial solution and draped. A sterile 1/16-in silicone sheet is stapled to the scalp over the area of the tumor, and the rigid acrylic template is secured to the frame (Fig. 1). Contrast-enhanced CT scans are made in planes 7.5 mm apart, corresponding to the successive rows of apertures in the template to permit planning of catheter placement. The target volume for implantation is the contrast enhancement, plus a 1-cm margin.

Using the CT scanning software, a line intersecting a portion of the tumor is projected through each appropriately positioned template aperture (Fig. 2). The implantation depth is determined by the scanning software from the distance along the line from the surface of the template to the deepest tumor

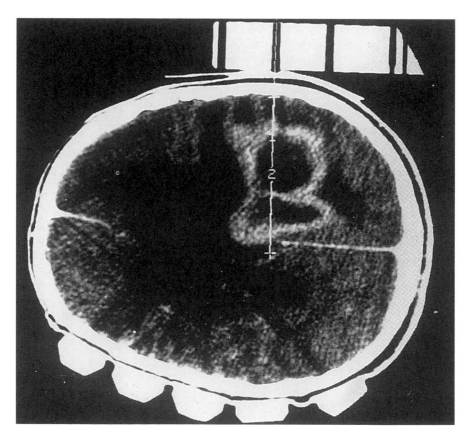

**Fig. 2.** Determination of catheter implantation depth and treatment length using CT scanning software.

(plus appropriate margin) point. The software is also used to determine the treatment length (active length of hyperthermia and brachytherapy implants) by measuring the distance traversed by the line across the tumor. Implantation depth and treatment length for a given aperture are both recorded on a template diagram.

Using the information recorded on the template diagram and guidance provided by the rigid acrylic template, the surgeon perforates the silicone sheet, scalp, skull, and dura with a sterile battery-operated twist-drill. The semirigid brachytherapy catheters and hyperthermia catheters of 1.8 mm and 2.2 mm in diameter, respectively, are implanted to the indicated depths, and the accuracy of their placement is verified by a CT scan (Fig. 3). Repeat CT scanning allows necessary adjustments and confirmation of hemostasis to be made immediately. Once the catheters are satisfactorily positioned, the template is carefully withdrawn, leaving the catheters protruding from the silicone sheet (Fig. 4).

Cyanoacrylate ester cement is used initially to anchor the catheters to the silicone sheet. The catheters are further secured by building a foam well and filling the center with silicone elastomer. The patient is then removed from the head stabilization frame and taken to the postanesthesia recovery unit.

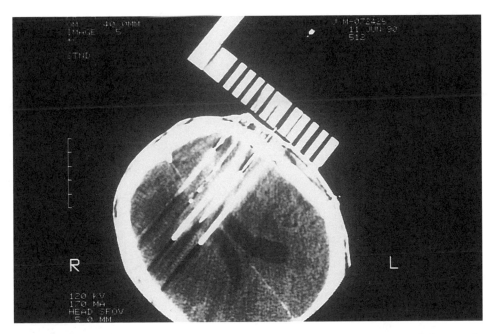

**Fig. 3.** A CT scan verifying the accuracy of catheter placement. From left to right, the catheters are hyperthermia, thermometry, brachytherapy, hyperthermia, and brachytherapy.

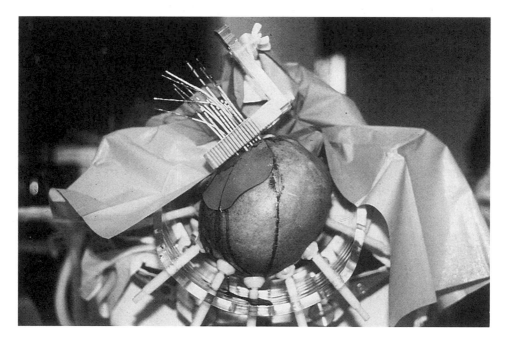

**Fig. 4.** Completed implant just prior to removal of the template.

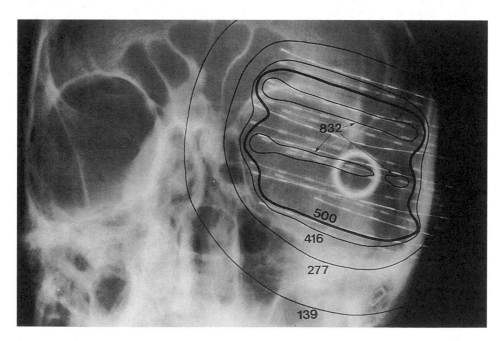

**Fig. 5.** Isodose curves imposed on simulation film showing an optimized plan for a prescription fraction of 500 cGy.

## Brachytherapy Treatment Technique

Once stabilized, the patient is brought to the radiation oncology department for simulation films (utilizing dummy sources within each catheter) required for computer-assisted brachytherapy treatment planning. After dummy sources are placed in each of the HDR catheters, an orthogonal set of films is taken. These films are used to determine the individual source positions, source travel length, and treatment volume relative to the tumor site. This information is digitized into the treatment-planning computer. The radiation dose distribution is optimized to the prescription dose points by adjusting the dwell times at each of the source positions. Proprietary optimization algorithms belonging to the Nucletron Corporation are used for these calculations (Fig. 5). Besides a printout of the best dwell times and positions, a plastic card is magnetically imprinted with the same information. This card can be used to transfer data to the HDR treatment console.

HDR treatments are administered with a spatially-programmed remote afterloaded $^{192}$Ir source. In the current protocol a total dose of 15 Gy at 1 cm, administered in 3 equal fractions, is given on 3 consecutive days.

## Hyperthermia Treatment Technique

With this technique HDR is given in combination with hyperthermia, which is delivered using a commercially-available, computer-controlled conductive heating system (Cook VH8500 Volumetric Hyperthermia Treatment System; Cook, Inc., Bloomington, Indiana). The protocol specification is 48 hours of moderate temperature hyperthermia (minimum tissue temperature, 41.5°C) to be delivered over a 64-hour period in 3-hour fractions every 4 hours. The 1-hour break between the 3-hour heating intervals allows patient mobility and nursing care.

## Explanation, Discharge, and Follow-up

Once treatment with hyperthermia and radiation is completed, catheters are removed in the CT suite, and scans are obtained to assess hemostasis, mass effect, and tumor status. Patients are discharged from the hospital when doing so is clinically indicated. Follow-up is performed every 2 months and includes neurological function tests and CT scans.

## Patient Characteristics

Between April 1990 and February 1992, 11 patients ranging in age from 23 to 65 years with newly diagnosed malignant gliomas were treated with external irradiation, followed by long-duration interstitial hyperthermia and interstitial HDR brachytherapy. Pretreatment Karnofsky scores ranged from 85 to 100 (median: 90). There were seven patients with GBM, three patients with AA, and one patient with an OLG. Tumor volumes determined from pretreatment CT scans ranged from 2 cc to 115 cc (mean: 27). Five of the 11 patients had undergone a subtotal surgical resection of the tumor prior to receiving external irradiation.

## Treatment Summary

An average of 11 brachytherapy catheters and nine hyperthermia catheters were implanted. The average duration of hyperthermia therapy was 34 hours. The average treatment temperature was 41.8°C, and the average maximum tissue temperature was 44.8°C. The average $T_{90}$ (temperature that was equalled or exceeded by 90% of measured points) was 39.9°C. Equivalent minutes at 43°C, a frequently used description of thermal dose[31] averaged 231 minutes.

Three patients required early treatment discontinuation at 3, 10, and 21 hours owing to increased intracranial edema and resultant deterioration in neurological condition. Of these three patients, two required craniotomy for debulking the necrotic tumor and mass effect within 1 week of implant. One additional patient required surgery 2 months after the implant. Complications arose in 6 of 11 patients. Two patients developed mass effect requiring craniotomy for decompression, two patients developed pulmonary emboli that cleared with medical management, and two patients developed scalp infections that were resolved with antibiotics.

## Survival

Six patients remain alive at 19 to 31 months follow-up. Three are alive free from local tumor progression (AFFP) with Karnofsky scores from 80 to 100, and three are alive with disease (AWD), with a mean Karnofsky score of 53. Five patients died of tumor progression. The length of follow-up now ranges from 8 to 31 months (mean: 20 months). Figure 6 shows actuarial survival for all patients and for the GBM subgroup. The patients with highly aggressive GBM have reached a median survival of 19.5 months (mean: 16.7 months) with two of seven remaining alive (21.8 and 22.7 months). Table 1 provides individual patient data.

## Tumor Response

CT analysis of tumor response included a quantitative evaluation of CT tumor volume. The pretreatment findings were compared to the findings on the follow-up examinations. Tumor response was classed as complete response (75–100% decrease), partial response (25–75% decrease), stable disease (± 25%), or progression ( >25% increase). Tumor-volume response evaluation on eight 3-month posttreatment CT scans showed complete response in one patient, partial response in two patients, stable disease in three patients, and progression in two patients. Three patients were not evaluated

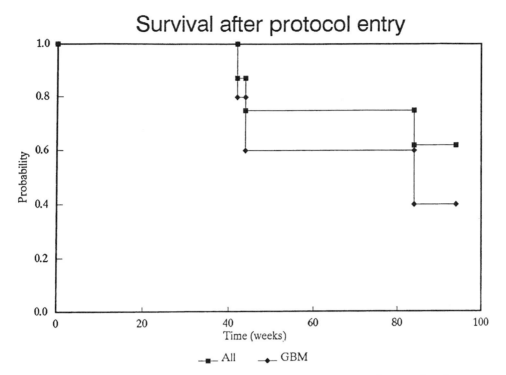

**Fig. 6.** Kaplan-Meier representation of the probability of survival in weeks after HDR brachytherapy with hyperthermia for newly diagnosed glioma patients (all) and for a subset of patients with GBM. Survival times are from initiation of external irradiation (protocol entry).

## Table 1

### HDR Brachytherapy and Long-Duration Interstitial Hyperthermia for Newly Diagnosed Malignant Gliomas

| Patient Age | Sex | Histology | Pre-TX Karnofsky | Post-TX Karnofsky (8 wks) | Survival from Protocol Entry (mos) | Current Status |
|---|---|---|---|---|---|---|
| 64 | M | GBM | 90 | 60 | 19.5 | DOD |
| 23 | M | AA | 100 | 100 | 30.9 | AFFP |
| 55 | F | GBM | 95 | 95 | 8.1 | DOD |
| 52 | M | GBM | 90 | 60 | 9.7 | DOD |
| 26 | M | GBM | 95 | 95 | 26.5 | DOD |
| 34 | F | AA | 90 | 60 | 25.5 | AWD |
| 32 | F | GBM | 100 | 100 | 23.9 | AWD |
| 35 | M | GBM | 85 | 40 | 22.7 | AWD |
| 26 | F | OLG | 90 | 80 | 21.8 | AFFP |
| 41 | F | AA | 100 | 100 | 19.0 | AFFP |
| 53 | M | GBM | 90 | 65 | 10.3 | DOD |

M = Male    TX = Treatment
F = Female    Surv = Survival
GBM = Glioblastoma Multiforme
AA = Anaplastic Astrocytoma

OLG = Oligodendroglioma
DOD = Dead of Disease
AFFP = Alive Free from Progression
AWD = Alive with Disease

using CT volume analysis owing to decompressive surgery in the early post-treatment period. Interestingly, these responses improved during the follow-up period, to the best responses of complete regression in four patients, partial regression in three patients, and progression in one patient. The interval from treatment to achieving best response varied with each patient and ranged from 3.5 to 28.8 months.

## Single and Multiple Catheters: Mundinger and Zamorano Experience

Techniques of HDR brachytherapy include the temporary implantation of isotopes and the use of remote afterloading devices. Intraoperative brachytherapy uses a remote afterloading device (GammaMed) constructed by Mundinger and Sauerwein[21] or the afterloading [125]I catheter system by Zamorano et al.[32]

If intraoperative or postoperative [192]Ir brachytherapy is indicated, the cannula is stereotactically introduced to the target point and radiographically checked. Depending on the size and geometry of the volume to be irradiated (e.g., square-shaped), several cannulas may be inserted through which [192]Ir is successively introduced. By shifting one cannula in the tumor axis to different positions, radiation periods of various lengths can be programmed in such a way that the peripheral tumor dose may be adapted to complicated geometrical tumor shapes (e.g., pear- or dumbbell-shaped). The dose for the tumor surface depends on the volume, 40–45 Gy in one sitting.

In cases where fractionation is planned over two to three sessions in combination with fractionated external irradiation, the single dose is reduced correspondingly. The additional peripheral tumor dose should not exceed 100–120 Gy. One radiation session lasts from a few minutes to about half an hour, depending on the present activity loading.

According to our clinical experiences, the application of high dose [192]Ir brachytherapy is limited to tumor volumes of under 125 cm$^3$ (5 cm in diameter). In applying the full dosage, this "radiosection" is only tolerated in tumors of the cerebral and cerebellar hemispheres. For larger hemisphere glioblastomas, however, the combination with external irradiation is, in any case, advisable and indicated. In tumors that infiltrate into the gray substance (basal ganglia), the tumor surface dose should not exceed 12 Gy per session. In such cases, a combination with permanent implantation is indicated for tumors of smaller volumes, whereas for larger volumes of AAs and GBMs external irradiation is advisable. In recurrences after external irradiation or insufficient regression of the tumor volume, HDR brachytherapy is additionally indicated for smaller volumes.

The technique for HDR brachytherapy with a single catheter was implemented in Germany initially by Mundinger et al. and employs a single steel tube (catheter) and remote afterloading unit.[21] The implant is performed as a primary treatment in patients with malignant AAs and GBMs as well as in recurrences.

**Implantation**

From the angiography, CT, and MRI films, the three-dimensional (3-D) volume and shape of the tumor are calculated.[33] On the basis of this information, an entry point and target point in the center of the tumor are chosen to define the main axis of the tumor. The target parameters are calculated (Riechert-Mundinger Stereotactic System and the Zamorano-Dujovny Multipurpose Localizing Unit: both made by Fischer Instrumentation, Freiburg, Germany). Under local anesthesia, a guide or probe is placed in the tumor using the standard stereotactic technique. Serial biopsies may be taken at different depth intervals. Finally, the probe is replaced by the metallic cannula or applicator that will follow the longitudinal axis of the tumor. In general, this is done under fluoroscopic control. The longitudinal placement is fundamental in achieving the desired isodose distribution curves.

The applicator is a metallic tube (or catheter), 3 mm in diameter, closed at the distal end. This tube replaces the probe and the middle point of the caudal border of the tumor is selected as the target point. From here the procedure varies in two ways. Mundinger treated the patients with a single dose of HDR done intraoperatively. Oppel et al. at the Steglitz University Clinic, Berlin, used fractionated HDR over a period of 7 to 14 days.[34] In the latter case, the applicator is fixed to the skull using a screw that is perforated in the middle allowing for passage of the tube. Finally, the tubes are cut about 5 mm over the limit of the screw, and the skin is sutured around it. Following this procedure and during the 2 weeks of radiotherapy, the patients are allowed to move themselves without any restrictions.

At Wayne State University, we have used one or multiple catheters depending on the tumor volume and shape. Our approach employs 3-D dosimetry using an image-based treatment-planning system (Stereotactic Treatment Planning, Fischer Instrumentation, Freiburg, Germany). Tumor volumes are drawn on multiple CT or MRI images. One or multiple catheters are placed within the tumor, and different seed activities of [192]Ir are entered at different space depths. Isodoses are displayed on the computer in axial, coronal, and sagittal views; 3-D images are generated, and intuitive and computerized optimization is performed. A final plan emerges when the isodose distribution follows the shape of the tumor, and the minimal dose involves the eloquent areas of the brain. At this moment, [192]Ir seed activities are replaced by "times" of exposure of a fixed [192]Ir activity of the remote afterloading unit, and the spacer between seeds is replaced by parameters of "position" of the fixed activity source. We then obtain the target parameters of the stereotactic unit to place the catheters.

**Afterloading Brachytherapy Treatment Technique**

A computerized remote afterloading unit with a highly radioactive [192]Ir source (70 curies) has been employed in all these studies. Isodose distribution curves are adjusted to the size and shape of the tumor by varying the source dwell time at different points in the tube. The total dose to be defined, whether as a single dose or a fractionated dose, varies according to the different approaches. Mundinger and colleagues delivered 20 Gy as a single intraoperative fraction (Fig. 7). Oppel and associates delivered a total dose of 30–60 Gy to the tumor border as fractionated doses (15 to 30 single 2 Gy doses) given once or twice a day. This fractionation allowed close clinical follow-up of the patients. Both Mundinger and Oppel deliver external irradiation 2 weeks after completing the afterloading therapy in the primary management of malignant gliomas. This allows irradiation of the tumor that is in the zone of rapid dose drop-off or in the parts of the tumor that cannot be reached because of the asymmetry of the tumor.

## Results

Table 2 shows the survival time of the patients evaluated until December 1967. Patients with GBM survived up to 49 months after treatment. A tendency toward increased survival was evident. A second evaluation was done of 150 patients treated from 1968 to 1979 with $^{192}$Ir brachytherapy, with or without radiosensitizing substances[25] (Table 3).

Table 4 demonstrates that in GBM and malignant OLG, the survival time of patients who had undergone surgery alone was significantly shorter than those of the $^{192}$Ir brachytherapy group ($P < 0.005$). Brachytherapy showed the longest mean survival times for all types of tumors, except for AAs.

In combination with radiosensitizers and metabolites, the average survival time in patients with GBM and OLG is better than with the postoperative $^{192}$Ir brachytherapy therapy alone. The death curves show a more favorable effect, with radiosensitizing and higher survival quotas for patients with AA and OLG. Only patients from the radiosensitized group were alive on the target day (Table 3).

A later analysis of 65 patients was done to calculate median survival (Table 5). For patients with recurrent GBM, median survival following brachytherapy was 4 to 7 months. It is evident that even in cases of tumor recurrences, such as GBM, an additional 5 to 7 months of life can be gained with brachytherapy (Table 6)(Fig. 8).

Oppel and coworkers reported on 30 patients treated with the fractionated afterloading technique and with case-control studies of 12 months or more.[34] Computed tomographic scans of these patients showed regression of the tumor, with radiation necrosis in the previous tumor area. These results correlate well with the continuous decrease of neurological deficit.

## Complications

Reported morbidity included cerebral abscess as a complication associated with the implantation of the tube, which was treated with stereotactic aspiration and antibiotics. Early complications from the stereotactic procedure

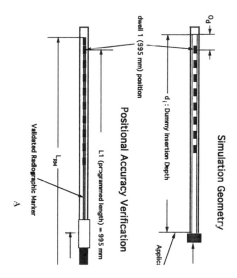

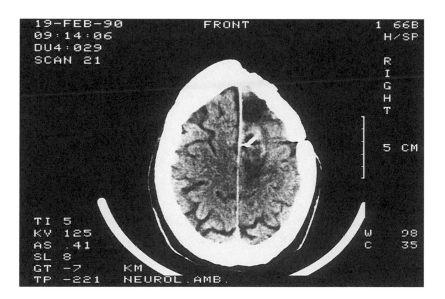

**Fig. 7.** (top) Preoperative CT of patient with GBM of right motor cortex (4.5 × 3.5 cm). Patient underwent HDR brachytherapy (15 Gy at 2.0 mm radius), followed by $^{125}$I permanent implantation (70 Gy at 2.0 mm) radius. (bottom) Postoperative CT 5 months later showing necrosis and regression of the tumor.

## Table 2

### Postoperative Survial Times of Malignant Brain Tumor Patients After Radiation with Interstitial ¹⁹²Ir HDR Brachytherapy (until December 1967)

| | Expired Patients | | | Surviving Patients | | |
|---|---|---|---|---|---|---|
| Classification | Months | Localization | Histology at Reoperation | Months | Localization | Reoperation |
| Glioblastoma | 23.7* | f | no tumor | 49.4 | p-t | no tumor |
| | 9.6 | f | tumor + necrosis | 39.6 | l-f | tumor |
| | 9.0 | c-p-t | — | 37.7 | f-c | no tumor |
| | 8.7 | t-o | — | 24.8 | t-o | — |
| | 6.0 | f-c-t | tumor + necrosis | 21.9 | l-t | — |
| | | | | 17.2 | f-c | no tumor |
| | 3.1 | c | — | 16.4 | — | — |
| | 2.7 | t-o | — | 14.9 | f | — |
| | 0.8* | f | — | 13.7 | c-p | — |
| Anaplastic Astrocytoma | 26.7 | c-p | tumor | 38.5 | f-t | — |
| | 18.7 | t-l | tumor + necrosis | 30.7 | f | tumor |
| | 17.4 | c-p | tumor + necrosis | 21.0 | f | — |
| | 2.9 | t-p-o-l | — | 14.7 | t-l | — |
| | | | | 12.1 | f | — |
| Oligodendroglioma (malignant) | 61.2 | f | tumor | 26.2 | f-c | no tumor |
| | 18.7 | f | tumor | 23.2 | f | no tumor |
| | 14.0 | p-o | tumor + necrosis | 24.3 | — | tumor + necrosis |
| | | | | 16.2 | f | — |
| | | | | 20.7 | c | — |

*dead of complication after reoperation
f = frontal, c = central, p = parietal, t = temporal, o = occipital localization, l = left hemisphere

## Table 3

### Survival After Interstitial ¹⁹²Ir HDR Brachytherapy with/without Radiosensitization (150 patients)

| Tumor Type | N+ | N− | Survival N+ (mos) | Survival N− (mos) |
|---|---|---|---|---|
| Glioblastoma | 62 | 9 | 9.6 ± 6.9 | 8.3 ± 6.8 |
| Anaplastic Astrocytoma | 43 | 4 | 22.1 ± 16.9 | 24.1 ± 16.7 |
| Oligodendroglioma | 25 | 7 | 37.2 ± 33.4 | 30.1 ± 18.5 |
| Total | 130 | 20 | | |

N+ = patients with radiosensitizers
N− = patients without radiosensitizers

## Table 4

### Differences in Three Methods of Treatment: Surgery, Surgery with External Radiation, Surgery with $^{192}$Ir HDR Brachytherapy

| Tumor Type | Surgery | | Surgery + External Irradiation | | Surgery + $^{192}$Ir HDR Brachytherapy | |
|---|---|---|---|---|---|---|
| | No. Cases | $t_s$ | No. Cases | $t_s$ | No. Cases | $t_s$ |
| Glioblastoma Multiforme | 10 | 4.2 ± 3.7 | 23 | 8.3 ± 7.8 | 71 | 9.4 ± 6.9 |
| Astrocytoma | 7 | 23.1 ± 20.6 | 10 | 24.8 ± 14.2 | 47 | 22.3 ± 16.7 |
| Oligodendroglioma | 7 | 10.5 ± 4.4 | 4 | 17.9 ± 17.6 | 32 | 35.7 ± 30.6 |

$t_s$ = survival time in months

## Table 5

### Survival from Time of Diagnosis and after Treatment with $^{192}$Ir and Afterloading HDR Brachytherapy

| Tumor Type | | Number of Cases | Median Survival after Diagnosis (months: min.–max.) | Median Survial after Brachytherapy | |
|---|---|---|---|---|---|
| | | | | + (mos) | * |
| Astrocytoma II | $^{192}$Ir | 6 | 16 (10–114) | 13 | 40 |
| | $^{125}$I | 2 | 8/58 | 12 | 7 |
| Astrocytoma III | $^{192}$Ir | 15 | 6 (1–50) | 7 | 7 |
| | $^{125}$I | 11 | 4 (1–24) | 4 | 26 |
| Oligodendroglioma III | $^{192}$Ir | 2 | 85/7 | 5 | 0 |
| | $^{125}$I | 1 | 27 | 7 | 0 |
| Glioblastoma IV | $^{192}$Ir | 17 | 2 (1–8) | 4 | 6 |
| | $^{125}$I | 11 | 2 (1–22) | 5 | 3 |

\* = still living
+ = dead

## Table 6

### Additive External Irradiation After $^{192}$Ir and $^{125}$I HDR Brachytherapy of 65 Cerebral Gliomas (1975–1984)

| Tumor Type | | Number of Cases | Brachy-therapy | Additive External Irradiation | Median Survival Time (months) |
|---|---|---|---|---|---|
| Astrocytoma II | $^{192}$Ir | 8 | 6 | 1 | 26 |
| | $^{125}$I | | 2 | 0 | 9 |
| Astrocytoma III | $^{192}$Ir | 26 | 15 | 5 | 7 |
| | $^{125}$I | | 11 | 7 | 5 |
| Oligodendroglioma III | $^{192}$Ir | 3 | 2 | 0 | 5 |
| | $^{125}$I | | 1 | 0 | 7 |
| Glioblastoma IV | $^{192}$Ir | 28 | 17 | 9 | 10 |
| | $^{125}$I | | 11 | 6 | 5 |

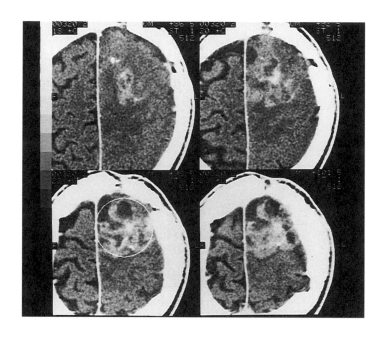

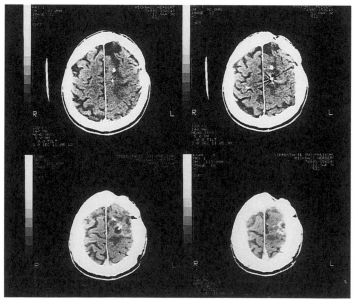

**Fig. 8.** (top) Preoperative recurrent malignant astrocytoma that underwent a combination of HDR brachytherapy followed by an [125]I permanent implant. (bottom) Postoperative CT 10 weeks after brachytherapy showing tumor regression.

or biopsy were not encountered. The most common complication of the after-loading therapy is brain edema. The use of corticosteroids during the 15 days of radiotherapy and in the posttreatment period is advised. It is important to note that fractionated afterloading therapy allows for follow-up of the clinical condition of the patient, making it possible to stop the radiation therapy at the onset of substantial edema. In about one-third of cases, radionecrosis takes place along with cystic liquefaction at a later time ("radioknife"). After 2 to 5 weeks, an increased perifocal edema occurs in many cases, requiring higher doses of dexamethasone.

## Discussion

In the single catheter technique, a very high activity (70 curie) [192]Ir source is used, thereby maximizing the dose penetration into the tissue. Practically speaking, if this source strength is not used, the dwell times required to adequately treat the entire tumor through one catheter may outweigh the benefits of the single catheter. Although this method was used as a primary treatment (60 Gy delivered), some patients with very irregular tumors required a post-implant course of external irradiation to cover the potentially undertreated margins. Unquestionably, the issue of adequate dose to the periphery is a critical one since most tumors recur at the margin.[1] This issue is also addressed in the St. Louis technique, and a limited course of external irradiation (46 Gy) was given before the HDR implant (15 Gy).

Complications associated with these therapies are not unlike those encountered with other brain tumor brachytherapy. Infectious complications are well managed with antibiotics. The development of brain edema is an expected event with indwelling brain catheters and is managed with appropriate steroid use and/or hyperosmolar agents. In extreme cases, therapy may need to be discontinued and decompressive surgery performed.

The decision regarding which method to use and which radioactive sources to apply depends on the histological diagnosis, the grading of the tumor, the localization within brain, the tumor volume, and the infiltration directions. HDR brachytherapy plays a role in recurrent hemispheric malignant gliomas or in primary hemispheric malignant gliomas in combination with external irradiation therapy. However, HDR brachytherapy should be limited to malignant tumors localized in the hemispheres. HDR brachytherapy is not indicated for tumors of the midline, except in anaplastic tumors where the dose is fractionated, possibly in combination with external irradiation and chemotherapy.

In some cases Mundinger and Zamorano have combined HDR brachytherapy (25–40Gy) with additional permanent implantation of [125]I or removable [192]Ir (79–90 Gy). Here the advantage is that the applied dose can be administered gradually over a period of time resulting in less-severe reactive perifocal edema. This combination is indicated for deep malignant tumors in the commissural systems and in the white matter near the third ventricle, that is, the corpus callosum, thalamus, basal ganglia, mediotemporal, and frontocaudal regions (Fig. 9).

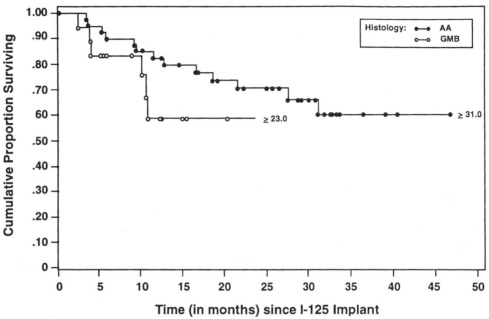

**Fig. 9.** Kaplan-Meier representation of the probability of survival for patients with GBM and anaplastic astrocytoma treated with permanent $^{125}$I implants and concurrent external radiation therapy.

There is an urgent need to improve survival in patients with malignant gliomas, especially GBM. Although therapeutic approaches employed to treat such tumors have utilized chemotherapy, hyperthermia, interstitial HDR brachytherapy, radiation sensitizers, and hyperfractionation, the "gold standard" of treatment remains some degree of surgery followed by postoperative external beam irradiation. Unfortunately, this standard approach yields a median survival of only 9 months for patients with GBM.[24,25] Median survival of newly-diagnosed GBM patients receiving HDR brachytherapy and interstitial hyperthermia was, at 21 months (St. Louis technique), improved over that reported for standard therapy.

Typically, endpoints for evaluation of therapies in brain tumor patients include, in addition to survival, CT scans and neurological evaluations. These measures are particularly useful for patients undergoing surgery or receiving chemotherapy. However, a CT scan and neurological evaluation are not easily interpreted for a brachytherapy patient because posttreatment mass effect and necrotic changes are slow to resolve, as seen by continued gradual improvement in CT tumor-volume responses. Therefore, it is often difficult to differentiate between radiation necrosis and persistent or recurrent tumors; in some cases, stereotactic biopsies have been used to make the distinction. In the future, even more importance may be attached to the kind of treatment in which radiation therapy is combined with radiosensitizers.

Experience with intraoperative HDR has shown that this therapy should be limited to either unresectable, persistent, or recurrent tumors of the white substance of the hemispheres. In other regions it should only be applied to 2–3 fractions of 8–10 Gy and in combination with permanent implants or external irradiation. The dose level depends on how far away from the midline structures the tumor is localized. The more peripheral, the higher the single dose can be (between 35 and 45 Gy of the peripheral tumor dosage).

## Conclusion

Fractionated HDR afterloading brachytherapy is a promising method of delivering relatively high intratumoral irradiation doses. Although the two techniques presented herein differ, the underlying theories are similar. An accepted principle evident in both techniques is the need to achieve a high dose in the 3-D target volume with only a minimal dose to the surrounding normal brain.

HDR brachytherapy in the treatment of malignant brain tumors with or without concomitant interstitial hyperthermia or other radiosensitizers offers several advantages. Among these advantages is the ability to deliver high intratumoral doses with only a minimal irradiation dose to the surrounding normal brain tissues. Preliminary results are encouraging; however, many questions are yet to be answered regarding the appropriateness of the therapy, criteria for use, and impact on survival.

*Acknowledgments:*
The authors would like to thank Deborah Welsh, R.N., Neuro-Oncology Coordinator at St. Luke's Hospital, St. Louis, Missouri for her contributions to the manuscript and Julie Bedore White for her valuable editorial assistance.

---

## REFERENCES

1. Bashir R, Hochbert F, Oot R. Regrowth patterns of glioblastoma multiforme related to planning of interstitial brachytherapy fields. Neurosurgery 23:127-130, 1988.
2. Choucair AK, Levin VA, Gutin PH, et al. Development of multiple lesions during radiation therapy and chemotherapy in patients with gliomas. J Neurosurg 65:654-658, 1986.
3. Davis RL, Barger GR, Gutin PH, et al. Response of human malignant gliomas and CNS tissue to brachytherapy: a study of seven autopsy cases. Acta Neurochir (suppl.) 33:301-305, 1984.
4. Hochberg FH, Pruitt A. Assumptions in the radiotherapy of glioblastoma. Neurology 30:907-911, 1980.
5. Walker MD, Alexander E Jr, Hunt WE, et al. Evaluation of BCNU and/or radiotherapy in the treatment of anaplastic gliomas. J Neurosurg 49:333-343, 1978.
6. Walker MD, Green SB, Byar DP, et al. Randomized comparisons of radiotherapy and nitrosureas for the treatment of malignant glioma after surgery. N Eng J Med 303:1323-1329, 1980.

7. Walker MD, Strike TA, Sheline GE. An analysis of dose-effect relationship in the radiotherapy of malignant gliomas. Int J Radiat Oncol Biol Phys 5:1725-1731, 1979.
8. Sheline GE, Wara WM, Smith V. Therapeutic irradiation and brain injury. Int J Radiat Oncol Biol Phys 6:1215-1228, 1980.
9. Frazier CH. Lesions of the hypophysis from the viewpoint of the surgeon. J Nerv Ment Disabil 41:103-109, 1914.
10. Leskell L. The stereotaxic apparatus for intracerebral surgery. Acta Chir Scand 102:316-319, 1951.
11. Mundinger F, Riechart T. Stereotaxic irradiation-procedure of brain tumors and pituitary adenomas by means of radio-isotopes and its results. Confin Neurol 22:190-203, 1962.
12. Mundinger F. The treatment of brain tumors with radioisotopes. Prog Neurol Surg 1:202-257, 1966.
13. Mundinger F, Metzel E. Interstitial radioisotope therapy of intractable diencephalic tumors by the stereotaxic permanent implantation of iridium-192, including bioptic control. Confin Neurol 32:195-202, 1970.
14. Mundinger F. The treatment of brain tumors with interstitially applied radioactive isotopes. In: Wang Y and Paoletti P, eds. Radionuclide Applications in Neurology and Neurosurgery. Springfield, Ill.: Charles C. Thomas Publishing Co.; 1970, 199-265.
15. Mundinger F. Interstitial curietherapy in the treatment of pituitary adenomas and for hypophysectomy. Prog Neurol Surg 6:326-379, 1975.
16. Mundinger F, Birg W, Klar M. Computer-assisted stereotactic brain operations by means including computerized axial tomography. Appl Neurophysiol 41:169-182, 1978.
17. Mundinger F, Birg W, Ostertag CB. Treatment of small cerebral gliomas with CT-aided stereotaxic curietherapy. Neuroradiology 16:564-567, 1978.
18. Mundinger F. Stereotactic interstitial therapy of nonresectable intracranial tumours with iridium-192 and iodine-125. In: Karcher KH, et al., eds. Progress in Radio-Oncology II. New York, NY: Raven Press, 1982, 371-380.
19. Mundinger F, Birg W. CT-stereotaxy in the clinical routine. Neurosurg Rev 7:219-224, 1984.
20. Mundinger F. Implantation of radioisotopes (curietherapy). In: Schaltenbrand G, Walker AE, eds. Textbook of Stereotaxy of the Human Brain. Stuttgart, Germany: Thieme Medical Publishers, Inc.; 1982, 410-435.
21. Mundinger F, Sauerwein K. "Gammamed", ein Gerat zur Bestrahlung von Hirngeschwulsten mit Radioisotopen. Acta Radiol Oncol Radiat Phys Biol 5:48-52, 1966.
22. Mundinger F. Imaging stereotaxic implantation of radionuclides in intracranial tumors (curietherapy and brachy-curietherapy). In: Sauer R., ed. Medical Radiology: Interventional Radiation Therapy Techniques—Brachytherapy. Heidelberg, Germany: Springer-Verlag, Inc.; 1991, 67-79.
23. Mundinger F, Braus DF, Krauss JK, et al. Long-term outcome of 89 low grade brainstem gliomas after interstitial radiation therapy. J Neurosurg 75:740-746, 1991.
24. Mundinger F, Busam B, Birg W, et al. Results of interstitial iridium-192-Brachy-curietherapy and iridium-192 protracted long-term irradiation. In: Szikla G, ed. Stereotactic Cerebral Irradiation. Elsevier North-Holland Biomedical Press (INSERM Symposium No 12); 1979, 303-320.
25. Mundinger F, Vogt P, Jobski C, et al. Klinische und experimentelle Ergebnisse der interstitiellen Brachy-Curietherapie in Kombination mit Radiosensibilisatoren bei infiltrierenden Hirntumoren. Strahlentherapie 143:318-328, 1972.
26. Zamorano L, Yakar D, Dujovny M, et al. Permanent iodine-125 implant and external beam radiation therapy for the treatment of malignant brain tumors. Stereotact Funct Neurosurg 59:183-192, 1992.
27. Moran CJ, Naidich TP, Marchosky JA. CT guided needle placement in the central nervous system: results in 146 consecutive patients. AJR 143:861-864, 1984.

28. Simpson JR, Marchosky JA, Moran CJ, et al. Volumetric interstitial irradiation of glioblastoma multiforme. ECHO 3:161-170, 1987.
29. Marchosky JA, Moran CJ, Fearnot NE, et al. Hyperthermia catheter implantation and therapy in the brain. J Neurosurg 72:975-979, 1990.
30. Garcia DM, Marchosky JA, Nussbaum G, et al. Interstitial HDR brachytherapy and long duration interstitial hyperthermia in the treatment of newly diagnosed malignant gliomas. Activity (Selectron Brachytherapy Journal) (6)2:70-74, 1992.
31. Sapareto SA, Dewey WC. Thermal dose determination in cancer therapy. Int J Radiat Oncol Biol Phys 10:787-800, 1984.
32. Zamorano L, Bauer-Kirpes B, Dujovny M. Dose planning for interstitial irradiation. In: Kelly PJ, Kall BA, eds. Computers in Stereotactic Neurosurgery. Boston, Mass.: Blackwell Scientific Publishing; 1992, 279-291.
33. Zamorano L, Dujovny M, Yakar D, et al. Multiplanar image guided stereotactic brachytherapy with iodine-125. In: Neurosurgery: State of the Art Reviews; vol. 4. Philadelphia, Pa., Hanley & Belfus, Inc.; 1989.
34. Oppel F, Pannek HW, Brock M. Die interstitielle Bestrahlung maligner inoperabler Hirntumoren nach dem Prinzip des "afterloading." Psychiatrie, Neurologie, und Psychotherapie fur Klinik un Praxis 5:2-4, 1985.

# Chapter 9

# High Dose Rate Brachytherapy for Cancer of the Head and Neck

*Peter C. Levendag, Bhadrasain Vikram, Albino D. Flores, and Wei-Bo Yin*

## Introduction

Brachytherapy has been used routinely in the past for a number of tumor sites in the head and neck. There is an abundance of literature regarding the local control rates and survival, mainly obtained by using low dose rate (LDR) techniques. For this material the reader is referred to standard textbooks. In recent years new technology dramatically changed the horizon of brachytherapy. New man-made isotopes (e.g., iridium-192, cesium-137, and iodine-125) were introduced, with iridium-192 being, at present, the most commonly used for cancers of the head and neck. Moreover, manual afterloading was replaced by computer-controlled afterloading devices, first with LDR afterloading machines and, more recently, with high dose rate (HDR) afterloaders. None of these developments was possible had not computer planning capabilities increased markedly as well. We have come from "implantation systems and rules," such as the Patterson-Parker and Paris systems used for LDR brachytherapy, to dose calculations for single-plane and volume implants using computer planning with optimization capabilities of planning systems that are used in HDR brachytherapy.

With the introduction of HDR brachytherapy, the radiobiology of tumor response and normal tissues changed. Unfortunately, there are no long-term data to date on the effectiveness of HDR brachytherapy for head and neck tumors. It is too early to substantiate the therapeutic window of HDR brachytherapy as compared to the standard LDR; if anything, HDR has become "less permissive" with respect to the tolerance of normal tissues. Pulse dose rate (PDR) has been suggested to cope with this radiobiological dilemma. To date, little is known about the optimal fraction size and interval between fractions for clinical practice with PDR. Moreover, the sophistication in technique of HDR and PDR brachytherapy (e.g., no source preparation, remote-controlled afterloaders, improvement in radiation protection, optimization of dose distribution, fractionation) has created the need for increased and intensive physics and personnel support. Finally, we would like to stress that computer power

From: Nag, S. (ed.): *High Dose Rate Brachytherapy: A Textbook*, Futura Publishing Company, Inc., Armonk, NY, © 1994.

and sophistication in planning systems and afterloading machines do not replace proper training in brachytherapy techniques with respect to the different sites of the head and neck. Close collaboration with a department of head and neck surgery remains essential.

This overview reports preliminary experiences of four different cancer centers around the world that have explored the use of PDR and/or HDR interstitial and endocavitary brachytherapy for treatment of cancer of the head and neck.

## The Rotterdam Experience—Peter Levendag, Peter Jansen, and Andries Visser

A total of 81 patients with cancer in the head and neck were treated, starting at the beginning of 1991 until June 1992. Crude local control rates of the implanted sites are summarized in Table 1. Treatment techniques and preliminary results on cancer of the nasopharynx (endocavitary) and oropharynx (interstitial) will be detailed.

## Preliminary Experience with Fractionated HDR-Endocavitary Brachytherapy of the Nasopharynx

### General Background of Endocavitary Brachytherapy

Some studies have demonstrated a dose-effect relationship for the primary tumor in the nasopharynx (or primary nasopharynx cancer (NPC)).[1] Also, it has been demonstrated that a local recurrence in the nasopharynx can be reirradi-

**Table 1**

**DDHCC/UHR (January 1991–June 1992): Summary of HDR/PDR Results**

| Implanted Site | Number (primary) | Control (crude) | Number (recurrence) | Control (crude) |
|---|---|---|---|---|
| Nasopharynx | 24 | 23/24 | 5 | 2/5 |
| Nasal Vestibule | 6 | 5/6 | — | — |
| Base of Tongue | 7 | 7/7 | 2 | 2/2 |
| Neck | — | — | 12 | 6/12 |
| Pharyngeal Wall | 1 | 1/1 | 1 | 0/1 |
| Tonsil and/or Soft Palate | 13 | 13/13 | 3 | 2/3 |
| Mobile Tongue | 5 | 5/5 | 0 | — |
| Skin | 0 | — | 2 | 2/2 |
| All Sites | 56 | 54/56 (94%) | 25 | 14/25 (56%) |

ated successfully to palliate symptoms or, in selected cases, to even attempt a cure. The nasopharynx, however, is a midline structure surrounded by many vital tissues, which prohibits the delivery of high doses of external beam radiation therapy (EBRT), particularly if previously irradiated. Therefore, people have initiated treatment programs that use endocavitary brachytherapy for boosting the nasopharynx after EBRT as part of their primary and recurrent tumor-treatment regimes. Wang,[2] for example, reported for 146 patients with primary T1-3 tumors of the nasopharynx, a 5-year actuarial local control rate of 91% for boost by means of brachytherapy versus 60% for boosting by means of EBRT ($P = 0.0002$). Pryzant et al.[3] reported that in 53 patients with recurrent NPC, a 5-year disease-free survival of 44% for brachytherapy versus 14% for EBRT ($p = 0.19$) and a 5-year overall survival of 60% for brachytherapy versus 16% for EBRT ($P = 0.029$) were observed.

## Daniel den Hoed Cancer Center/University Hospital of Rotterdam(DDHCC-UHR) Protocol and Treatment Techniques for Fractionated HDR-Endocavitary Brachytherapy

The treatment protocol of the Rotterdam Head and Neck Cooperative Group for patients with T1-4N0, + cancer of the nasopharynx is shown in Table 2.

To perform endocavitary brachytherapy on an outpatient basis in a busy clinic in conjunction with the microSelectron HDR and the Nucletron Planning System (NPS)/PLATO optimization-computer planning system, a simple

---

### Table 2
### NPC Treatment Protocol (DDHCC/UHR)

| | Cumulative Dose |
|---|---|
| Primary tumor and neck: External Beam Radiation | 46 Gy |
| Primary tumor and positive neck nodes: External Beam Radiation | 60 Gy |
| Positive neck nodes and parapharyngeal mass: External Beam Radiation | 70 Gy |
| Primary tumors: microSelectron HDR; 2 fractions of 3 Gy/day, 6-hour intervals, 4 (*) or 6 times 3 Gy. Brachytherapy | 78–82 Gy |

* If the primary tumor has been treated by EBRT 70 Gy (parapharyngeal extension and/or T4 tumor), 4 fractions of 3 Gy will be given (cumulative dose, 82 Gy). In other cases, EBRT 60 Gy plus 6 fractions of 3 Gy (cumulative dose, 78 Gy) are applied.

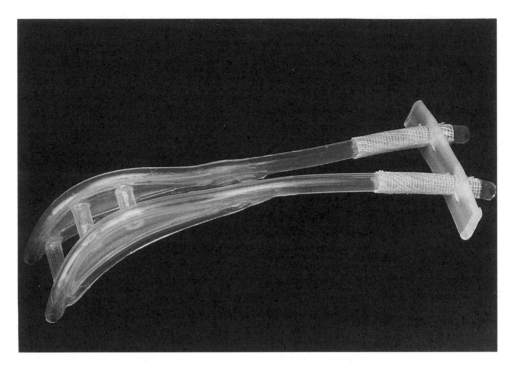

**Fig. 1.** The silicone Rotterdam Nasopharynx Applicator (outer diameter 5.5 mm, inner diameter 3.5 mm).

silicone mould, the so-called Rotterdam Nasopharynx Applicator (Fig. 1) was designed. This device can be easily introduced under topical anesthesia (Fig. 2).

Subsequently, anterior/posterior and lateral x-ray films (Fig. 3) are taken, and the dose is calculated in different patient points ("tumor tissue" and "normal tissue" points (Table 3). The dose in the nasopharynx is prescribed to the so-called "nasopharyngeal-point" (Na). This Na-point lies on the bony surface of the nasopharynx, that is, on the crossing of a line connecting the soft palate-point (Pa) and the base of skull-point (BOS) (Fig. 3). Generally, the distance of Na to the source axis varies from 0.75 cm to 1 cm, depending on the position of the mould relative to the bony anatomy. In case of a nonsatisfactory dose distribution in a number of dose points (see Table 3), a recalculation, that is, an optimization of the dose distribution, can be performed by changing the dwell times for the iridium-192 point source.

High dose rate irradiation can be started by simply inserting standard afterloading catheters into the Rotterdam Nasopharynx Applicator and connecting the catheters to the microSelectron HDR (Fig. 4). For twice-daily ease of insertion of the afterloading catheters in the silicone mould, a lubricant spray (R /Silisonde) is preferred.

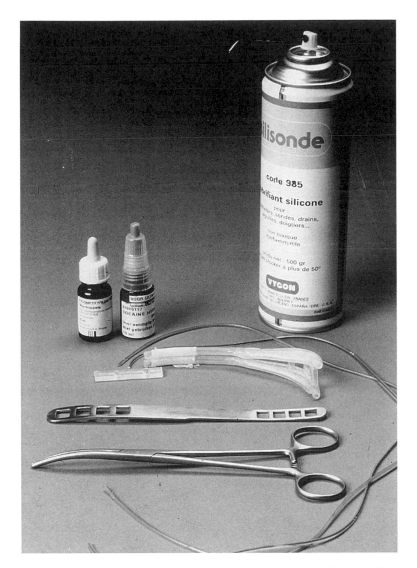

**Fig. 2a.** Silicone spray for easy insertion of standard flexible after-loading catheters into the Rotterdam Nasopharynx Applicator. Also shown are the Rotterdam Nasopharynx Applicator, forceps, decongestants (R/Xylometazoline HC1 1%) and anesthesia (R/Cocaine Hydrochloride 7%) used for introduction of the applicator into the nasopharynx.

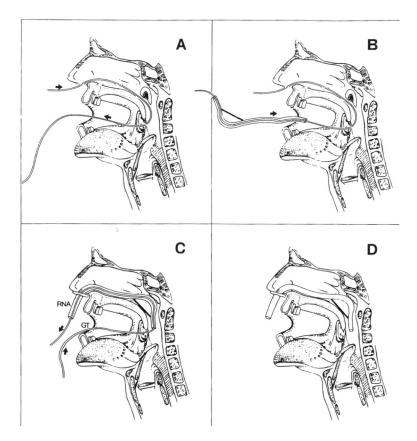

**Fig. 2b.** After decongestion (R/Xylometazoline HCl 1%) and topical anesthesia (R/Cocaine Hydrochloride 7%) of the nasal mucosa and nasopharynx, guide tubes (outer diameter: 2 mm) are introduced through the nose and withdrawn through the mouth. The Rotterdam Nasopharynx Applicator is guided intraorally over the guide tubes (GT); by pulling on the nasal part of the guide tubes, the applicator is finally placed in situ into the nasopharynx and nose. To facilitate positioning of the applicator into the nasopharynx, gently pushing the oral parts of the guide tubes intraorally by a standard type of forceps can sometimes be of some additional help (panel C). By using a silicone flange, the Rotterdam Nasopharynx Applicator is secured in the right position for the duration of the treatment (e.g., 3 to 4 days).

## Preliminary Results of Fractionated HDR-Endocavitary Brachytherapy

Twenty-nine patients were treated, 24 because of a primary cancer and 5 after local recurrence in the nasopharynx (reirradiation). With regard to the primary cancers, the mean follow-up was 261 days (range: 114–481 days); only one patient (4%) failed locally. Of the 5 patients treated for a recurrence, 3 (60%) experienced a local failure after fractionated HDR, with a mean follow-up of 278 days (range: 217–386 days). Figure 5 shows the actuarial local relapse free survival and overall survival, respectively, for patients with primary and recurrent cancers of the nasopharynx.

## Table 3
### Dose Optimization Nasopharynx Fractionated HDR

| | Dose (cGy) | | | | | |
| | Right | % | Left | % | Midline | % |
|---|---|---|---|---|---|---|
| Pituitary Gland (P) | — | — | — | — | 35 | 18 |
| Optic Chiasm (OC) | — | — | — | — | 35 | 12 |
| Retina (Re) | 50 | 17 | 57 | 19 | — | — |
| Base of Skull (BOS) | 164 | 55 | 163 | 54 | — | — |
| Nasopharynx (Na) | **302** | 101 | **298** | 99 | — | — |
| Nose (N) | 176 | 59 | 207 | 69 | — | — |
| Palate (P) | 214 | 71 | 232 | 77 | — | — |
| Rouviere Node (R) | — | — | — | — | 319 | 106 |
| Cord (C) | — | — | — | — | 67 | 22 |

Dose calculation example in different tumor tissue and normal tissue points. See also Figure 3. In case of nonsatisfactory dose distribution in a number of dosepoints, a recalculation (optimization) could be performed using the NPS/PLATO planning system for the microSelectron HDR by changing the dwell times for the iridium-192 point source. Explanation of normal tissue points (OC, P, Re, N, Pa, C) and tumor tissue points (Na, BOS, R) is given in the legend for Figure 3a.

For all brachytherapy patients with a minimum follow-up of 3 months, acute and late side effects were scored according to a modified Radiation Therapy Oncology Group (RTOG) scoring system (grade 0–4). For the purpose of this review, only M (mucosa) scores are displayed in relation to the total dose for primary cancers (Fig. 6). For the period after 3 months following treatment, all side effects were considered as "late" effects. Figure 7 shows late effects in M (mucosa; panel A) and S (skin; panel B) related to the total dose for primary tumors. Although the follow-up period is much too short with regard to the scoring of the late side effects, so far no obvious detrimental side effects were observed for these new brachytherapy fractionation regimes. Some patients, however, experienced synechia of the mucosal linings in the nose, which may be attributed to the so-called hyperdose sleeve (defined as the volume receiving 200% of $D_{reference}$) around the source axis (Fig. 8). To prevent this type of side effect, one could either change the dose-prescription point (i.e., the distance from source axis to the Na-point) and/or insert fatty gauzes (R/optule) in the nose temporarily after having removed the Rotterdam Nasopharynx Applicator.

## Dosimetry

Previously, with LDR brachytherapy, we used iridium-192 wire sources, manually afterloaded into Foley catheters inserted into the nasal cavity and nasopharynx proper. Because uniform iridium wires were used, a dose distribution very similar to using an iridium-192 point source of the microSelectron HDR with constant dwell times and dwell positions with a constant spacing would be obtained (Fig. 9). This LDR procedure had severe limitations with re-

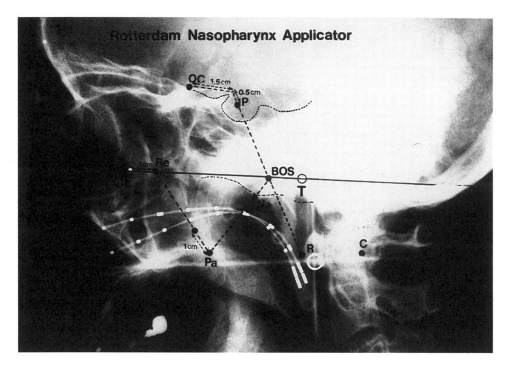

**Fig. 3a.** Lateral x-ray film of target volume in case of an endocavitary brachytherapy booster dose to the nasopharynx. On the lateral (Fig. 3a) and anterior/posterior (Fig. 3b) x-ray films, a number of tumor tissue points (Na, R, BOS), as well as normal tissue points (OC, P, Re, N, Pa, C) are depicted. The first base line is drawn on the lateral x-ray film from a Pb-marker placed on the bony canthus lateralis (CL) to the tragus (T). The retina-point (Re) is depicted on the baseline 1 cm posterior to CL. At the anterior border of vertebra C-I lies the node of Rouviere (R); the cord (C) is depicted posterior to R. The pituitary gland-(P) and base of Skull-point (BOS) can be found on a line from anterior clinoid process to R. Optic chiasm (OC) is situated 1.5 cm from the anterior clinoid process. The palate-point (Pa) lies at the junction of the hard and soft palate; the Nose-point is depicted 1 cm from Pa on line Re-Pa.

gard to dose distributions: that is, manipulation of these dose distribution patterns could sometimes be necessary due to the position of the applicator (anatomical constraints) relative to important normal tissue structures. When the Rotterdam Nasopharynx Applicator is being used for endocavitary brachytherapy in conjunction with the microSelectron HDR, planning of the dose distribution is performed using dwell-time optimization and dose prescription on so-called patient points (Table 3). For optimization purposes, usually the Na, N, and R points are used; that is, the dose distribution is optimized to deliver 100% of the reference dose to these 5 patient points (Na-r, Na-l, N-r, N-l, R) (Table 3). The node of Rouviere (R) is also included in this procedure because use of this "patient point" for dose prescription limits the dose in the spinal cord. Depending on the resulting dose distribution, one is able to vary

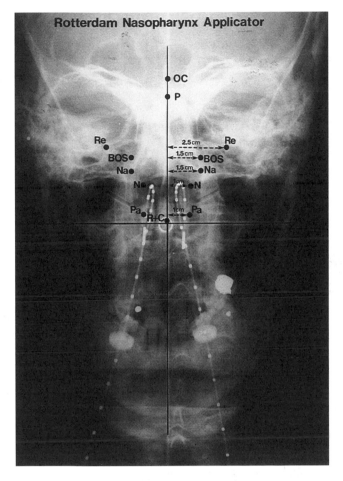

**Fig. 3b.** Anterior/posterior x-ray film showing tumor tissue and normal tissue points. See also legend to Fig. 3a.

the relative weight of each patient point in the optimization procedure to arrive at the desired doses as shown in the example depicted in Table 3 and Fig.10.

## Fractionated HDR Interstitial Brachytherapy for Tumors in the Head and Neck

### General Background of HDR-Interstitial Brachytherapy

In advanced cancers of the base of the tongue (BOT) and in case of reirradiation of tumors in the head and neck, improvement in local control and (for

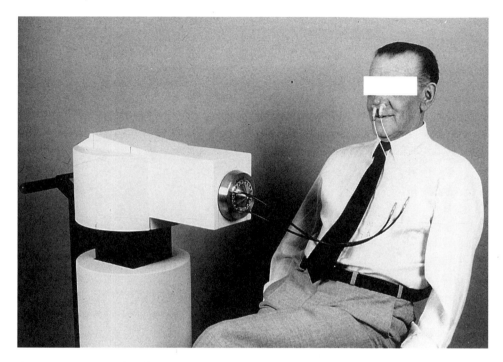

**Fig. 4.** Patient with silicone Rotterdam Nasopharynx Applicator in situ and connected to the microSelectron HDR for outpatient endocavitary brachytherapy of the nasopharynx.

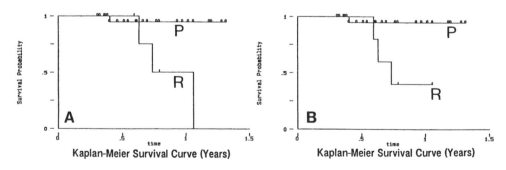

**Fig. 5.** Actuarial local relapse free survival (panel A) for primary (P) and recurrent (R) tumors of the nasopharynx, treated between January 1991 and June 1992 at the DDHCC/UHR by external beam radiation and fractionated HDR-endocavitary brachytherapy. Panel B shows actuarial overall survival for the same patient groups.

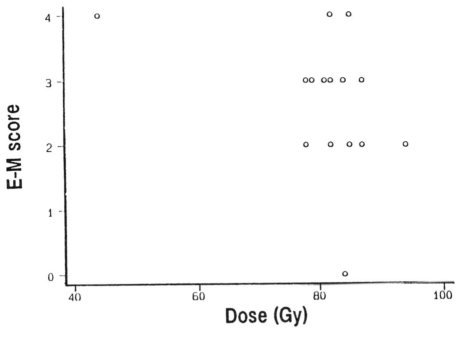

**Fig. 6.** Examples of distribution of early side effects (grades 0–4) for mucosa in relation to the dose for primary cancers of the nasopharynx.

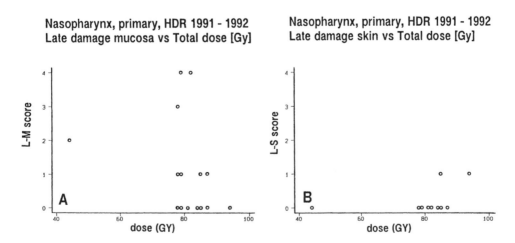

**Fig. 7.** Examples of distribution of late side effects (grades 0–4) for mucosa (panel A) and skin (panel B) in relation to the dose for primary cancers of the nasopharynx.

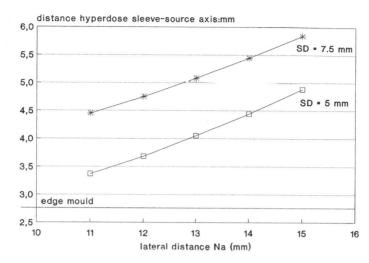

**Fig. 8.** Diameter of hyperdose sleeve (200%) as a function of dose prescription distance (∂). ∂ in sagittal plane fixed at 5 and 7.5 mm. Edge mould: surface Rotterdam Nasopharyngeal Applicator.

BOT tumors) survival has been observed in some series by using LDR brachytherapy techniques in combination with EBRT as opposed to EBRT only.[4,5] However, being immobilized and connected for extended periods of time to a microSelectron LDR can be extremely cumbersome to a patient. Moreover, the dosimetry of large-volume implants is complicated, and the obtained dose distributions are far from being optimal; in our view, this is to some extent even reflected in the morbidity some of our patients experienced (e.g., severe mucositis, pain, ulceration). It was anticipated at the time that, by modern brachytherapy technology (e.g., HDR/PDR afterloading machines, optimization capability of computer planning systems), a gain in terms of patient welfare can be obtained. That is, more flexibility in doctor/nursing/family care, more freedom of movement for patients since they can be disconnected from the afterloading machines between fractions, and a decrease in side effects of optimization because of improvement in dose distribution and elimination of "hotspots," can be expected.

## Fractionation Regimes: HDR- and PDR-Interstitial Brachytherapy

In Rotterdam, HDR and PDR brachytherapy is given in 2 fractions (fractionated HDR) or 4–8 fractions (PDR) per day. The fractionation regime and the total number of fractions (i.e., total dose brachytherapy) depend on site and T-stage as well as on whether a full course or booster dose (interstitial radiation therapy (IRT) combined with EBRT) is to be given by brachytherapy according to the protocol of the Rotterdam Head and Neck Cooperative Group). In the DDHCC/UHR we defined the following regimes.

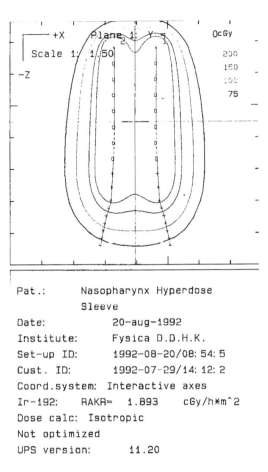

**Fig. 9.** Using iridium-192 wire sources, a dose distribution in the posterior part of the nasal cavity (septum) and the nasopharynx proper very similar to using an iridium-192 point source of the microSelectron HDR with constant dwell times and positions with a constant spacing would be obtained. Compare also to Fig. 10.

*Fractionated HDR*: Schemes delivering 2 fractions of 3 Gy per day with a minimum interval of 6 hours between the fractions. This type of treatment can sometimes be given on an outpatient basis (e.g., nasopharynx) during the day.

*PDR (Pulsed Dose Rate)*: Treatment schemes with either 4 fractions ("day-time regime," i.e., 4 fractions with 3-hour intervals between fractions used in

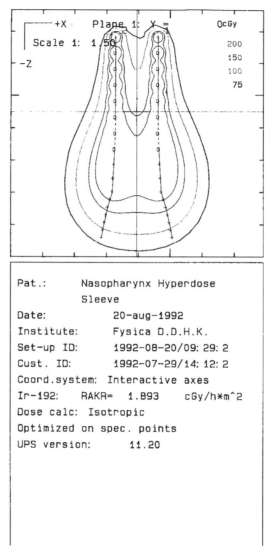

**Fig. 10.** Coronal section through the region of the nasopharynx proper and posterior part of nasal cavity, showing the optimized dose distribution. Compare also to Fig. 9.

the start-up phase of PDR to test the reliability of the PDR microSelectron with qualified radiotherapy personnel present during the day) or 8 fractions ("pulses") per day (24 hours), with 3-hour intervals between fractions. The 8 fractions per day will be the regime of preference after extensive testing and is now implemented in routine clinical use. PDR is given in a dedicated (shielded) room on the ward. The patient can be either permanently connected to the PDR afterloading machine or disconnected between fractions.

For calculations of the total number of fractions to be given, the linear quadratic (LQ) model is used, taking into account incomplete repair of sublethal damage in the limited time between fractions and also the finite duration of each radiation fraction. Specifically, the formulation as cited by Brenner and Hall has been used.[6] In one aspect, the method of Brenner and Hall has not been followed; that is, the total PDR dose has not been chosen to equal the total LDR dose. In contrast, the following procedure was used.

(1). The total LDR (50 cGy/h) dose that should be equivalent to a chosen fractionation scheme (dose) as used for conventional external beam irradiation (i.e., EBRT with 1 fraction of 2.0 Gy per day, 5 days per week; reference schedule) was calculated. For this step the incomplete repair model (Dale) was used.

(2). After the PDR fraction size (1 Gy for boost or 1.5 Gy in case of full-course brachytherapy) and the interval between PDR fractions (3 hours) was chosen, the number of fractions that would result in the same extrapolated tumor dose (ETD) as with the EBRT (or LDR scheme) was calculated.

In our fractionation regime, the PDR (HDR) dose does not necessarily have to equal the LDR dose; therefore, there is less need for extreme fractionation (i.e., less need for small fraction doses and very short intervals between fractions). However, to keep the probability of late effects in normal tissues as low as possible, it remains essential to choose an overall treatment time of the PDR (HDR) scheme comparable to or longer than the application time of the corresponding LDR scheme. The overall treatment time should not be shortened. With regard to the calculations, the parameters shown in Table 4 were used.

**Treatment Techniques—Fractionated HDR and PDR**

In one plane (subjectively the most representative plane with regard to tumor volume, the so-called central plane), through the center of the tumor and

---

### Table 4

### Parameters Used for Calculations of HDR and PDR Schemes of Equivalent Fractionation

Tumor effect: $\alpha/\beta = 10$ Gy, $\alpha = 0.3$ Gy$-1$

Late effects (normal tissues): $\alpha/\beta = 3$ Gy, $\alpha = 0.3$ Gy$-1$

Half-time for repair of sublethal damage: $T1/2 = 1$ hour for early effect (=tumor effect) and 3 hours for late effects (damage to normal tissues).

Pulse duration: 5 minutes. This choice is not very relevant as long as the chosen repair half-time is long compared to the pulse duration. For small PDR pulses, this will mostly be the case.

perpendicular to the main direction of the source trains/source axes, the dose distribution is computed. Specifically, the doses are determined in the geometrical centers of triangles formed by neighboring intersections of the source trains with the central plane. The prescribed dose is then delivered by taking 85% of the average dose over the geometrical centers (Fig.11). In fact, this procedure is a generalization of the dose prescription method of the Paris system. At present, the HDR or PDR microSelectron is used for all our head and neck implants. Examples of optimization procedures are discussed in chapter 6. Us-

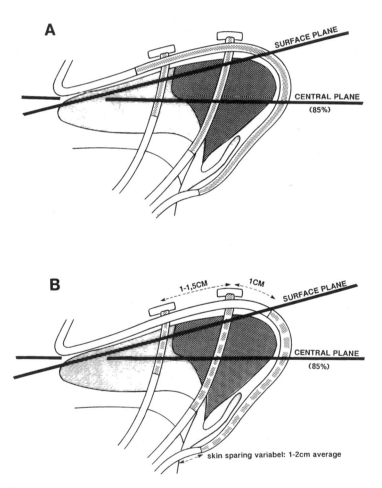

**Fig. 11.** Schematic representation of the base of tongue (BOT) implant, showing parts of the implanted catheters actually loaded with an iridium-192 wire source (continuous gray zone, A) or point sources (stipulated gray zone, B) and some of the planes for dose calculation. Note the catheter running over the dorsum of the tongue. The part of the dorsum catheter forming the intersection between the other two "vertical" catheters (with buttons) in each sagittal plane is loaded (in case of continuous iridium-192 wires; panel A, LDR-IRT) or unloaded (in case of iridium-192 point source; panel B, HDR-IRT).

ing the optimization program, we readily found clinical advantages. For example, in the past, long-lasting (severe) mucositis and pain in the mucosal surface of the BOT were frequently observed. This was undoubtedly due to large hot spots resulting from the loading patterns (long trajectories of catheters across the mucosal surface). Now, by routinely not loading some parts of the catheters running over the dorsum of the tongue (Fig.11), this side effect has been eliminated. Possible underdosage of the surface of the tongue (tumor) should be investigated but can be prevented by using longer dwell times in the top positions of other catheters. However, dosimetry checks, particularly in the sagittal planes, should be performed routinely (see physics section in "Optimization of Interstitial Implants of the Base of the Tongue," Chapter 6).

### Preliminary Results—Fractionated HDR and PDR

As of January 1991, 46 patients with a variety of tumors in the head and neck were treated by interstitial HDR or PDR brachytherapy, with or without EBRT and surgery (Table 1). Twenty-six had a primary cancer, and 20 had a recurrent tumor after previous irradiation. With regard to the primary cancer, the mean follow-up was 132 days (range: 101–152 days). One patient failed at the implanted site. Among the 20 patients experiencing recurrence after previous irradiation, the mean follow-up was 187 days (0–483 days); 8 patients (40%) experienced a local failure. Figure 12 shows the actuarial local relapse-free survival and overall survival, respectively, for patients with primary and recurrent cancers in the head and neck region.

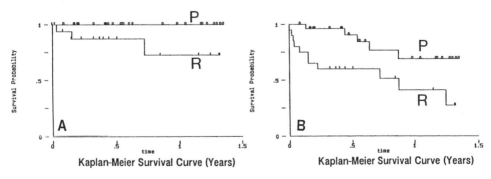

Left: local control – Right: overall survival
Primary [0] and recurrent [1]  Other Head and Neck tumors,  HDR/PDR 1991 - 1992

**Fig. 12.** Actuarial local relapse free survival (panel A) for primary (P) and recurrent (R) tumors in the head and neck, treated between January 1991 and June 1992 at the DDHCC/UHR by external beam radiation and/or HDR- or PDR-interstitial brachytherapy (see text). Panel B shows actuarial overall survival for the same patient groups. For all brachytherapy patients with a minimum follow-up of 3 months, acute and late side effects were scored according to a modified RTOG scoring system (grade 0–4). Although the follow-up period is (too) short, no obvious (extreme) acute and late side effects were observed so far.

# The New York Experience—Bhadrasain Vikram and Lio Yu

## Introduction

Between November 1988 and July 1992, 27 patients were treated by means of HDR brachytherapy in the department of Radiation Oncology at Beth Israel Medical Center in New York City. Fifteen patients were treated to palliate or prevent distressing symptoms of recurrent cancer (either alone or in conjunction with EBRT), and 12 were treated for a primary cancer (usually as a boost). Relative contraindications for the use of HDR brachytherapy include (1) large and ill-defined tumor masses (unfavorable geometry), (2) medical inoperability or poor operative risk, (3) sharp catheter curvatures or angles that the HDR source might be unable to negotiate. It was previously thought that HDR brachytherapy was contraindicated for tumors near major blood vessels such as the carotid artery. However, recent experimental studies in which HDR brachytherapy was employed have indicated a rather high tolerance of these blood vessels to radiation (Alfieri A, personal communication, 1992).

The equipment needed for HDR brachytherapy includes the HDR unit with its source and connections and catheters of specified gauge and length. We now most commonly use flexiguide catheters (Best Industries, Arlington, Virginia), which are closed and sharp tipped at one end. The flexiguide catheters come in various lengths and include a metal stylet that facilitates interstitial insertion. When the stylets are removed, significant flexibility of the catheters can be achieved, allowing for a customized fit to the area of interest with a minimum of trauma. These catheters are sutured in place within the tumor bed and are secured to the skin or mucosa by metal buttons. The catheters are placed in a parallel fashion 1.0–1.5 cm apart in a single plane, multiple plane, or volume arrangement, as appropriate. Uniform spacing is used, and the dose distribution is optimized by varying the dwell times.

The optimal time dose fractionation for HDR brachytherapy in the head and neck has not been determined. Hyperfractionation, hypofractionation, and accelerated fractionation all have been used. Various methods and formulae attempting to define the radiobiological dose equivalent of HDR brachytherapy to external beam radiation as well as LDR brachytherapy have already been suggested. Clearly, however, clinical data from HDR irradiation need to be obtained.

## Patients Treated by HDR Interstitial Radiation[7,8]

During the study, 27 patients were treated; the tumors included 23 epidermoid cancers, 1 adenocarcinoma, 1 muco-epidermoid carcinoma, 1 anaplastic carcinoma, and 1 desmoid tumor. The male to female ratio was 20:7 and the age range was 21–94 years (median: 60 yr). The sites of implant are listed in Table 5.

Fifteen patients had recurrent cancer: 11 of 15 had previously received EBRT doses of 50–65 Gy (median 60 Gy) and had recurrent cancer, while 4 out

**Table 5**

**Site and Number of Patients Treated by Interstitial Radiation Using HDR Regime**

| Sites of Implant | Number of Patients |
|---|---|
| Oral Cavity | 6 |
| Oropharynx | 5 |
| Nasal Cavity | 5 |
| Neck | 4 |
| Nasopharynx | 2 |
| Parotid | 2 |
| Miscellaneous | 3 |

of 15 had a recurrence after surgery alone. These patients received HDR to doses of 15–47 Gy (median: 28 Gy) in 2–10 fractions (median: 7 fractions) of 2–10 Gy each (median: 4 Gy) (Fig. 13). Seven out of 15 patients also received EBRT in conjunction with the HDR (4 patients without prior EBRT received EBRT of 40–71 Gy in 4–7 weeks and 3 patients with prior radiation therapy received an additional 20–30 Gy of EBRT). These patients have been followed for 4–30 months after treatment (median follow-up: 6 months). Twelve patients who

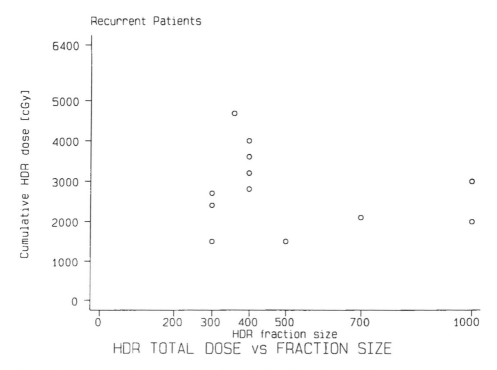

**Fig. 13.** HDR total dose versus fraction size for 15 patients with recurrent cancers.

were previously untreated received HDR doses of 12–64 Gy (median: 16 Gy) in 3–8 fractions (median: 6 fractions) of 2–5 Gy each (median: 3 Gy) (Fig. 14). In addition, all 12 patients received planned EBRT to 36–60 Gy (median 50.4 Gy) in 1.8–2.0 Gy fractions. Thus, the total dose received by these 12 patients ranged from 52–92 Gy (median 69.5 Gy) over 7–14 weeks (median: 12 weeks) (Fig. 15). These patients have been followed for 4–48 months (median: 12.5 months).

## Results of HDR—Interstitial Radiation

The observed survival rate of patients with recurrent disease is 39% at 1 year and 29% at 2 years (Fig. 16). The actuarial rate of local control is 47% at 2 years (Fig. 17). Eight of 15 patients have developed local recurrence, and 6 have developed serious complications. Among patients who received HDR with fractions of 3 Gy or less, 3 of 4 (75%) have local control without complications. In contrast, only 1 of 11 (9%) of the patients treated with larger fractions obtained uncomplicated local control. Among patients with previously untreated disease, the survival rate is 68% at 1 year and 45% at 2 years (Fig. 16). The actuarial local control rate is 80% at 2 years (Fig. 17). No patient has developed complications; thus, 10 of 12 patients (83%) have local control without complications.

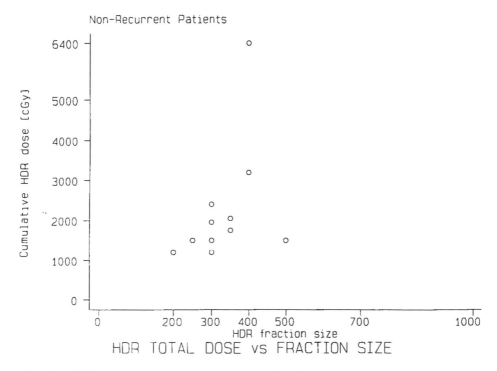

**Fig. 14.** HDR total dose versus fraction size for 12 previously untreated patients.

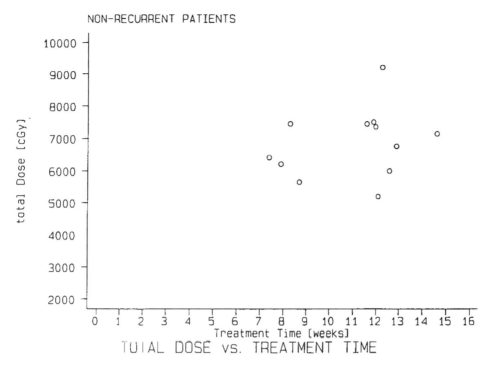

**Fig. 15.** Total (EBRT plus brachytherapy) dose versus treatment time (in weeks) for 12 previously untreated patients.

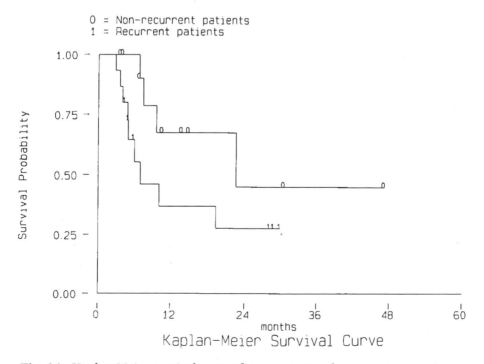

**Fig. 16.** Kaplan-Meier survival curves for recurrent and nonrecurrent patients.

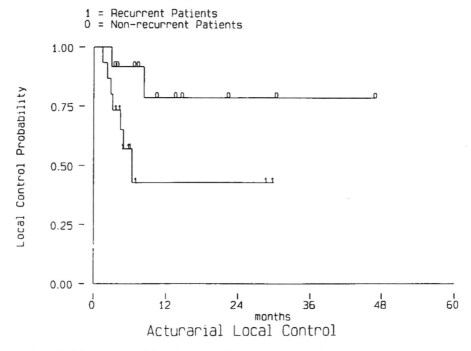

**Fig. 17.** The actuarial local control for recurrent and nonrecurrent patients.

## The Vancouver Experience—Albino Flores

### Introduction

From the philosophical point of view, in Vancouver we would consider almost all patients with squamous cell carcinomas in the head and neck region as potential candidates for brachytherapy, either as a complement to EBRT or as a single primary treatment, depending on the extent of the disease at presentation. However, if bone invasion has already occurred, complications following primary radiotherapy are usually high, and, for that reason, primary surgical treatment is the treatment of choice in our institution. Adjuvant radiotherapy is given postoperatively for microscopic residual disease left behind either at the primary or regional level (e.g., extranodal disease). We believe that interstitial irradiation alone is the treatment of choice for early cancers of the mouth mucosa (T1-T2 NO) provided they are (1) accessible, (2) well differentiated, (3) well defined, and (4) small. The value and effectiveness of this treatment (brachytherapy alone) diminishes proportionally if any of these parameters are not met (concurrent EBRT is given in these cases). In our institution, brachytherapy has been constantly changing mainly because of technological advances (new radioisotopes with better specific activity and remote afterloading systems) and as radiobiological principles are better understood and applied.

LDR radioactive material (radium and cesium) were replaced by HDR iridium-192, and, since 1988, remote afterloading has replaced manual loading in all cases, except for the radioactive gold seed implant, which is only used in elderly patients.

For bulky T2 (3 cm or more), T3, or T4 tumors of the mouth, we prefer EBRT initially since it includes the regional lymphatics, even if they are not clinically involved. Five thousand cGy in 20 fractions in 4 weeks is given to the primary site and regional lymphatics with multiple fields or, at least, a wedged pair of fields. Since 1978 a linear accelerator (4 or 6 MeV unit) has been used for this purpose; a shell-fixing device is used to reproduce daily treatment set-ups. All these patients receive a complementary treatment boost brachytherapy if the treatment volume is acceptable (4 × 4 × 3); otherwise, an EBRT boost may be preferred.

For patients with carcinomas in the nasopharynx, postcricoid region, or cervical esophagus, an intracavitary brachytherapy boost is employed after external irradiation in all cases. Our past experience using LDR radioactive materials (radium, cesium) at these sites have been reported previously.[1,2]

## HDR Brachytherapy for Cancer of the Nasopharynx

Before 1980, brachytherapy was used only to treat patients with recurrent disease. Radium and, subsequently, cesium tubes were placed in the nasopharynx, and a dose of 6,000 cGy at 1.5 cm from the axis of the 2 sources was given in 48 hours. From 1980 to 1988, 21 patients were treated with similar intranasal devices (Figs. 18 and 19), but these were modified to allow their connection to a remote afterloading system containing radioactive cesium pellets. These produced a dose rate of 1,000 cGy per hour so that treatment time at the same point of reference (1.5 cm from the axis) was only 1.77 hours for 2,500 cGy. Eleven out of 21 patients treated for a recurrence were alive with no evidence of disease (NED) 4 years or more after retreatment. Surprisingly, there were only minor complications, and the quality of life of all the survivors was excellent.

Good tolerance to this type of brachytherapy prompted us in 1988 to consider a brachytherapy boost as a regular complement to EBRT in the treatment of all new patients with NPC, with the exception of those with bone invasion. Since that time, an HDR brachytherapy boost has been given concurrently with radiation therapy in more than 50 new patients with NPC. The external irradiation consists of 6,000 cGy for T1 lesions and 6,500 cGy for T2, T3, and T4 lesions, with CT planning for the primary site and shielding of the spinal cord at 4,000 cGy. A brachytherapy boost of 2,500 cGy was given to the first 9 patients 4 weeks after completion of EBRT to allow sufficient healing of radiation mucositis. In the following 41 patients, a brachytherapy boost of 1,000 cGy was given just before or concurrently to EBRT. All 50 patients were treated using the iridium-192 HDR microSelectron unit.

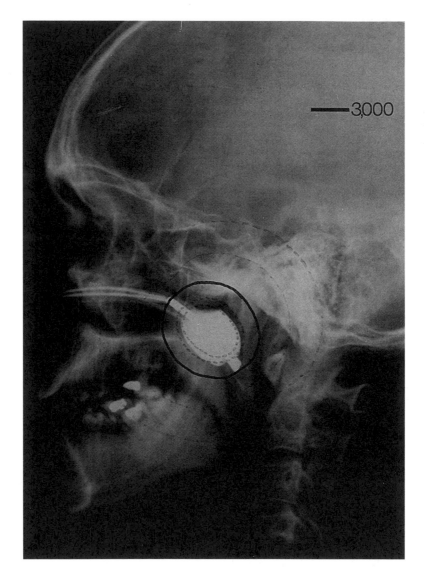

**Fig. 18.** Two nasopharyngeal devices containing cesium to be in tandem to generate LDR 125 cGy/hr manual loading.

## Radiobiological and Technical Aspects for HDR Brachytherapy of the Nasopharynx

In view of the still uncertain radiobiological effect of HDR, we felt that it was reasonable to use mathematical models and a linear quadratic formula to estimate radiobiologically equivalent doses to our historical LDR brachytherapy for NPC (Fig.20). From these models, higher biological effects should be expected with changes in dose rates from the standard LDR of 60 cGy/hr to

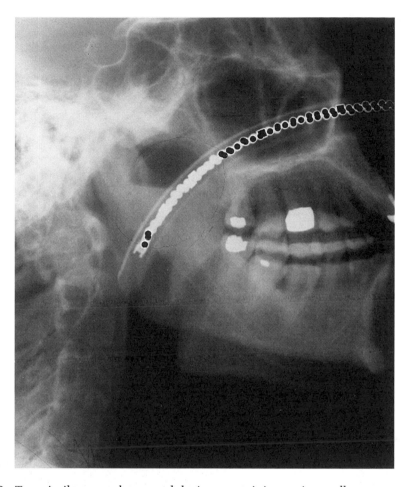

**Fig. 19.** Two similar nasopharyngeal devices containing cesium pellets to generate an MDR 1,000 cGy/hr with remote afterloading. The same devices are used with HDR Ir to generate a 30,000 cGy/hr with remote afterloading. Note the inflated balloon and water level used to improve treatment distance and depth dose.

1,200 cGy/hr. One can see, however, that dose rates higher than 1,200 cGy/hr do not produce any significant change in the slope and that the expected effect appears to be similar. From our previous data, 6,000 cGy at 1.5 cm from the axis of the LDR isotope (radium, cesium) is equivalent to 2,500 cGy at the same point using cesium-137 pellets, producing a dose rate of 1,000 cGy/hr, which is practically similar to 2,200 cGy required by iridium-192 that produces dose rates higher than 30,000 cGy/hr.

The treatment site and volume for NPC brachytherapy is determined by fiber optic endoscopy and scanning. It is an out-patient procedure, and the placement of the nasopharyngeal catheters is verified under fluoroscopy using dummy sources. Optimization with CT three-dimensional (3-D) reconstruction is also possible (Figs. 21 and 22).

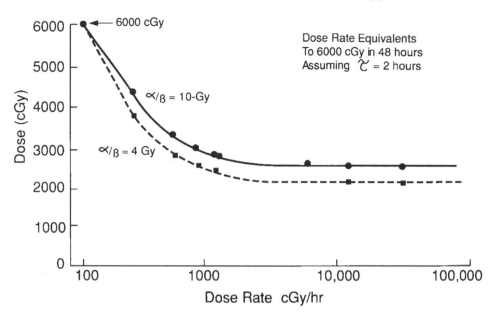

**Fig. 20.** Theoretical model of isoeffects curves for different dose rates for NPC brachytherapy.

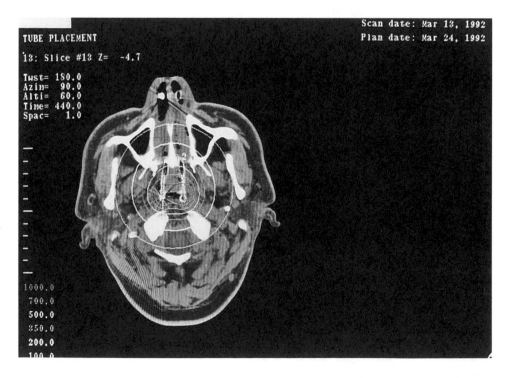

**Fig. 21.** CT (3D) in NPC patient outlining dose distribution with [192]Ir in place.

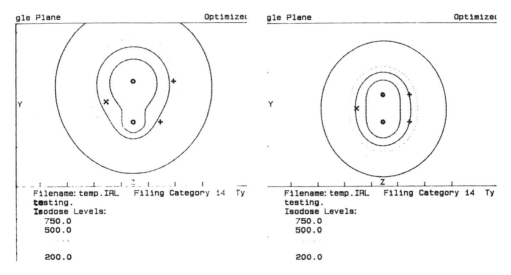

**Fig. 22.** Optimization of dosimetry for NPC with two linear sources. Note even and uneven dose distribution.

## Treatment Results and Complications for Cancer of the Nasopharynx

All 50 NPC patients treated with concurrent brachytherapy and EBRT tolerated this combined treatment quite well. All had transient radiation mucositis, but this was not more severe than in patients treated by EBRT alone. Twenty percent of the patients required nasogastric tube feeding after completion of therapy, and, as expected, some degree of xerostomia was present in all of them. Not a single case of severe complication has been observed (i.e., soft tissue or bone necrosis). Forty NPC patients treated with HDR and EBRT are eligible for a preliminary follow-up analysis for at least 6 to 40 months from therapy. One patient has died with local, regional, and distant metastasis. Three other patients are still alive with regional and distant metastasis but without local recurrence. The remainder of patients are apparently alive NED.

## HDR Brachytherapy for Mouth Cancer

Since 1988 all cancers of the mouth suitable for interstitial irradiation have been treated with HDR iridium-192 remote afterloading. The basic reasons for this change from LDR manual loading were (1) to improve radiation dosimetry by optimization, (2) to improve radiation protection, and (3) to study therapeutic effect and benefits.

As per our treatment protocol, a decision was made to treat all T1 and early T2 N0 (3-cm) carcinomas of the tongue and floor of the mouth by means of interstitial HDR brachytherapy alone. For bulky T2, T3, and T4 tumors, an HDR brachytherapy boost was given concurrently or just before the EBRT. The

EBRT treatment volume included the ipsilateral regional neck. The EBRT dose was 5,000 cGy given in 20 fractions in 4 weeks. The interstitial HDR brachytherapy boost in these cases consisted of 3 fractions, each 650 cGy, given b.i.d. (1 1/2 days) and a total boost of 1,950 cGy.

For T1 and early T2 (3-cm) NO tumors of the tongue and floor of the mouth, the primary HDR brachytherapy consisted of 7 fractions each of 650 cGy given b.i.d. in 3 1/2 days for a total of 4,500 cGy. No EBRT was used in these early cases.

### Radiobiological and Technical Aspects of Mouth HDR Brachytherapy

A mathematical model was also used to estimate equivalent doses for HDR (Fig. 23) for mouth cancer. The standard 6,000 cGy of continuous LDR in 6 days was the chosen parameter. As can be seen in the scheme, this amount of LDR is equivalent to 4,500 cGy with HDR. Although we would have preferred to use at least 10 fractions b.i.d. for 5 days as the theoretical model suggested (Fig. 24) to achieve the same therapeutic ratio, this was not possible at that time in our hospital for logistic reasons. For example, since an operation theater was not available on Mondays, implants could only be done on Tuesdays. Moreover, the radiotherapy department did not work on weekends. Therefore, 7

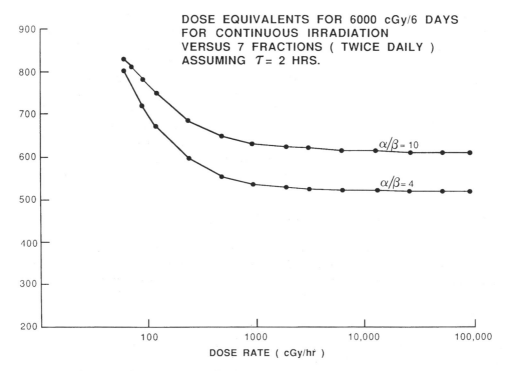

**Fig. 23.** Theoretical model of isoeffects curves for different dose rates for interstitial implant mouth cancers.

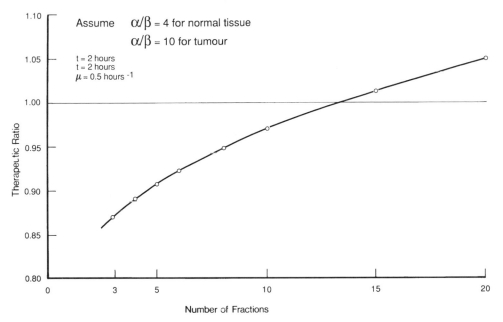

**DOSE RATE vs NUMBER OF FRACTIONS**
Reference Dose = 3 x 1550 @ 100 CGy/hour

**Fig. 24.** Theoretical model for therapeutic ratio isoeffects and number of fractions.

fractions b.i.d. in 3 1/2 days of treatment were chosen. To allow a repopulation of normal tissues and to reduce potential radiation damage, the interval of time chosen between fractions was to be 6 hours (experimental repair of sublethal radiation damage is less than 2 hours). Since the real biological effects of HDR are not very well known, these mathematical models gave us at least a good starting point, and subsequent preliminary analysis seems to have confirmed this. The technical aspects of HDR brachytherapy are the same as in LDR continuous irradiation. At our hospital, all treatments are preplanned. The treatment volume is outlined, and the number of catheters to be used is chosen. A dental assessment is made, and a prosthetic appliance is fabricated (Fig. 25). In particular a space of 1 cm is created between the alveolus and the implanted area to reduce unnecessary irradiation to the bone and tissues. A geometric optimization is done in all cases to ensure even dose distribution prior to treatment (Figs. 26, 27, and 28).

**Material, Treatment Results, and Complications**

Since 1988, 45 patients with carcinomas in the mouth have been treated by a form of HDR brachytherapy (4 had carcinomas in the dorsum of the tongue, 3 had carcinomas in the floor of the mouth, and 38 had carcinomas in the lateral aspect of the anterior tongue). Thirteen patients had an HDR

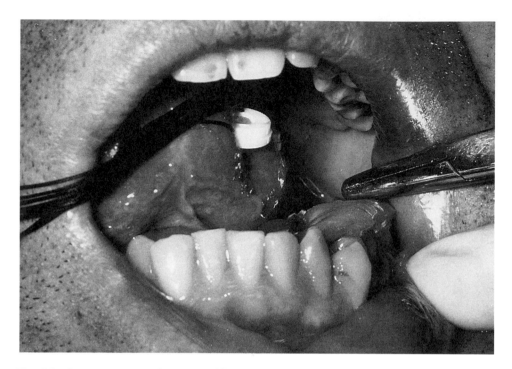

**Fig. 25.** Forceps on top of a removable dental prosthetic device to widen the separation between the implanted catheters and the alveolus to reduce unnecessary irradiation.

brachytherapy boost as a complement to radiation therapy, and 32 had HDR primary treatment only. Forty patients are eligible for a preliminary analysis of acute and late effects and a response from 6 to 40 months. All patients had an acute transient confluent mucositis in the local area of the implant. This was similar to what we had experienced with LDR continuous irradiation. Late effects were, however, more significant, as seen in Table 6. Severe complications did occur in 3 out of 40 patients (8%) and led to hospitalization and some degree of surgical intervention. Although late complications were slightly higher, local control and survival to the present time seem to be similar to, if no better than, historical controls using LDR (Table 7).

## HDR Brachytherapy for Nasopharyngeal Carcinoma in China—Wei-bo Yin

### The Beijing Experience

From April 1989 to May 1992, 101 patients with carcinoma of nasopharynx were treated by a microSelectron HDR.[9,10] There were 66 males and 35 females (median age: 50; range: 15–70). All had histopathologically proven carcinoma of the nasopharynx. The neck nodes were controlled by external

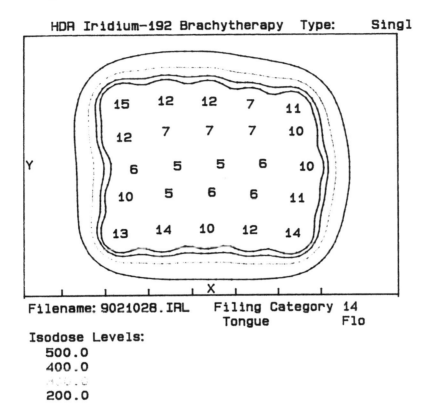

**Fig. 26.** Geometric optimization of an interstitial implant. Numbers in circles indicate the time of exposures at each point as provided by the HDR $^{192}$Ir.

beam irradiation only. Treatment characteristics are presented in Table 8. Patients were followed for 6–42 months (median follow-up: 24 months).

EBRT was carried out by 8 MV or 6 MV x-rays. Twenty-six patients with T1, T2, or T3 lesions were included in a randomized study in which they were randomly assigned to EBRT plus brachytherapy versus EBRT alone (Table 8). The brachytherapy group was given a dose of 60 Gy in 6 weeks (30 fractions of 2 Gy) by means of EBRT; subsequently, 2–3 applications of brachytherapy were given at weekly intervals. A microSelectron HDR iridium-192 afterloader with a

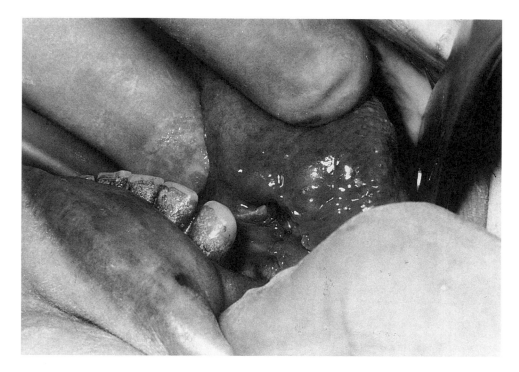

**Fig. 27.** Patient with a $T_2$ (4-cm) ulcerated cancer in the lateral aspect of tongue and floor of the mouth prior to implant with HDR $^{192}$Ir.

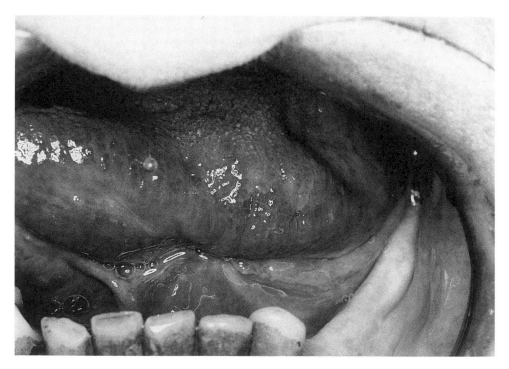

**Fig. 28.** Same patient as Fig. 27, 2 years after a 2-plane implant with HDR $^{192}$Ir. Note only a retracted scar but no ulceration or evidence of disease.

### Table 6
### Late Effects of HDR Brachytherapy in Mouth Cancers

|  | Brachy. Boost (3F)* | Brachy. (7F) |
|---|---|---|
| Mild (0–1) | 6 | 14 |
| Moderate (2) | 6 | 11 |
| Severe (4) | 1 (8%) | 2 (16%) |
| All | 13 | 27 |

*3 fractions

### Table 7
### TNM Distribution of Mouth Cancer Cases and Local Control

|  | N0 | N1 | N2 | N3 | NED | ALIVE NED |
|---|---|---|---|---|---|---|
| T1 | 11 | — | — | 1 | 11/11 | 11/11 |
| T2 | 22 | | 1 | — | 21/23 | 19/23 |
| T3 | 4 | 2 | — | — | 5/6 | 3/6 |
|  | 36 | 2 | 1 | 1 | 37/40 (92%) | 33/40 (83%) |

### Table 8
### Patient Status Before HDR Brachytherapy

| No. Previous Courses of Radiotherapy | Number of Patients | Primary Sites | | | |
|---|---|---|---|---|---|
|  |  | Residual Disease | Local Recurrence | Boost* | Randomized Trial |
| One | 59 | 38 | 13 | 8 | — |
| Two and three | 16 | 6 | 6 | 4 | — |
| Randomized trial | 26 | — | — | — | 26 |
| Total | 101 | 44 | 19 | 12 | 26 |

*: Brachytherapy boost given to primary lesion for slow resolution after radical external-beam radiation therapy.

brachytherapy planning system was used for intracavitary brachytherapy; 101 patients were treated with a total of 232 applications at intervals of 7 to 20 days between the external beam and the brachytherapy parts of the treatment.

Flexible rubber tubing was used as the nasopharyngeal applicator; this proved to be a simple and painless procedure. The applicators could be easily fixed in treatment position. Computer planning was used, and orthogonal x-ray films were taken for every treatment for all patients in this series.

The dose reference point varied with tumor site and the size and position of the applicator in the nasopharyngeal cavity. In this series, the dose reference point distance was 10–12 mm from the applicator in most patients (90% of treatment). The dose in the reference point was 8 Gy per fraction for most patients (178 of 232 fractions, 76.7%), less than 8 Gy per fraction in 28 patients (12%), and more than 8 Gy per fraction in 34 patients (15%; mainly in cases of larger tumors). In addition to a series of tumor dose points, 8 other anatomical points were used in our department to evaluate the dose distribution in the tumor and in surrounding radiation-sensitive structures (Fig. 29).

The local control rate proved to be 95% (96 of 101) (Table 9). Local failure was observed in 5 patients. Three patients experienced local recurrence after

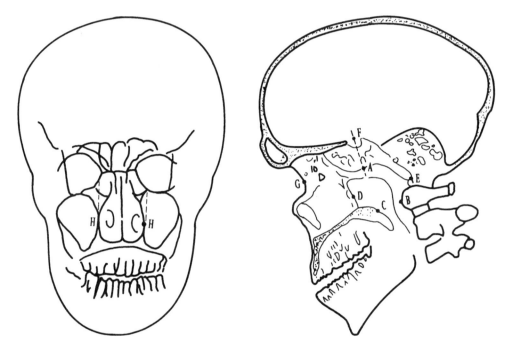

**Fig. 29.** Normal tissue points nasopharynx in which the dose is calculated for endocavitary brachytherapy nasopharynx.

### Table 9

#### Local Control Rates of 101 Nasopharyngeal Carcinomas Following Brachytherapy

| Follow-up (mos) | After 1 course of EBRT | | After 2 courses of EBRT | | | Randomized | |
| | Residual | Recurrence | Residual | Recurrence | Boost | Trial | Total |
|---|---|---|---|---|---|---|---|
| 6 | 5/5 | 2/2 | 1/1 | — | 2/2 | 8/8 | 18/18 (100) |
| 12 | 9/9 | 5/5 | 1/2 | — | 2/2 | 15/15 | 32/33 (97) |
| 24 | 13/13 | 4/4 | 1/1 | 1/3 | 3/3 | 3/3 | 25/27 (93) |
| 36 | 11/11 | 2/2 | 2/2 | 2/3 | 4/5 | 0 | 21/23 (91) |
| Total (%) | 38/38 (100) | 13/13 (100) | 5/6 (83) | 3/6 (50) | 11/12 (92) | 26/26 (100) | 96/101 (95) |

EBRT = external beam radiation therapy

previous EBRT; these patients were treated by brachytherapy alone. One patient experienced relapse in the parapharyngeal space and oropharynx. Another was treated for a recurrent tumor in another hospital; no details were available.

Transient side effects, such as nasal obstruction and mild mucositis of the nasopharyngeal mucosa, were seen in most patients. Three patients developed patchy mucositis on the soft palate, which subsided completely within 1 or 2 weeks after completion of the brachytherapy. Four patients who were treated during the earlier phase of brachytherapy protocol developed perforation of the soft palate (Table 10).

## The Hunan Experience

Dr. Lei Yan-fan of Hunan Medical University reported on 390 patients treated by a cobalt-60 machine and intracavitary brachytherapy with a cumulative dose of 80–85 Gy; 302 patients treated by EBRT only served as a control series. The results are shown in Table 11. Ninety-nine patients with recurrent tumor after radiotherapy were retreated by EBRT and intracavitary treatment.

### Table 10
#### Clinical Materials of the Patients with Soft Palate Perforation

| Points | External Beam Irradiation | Intracavitary Irradiation | Interval Between Last Treatment and Perforation (mos) | Present Status | Survival (yrs) |
|--------|---------------------------|---------------------------|------------------------------------------------------|----------------|----------------|
| 1 | 155 Gy/3 courses/25 yr | 40 Gy/ 4F/4W | 6 | hemorrhage | 6.5 |
| 2 | 150 Gy/2 courses/5.5 yr | 32 Gy/ 4F/4W | 4.5 | multiple metastasis | 5.5 |
| 3* | 70 Gy/53 days | 23 Gy/3F/3W | 9 | free from tumor | 3 |
| 4+ | 70 Gy/50 days | 30 Gy/3F/3W | 30 | free from tumor | 3 |

*Residual tumor on soft palate
+Residual tumor

### Table 11
#### Survival Rates of Carcinoma of Nasopharynx Treated by Telecobalt Alone or in Combination with Intracavitary Treatment

| Survival | External Beam Irradiation Plus Intracavitary Treatment | | External Beam Irradiation Alone | |
|----------|------------------|--------|------------------|--------|
| > 1 yr | 292/316 | 92.4% | 225/245 | 91.8% |
| > 2 yrs* | 189/260 | 72.7% | 102/173 | 59% |
| > 3 yrs | 43/70 | 61.4% | 45/95 | 47.4% |

*p< 0.05

A 1-year survival rate of 76.7% (56 of 73 patients), a 2-year survival rate of 48.8% (20 of 41 patients), and a 3-year survival rate of 37.9% (11 of 29 patients) were observed. The response rates after treatment are shown in Table 12. Complications were perforation of the soft palate (1 patient) and fibrosis and stenosis of the nasal cavity (2 patients).

## The Sichuan Experience

Dr. Wang Jong-bo of Sichuan Cancer Hospital reported on T1 and T2 lesions treated with an EBRT dose of 50 Gy for 5 weeks and T3 and T4 lesions with 56 Gy for 5.5 weeks. Subsequently, the patients were treated by intracavitary HDR at a dose of 6 Gy twice weekly; for T1 and T2 cancers 24 Gy was given; for T3 and T4 tumors 18 Gy was given. Sixty-one patients had been followed for more than 2 years. The 2-year survival rate was 80% (49 of 61 patients); the 2-year disease-free survival rate was 78.6% (48 of 61 patients), and the local control rate at 2 years was 92% (56 of 61 patients). Complications included fibrosis of the uvula in 2 patients and perforation of the soft palate in one.

## Conclusion

It is too early to make definitive statements with regard to tumor control and side effects for patients treated by interstitial or endocavitary fractionated HDR or PDR brachytherapy as opposed to our previous experience with LDR brachytherapy. Preliminary results, however, show excellent control rates and do not warrant a change of policy. The group at DDHCC/UHR will preferentially treat cancers of the head and neck by HDR or PDR brachytherapy. For IRT brachytherapy, a PDR regime is preferred. However, since there is only one microSelectron PDR in this center, logistic reasons (i.e., unavailability of the microSelectron) may dictate that patients be treated according to the fractionated HDR protocol. It should be emphasized that both treatment protocols are experimental and should be evaluated cautiously and prospectively relative to

### Table 12

#### The 3-Month Complete Response Rates of Carcinoma of Nasopharynx After Treatment

|  | Complete Response Rates | | | | Total |
|  | Stage I | Stage II | Stage III | Stage IV | |
|---|---|---|---|---|---|
| External + Brachytherapy | 25/25 100% | 93/95 97% | 207/230 90% | 36/40 90% | 361/390 92.6% |
| External Alone | 21/22 95.5% | 41/45 91.1% | 133/170 78.2% | 54/64 84.3% | 249/301 82.7% |

the worldwide experience with LDR brachytherapy, both with regard to tumor control and with respect to late side effects. Also, it should always be remembered that technological progress such as optimization of dose distributions is no substitute for poor implants.

High dose rate brachytherapy at fractions of 3 Gy or less appears safe and effective in the dose range used by the New York group. It provides reasonable palliation for patients with recurrent disease and, thus far, a high rate of local control without complications in the limited number of previously untreated patients.

The British Columbia experience shows that a single HDR brachytherapy boost concurrent to EBRT for NPC is safe and appears to enhance local control and that acute and late effects of HDR can be reasonably predicted by the linear quadratic equation. Although HDR brachytherapy alone is feasible, more than 7 fractions may be required with HDR to achieve a similar therapeutic ratio as LDR continuous irradiation for the primary treatment of mouth cancer.

## REFERENCES

1. Perez CA, Venkata RD, Marcial-Vega V, et al. Carcinoma of the nasopharynx: factors affecting prognosis. Int J Radiat Oncol Biol Phys 23:271-280, 1992.
2. Wang CC. Improved local control of nasopharyngeal carcinoma after intracavitary brachytherapy boost. Am J Clin Oncol 14(1):5-8, 1991.
3. Pryzant RM, Wendt CD, Delclos L, et al. Retreatment of nasopharyngeal carcinoma in 53 patients. Int J Radiat Oncol Biol Phys 22:941-947, 1992.
4. Levendag PC, Meeuwis CA, Visser AG. Reirradiation in recurrent head and neck cancer: external and/or interstitial radiation therapy. Radiother Oncol 23:6-15, 1992.
5. Levendag PC, Putten WLJ. Brachytherapy in head and neck cancer: Rotterdam low dose rate experience. In: Martinez AA, Orton CG, Mould RF, eds. Brachytherapy HDR and LDR. Columbia, Md.: Nucletron Corp.;1990, 325-344.
6. Brenner D, Hall E. Conditions for the equivalence of continuous to pulsed low dose rate brachytherapy. Int J Radiat Oncol Biol Phys 20:181-190, 1991.
7. Flores AD, Dickson R, Riding K, et al. Cancer of the nasopharynx in British Columbia. Am J Clin Oncol 9:281-291, 1986.
8. Flores AD, Nelems B, Evans K, et al. Impact of new radiotherapy modalities on the surgical management of cancer of the esophagus and cardia. Int J Radiat Oncol Biol Phys 17:937-944, 1989.
9. Yin Wei-bo. Brachytherapy Working Conference, 2nd People's Republic of China Selectron User's Meeting, April, 1992. The Development of Modern Brachytherapy in China and Its Problems. Shanghai, China: Nucletron Far East; in press.
10. Gao Li, Xu Guo-zhen, Yin Wei-bo, et al. Preliminary experience in HDR brachytherapy for 72 nasopharyngeal carcinoma patients. In: Mould RF, ed. Brachytherapy in the People's Republic of China. Kowloon, China: Nucletron Far East; 1992, E76-81.

# Chapter 10

# High Dose Rate Brachytherapy for Carcinoma of the Esophagus

*Albino D. Flores, Chris G. Rowland, and Wei-bo Yin*

## Introduction

Cancer of the esophagus comprises approximately 1.5% of all cancers in North America, and the incidence rates for males and females have been 4.5 and 1.5 per 100,000 males and females in the population, respectively. Although squamous cell carcinomas have predominated in the past, the incidence of adenocarcinomas has significantly increased in North America during the last decade.[1] Cancer of the esophagus is found in many regions of the world, and higher incidence rates have been observed in certain specific regions of Iran, the former Soviet Union, South Africa, and China. Many environmental factors have been associated with the disease, including alcohol intake, smoking, and dietary factors. Achalasia, lye ingestion, and Barrett's esophageal epithelium have long been recognized as precursors. Previous gastrectomy, hiatus hernia, or conditions associated with esophageal reflux also appear to be conditioning factors. All of these factors suggest that prevention and screening for early detection of the population at higher risk is possible and may need to be pursued. This may be particularly important as the majority of patients with carcinoma of the esophagus are usually diagnosed late and with an already incurable disease. This chapter will review the natural history of the disease patterns of failure, past and present therapeutic trends, and experiences and treatment results with high dose rate (HDR) brachytherapy in three different institutions around the world.

## Background

An extensive review of the world literature in 1980[13] showed that only 4–6 patients out of 100 diagnosed with carcinoma of the esophagus survived 5 years. The treatment results were equally poor in patients treated by either radiotherapy or esophagectomy. The improvements in operative techniques, operative mortality, and/or technological advances during the last 4 decades has not translated into better survival for these patients. During the last decade, conscious efforts have been made to improve these poor results by combining

From: Nag, S. (ed.): *High Dose Rate Brachytherapy: A Textbook*, Futura Publishing Company, Inc., Armonk, NY, © 1994.

different treatment modalities. Although encouraging preliminary results have been reported, using chemotherapy as an adjuvant treatment to radiotherapy and/or to surgery,[4-10] unfortunately, overall statistics are still poor,[11-14] and combined therapies have been associated with significant increased morbidity and even mortality.[8,9]

The last decade has also seen the renascence of brachytherapy, the introduction of new and better radioisotopes, and improved technology that has facilitated delivery and optimization of radiotherapy.

## Natural History and Pattern of Failures

Since dysphagia is the main presenting symptom, most patients are diagnosed when the disease is already locally advanced and metastatic. Most of them are old, frail, malnourished, and in very poor condition. Since the esophagus does not have serosa, the disease can extend readily into the adjacent periesophageal tissues and through the rich submucosal lymphatics to the most proximal and distal esophageal wall and perigastric and mediastinal lymph nodes. An analysis of the patterns of failures at several institutions including our own[15-19] shows that most patients die with local recurrence or local recurrence and metastasis as a consequence of esophageal obstruction. In British Columbia, Canada, 83% (401 of 483) of the patients had tumors larger than 5 cm at presentation, and in 60% (288 of 483) the disease had extended beyond the esophageal wall. Even in early and operable cases, lymphatic spread is recognized in 75% of the resected specimens.

## New Therapeutic Trends

The theory behind systemic chemotherapy as an adjuvant treatment to radiation was the hope that it could improve local control by radiosensitization and also could affect microscopic systemic metastatic disease. In recent reports,[6,20] an improvement in local control and even survival has been suggested using adjuvant chemotherapy to radiotherapy. These conclusions have not been shared by others.[11,21,22] There is, however, a consensus among authors that present chemotherapy regimens have not affected metastasis or the development of metastasis in esophageal malignancies.[4-11] Better systemic therapy is clearly needed to enhance tumor response and survival.

Preoperative external irradiation has also been used in the past, and the treatment results have also been mixed. Two phase III European studies[23,24] comparing esophagectomy alone versus preoperative external irradiation suggested no advantage with the treatment combination. In these trials, however, the radiotherapy schedule was short and unusual, and complications (even perioperative mortalities) were high. Three more recent phase III studies, comparing esophagectomy alone with a more standard preoperative external irradiation, reported significant benefit in the group receiving preoperative irradiation.[25-27]

Brachytherapy, using low dose rate (LDR) radioactive materials, alone or in combination with external irradiation has been employed only sporadically in the past. Because of the long treatment time, patients had to be admitted to the hospital, and there was the inevitable problem of radiation exposure to the staff.

In the last few years, the development of safer and higher specific activity radioactive sources has permitted the fabrication of better miniaturized sources; this, in turn, has translated into a shorter treatment time and an improved treatment delivery by remote afterloading systems (Table 1). This technology has made intracavitary irradiation a feasible, easy, and attractive complement to external irradiation in esophageal malignancies.

The rationale of adding brachytherapy to radiotherapy is based on the fact that the amount of irradiation that can be safely given by external irradiation is limited by the tolerance of the periesophageal tissues; brachytherapy, on the other hand, owing to its rapid dose fall-off, can increase the amount of irradiation to the intraluminal disease without significantly affecting the adjacent normal tissues. In other words, brachytherapy can enhance the therapeutic ratio of external irradiation.

## The Vancouver Experience with HDR Brachytherapy— Albino D. Flores

### Materials and Methods

Before 1984, intracavitary irradiation for cancer of the esophagus was used sporadically and used only for recurrent disease. It consisted of LDR radium or cesium tubes that were placed in tandem in an esophageal tube to deliver a dose of 3,000 cGy at 1 cm from the axis in 48 hours (Fig. 1). This treatment time required the patient to be hospitalized but was well tolerated. The palliative effect was brief since patients had advanced recurrent disease. An esophageal applicator[28] became available to us in February of 1985. This device could be connected to a remote afterloading system containing radioactive cesium-137 pellets 4 mm in diameter. These pellets each had 40 MCi of Ra equivalent and, when placed in tandem (40 pellets for a 10-cm linear source),

---

### Table 1
### Linear Activities for Different Radioactive Isotopes

| Source | Linear Activity | |
|---|---|---|
| ¹³⁷Cs tubes | 21 MCi/cm | 770 MBq/cm |
| ¹³⁷Cs selectron pellets (4 pellets per cm) | 126 MCi/cm | 4660 MBq/cm |
| ¹⁹²Ir (10 Ci/4mm) | 20 Ci/cm | 74,000 MBq/cm |

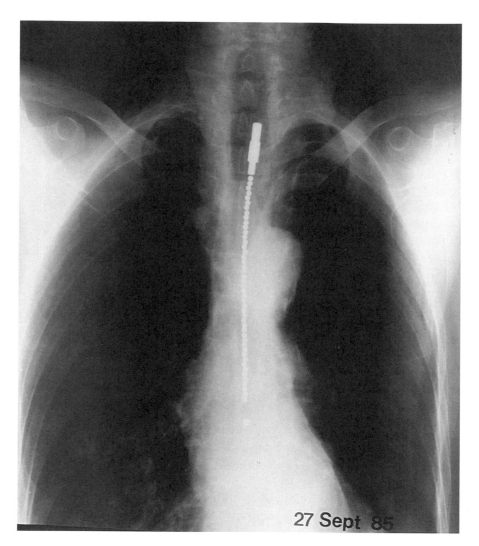

27 Sept 85

**Fig. 1.** Esophageal tube with dummy sources to simulate cesium-137 pellets (HDR 1,000 cGy hr).

could generate a dose rate of 1,000 cGy per hour at 1 cm from the axis of the source. A similar device is used now with HDR iridium-192 (Fig. 2).

Because higher biological effects are expected with higher dose rates, it was necessary in designing new treatment protocols to estimate equivalent doses for higher dose rates against safer and well-tried LDR regimens. This was accomplished using a linear quadratic model.[29] Figure 3 shows that 3,000 cGy given with LDR radioactive materials is equivalent to 1,500 cGy given with HDR if one assumes an a/b ratio of 4 for late effects and 10 for acute effects. It also can be seen that while the biological effect changes significantly from a dose rate of 100 cGy/hr to 1,000 cGy/hr, the isoeffect curve flattens and there

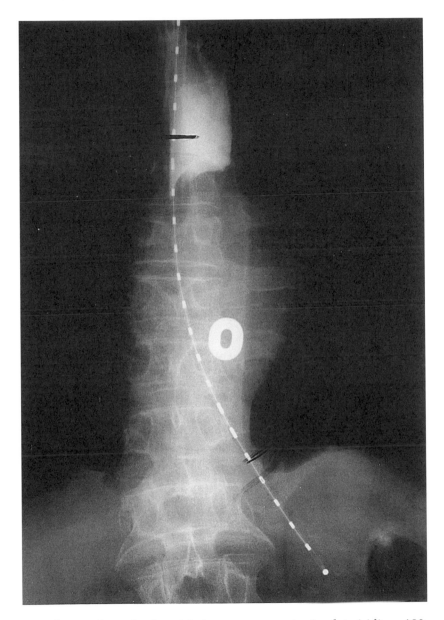

**Fig. 2.** Similar esophageal tube with dummy sources to simulate iridium-192 source positions (HDR > 20,000 cGy/hr).

is practically no change in effect beyond 1,000 cGy/hr. In 1975 a phase I study was started in Vancouver to evaluate external irradiation of 4,000 cGy in 3 weeks plus brachytherapy of 1,500 cGy at 1 cm from the axis (Fig.4). The main goals of this initial program were to evaluate the toxicity and effectiveness of this treatment and to assess the quality of life of the patients treated. Only pa-

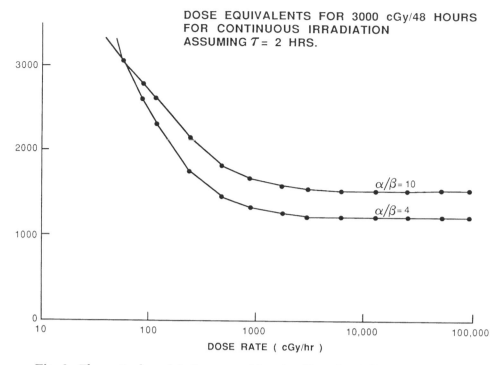

**Fig. 3.** Theoretical model of acute and late isoeffects for different dose rates.

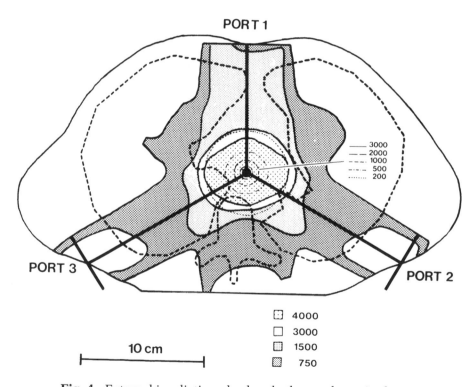

**Fig. 4.** External irradiation plus brachytherapy boost isodoses.

tients with bronchial or tracheal fistulas or impending bronchial or tracheal fistulas were excluded from the study. The results of treatment in 171 patients have already been reported.[19]

Because dysphagia was the major symptom these patients have, there is a practical advantage to starting treatment with intracavitary irradiation in patients who have severe obstruction. The esophageal applicator is also a mild dilator, and dysphagia can immediately improve after brachytherapy. On the other hand, brachytherapy may be more effective after an initial course of external irradiation, since shrinkage of the tumor bulk allows a better dose at the base of the tumor.

To determine the best timing of brachytherapy, a phase III study was started in 1987 to compare two groups of patients: one group of patients receiving brachytherapy before radiotherapy and a second group receiving brachytherapy after radiotherapy. The brachytherapy dose was 1,500 cGy at 1 cm from the axis, and the external irradiation component was 4,000 cGy given in 15 treatment days in 3 weeks overall time. The objective of this study was to compare local control, survival, and quality of life of the patients. This trial has now accrued 200 patients and has been closed. However, an interim analysis is not yet possible.

## Treatment Results

An analysis of the first 171 patients treated[19] showed that intracavitary irradiation was a feasible outpatient treatment with acceptable morbidity and no mortality. The quality of life of the patients treated by brachytherapy, as measured by their performance status, swallowing ability, and pain, was significantly better after treatment. From 1985 to 1992, more than 600 patients with carcinomas in the esophagus and/or cardia have been treated at the Cancer Agency in Vancouver with intracavitary irradiation. Of these patients, the first 150 patients were treated with radioactive cesium pellets generating a dose rate of 1,000 cGy per hour. All subsequent patients (450) received treatment with an HDR iridium source producing between 20,000–50,000 cGy per hour (Fig. 5). However, the dose given at 1 cm from the source was the same as estimated by the linear quadratic model, or 1,500 cGy (given in an overall time of a very few minutes).

Since we have not seen any significant difference in acute or late effects among patients treated with either LDR (radium, cesium), medium dose rate (MDR) (cesium pellets) or HDR (iridium), we have to assume that the linear quadratic formula has reasonably predicted the isoeffect values for different dose rates.

From 1985 to 1989, 297 patients with carcinomas of the esophagus and cardia were treated with radiotherapy and brachytherapy at our institute and were eligible for an analysis with a minimum follow-up of at least 3 years from treatment. The site distribution, clinical status at presentation, type of treatment, and outcome of all these cases is shown in Table 2. Thirty-one percent (93 of 297) of the patients had their tumor located above the tracheal bifurca-

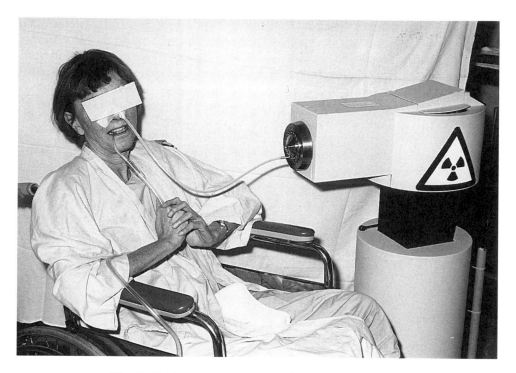

**Fig. 5.** Patient on treatment with HDR iridium-192.

tion and were treated only by radiotherapy, as is the policy in our center. Forty had only palliative treatment, and 53 had radical treatment by radiotherapy and brachytherapy. Only 2 of these patients survived the disease at 5 years. Most patients (204 or 68%) had their tumor located below the tracheal bifurcation. The majority of them had an inoperable, locally advanced, or metastatic disease, and received only radiotherapy (radiation therapy plus brachytherapy). Eight out of 85 or 9.4% were alive with no evidence of disease (NED) at the time of the analysis. Only 90 (30%) of patients had a potentially resectable lesion, and 66 of them had their tumor actually resected following radiotherapy and brachytherapy. Only one patient died because of complications related to this treatment. Three of the patients had liver metastasis at the time of the operation, and none of them survived more than 4 months. Of the 63 patients who had a resection with curative intent, 32 are still alive NED for more than 3 years (median survival time of 43 months).

## The Exeter Experience: Palliative Brachytherapy— Chris G. Rowland

The sometimes encouraging reports on survival impact in cancer of the esophagus tend to be highly anecdotal in very selected series. A more realistic picture can be seen in larger series drawn from experience in the overall man-

**Table 2**

**Distribution Analysis of Esophageal and Cardia Carcinomas,
Treatment, and Outcome**

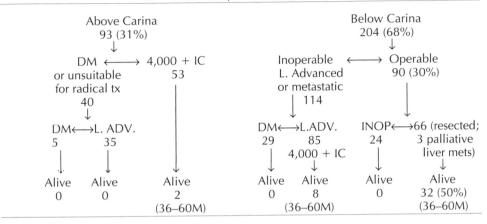

agement of esophageal cancer in larger hospitals with thoracic surgery and radiation/medical oncology services (in Britain referred to as "clinical oncology"). In the majority of cases, the patients are elderly, of poor performance status, socially deprived, and with stage 3 or 4 disease (at times I wonder whether there is need for a stage 5 category). The inability to swallow even saliva must surely be one of the most awful symptoms of any cancer to be inflicted during what is often the dying process.

The cancerous esophagus is pragmatically best considered as a blocked tube that needs to be effectively reamed out as simply and quickly as possible with minimal morbidity or mortality. The treatment should relieve dysphagia until death and should require only a single application. Many techniques exist (external beam, laser, tube, electrocoagulation, ethanol injection), but the criteria are best met by intraluminal brachytherapy.

The history of esophageal applicators dates to around 1907 when Hartigan's applicator was described for use in inaccessible situations. Other well-known exponents were Guisez and Finzi.[30] Gold-198 wire encased in a plastic tube wrapped around Souttar's tube was used in the 1960s by Ledermann et al.[31]

Modern radiological protection legislation would have referred this technique to the history books had it not been for the development of modern afterloading equipment such as the Selectron and GammaMed machines. Our Exeter experience lies with the former, initially in its LDR guise and more recently in its HDR guise.

## Technique

Investigative procedures such as a barium swallow may be used as an adjunct to flexible endoscopic measurement of the extent of the tumor and placement of a guide wire to allow applicator insertion. Dilatation was rarely used and is of doubtful benefit in relieving symptoms especially in view of the later data with nasogastric tubes (no dilatation). The original applicator was 8 mm in diameter to transmit the Cs[137] sources.[28] It allows treatment of a 13-cm length or, after movement, a further 13 cm, giving an overall length of 26 cm. Radiological screening allows confirmation of the length to be treated. This procedure is carried out under general anesthesia, a possible disadvantage in certain circumstances. The applicator exits through the mouth (an insert is vital to protect against unwitting biting of the tube) and is fixed in place by a plastic face mask.

The patient is connected to the LDR Selectron and observed via closed circuit television (CCTV) during treatment. Using cesium sources, a dose of 15 Gy at 1 cm off axis is given, the treatment time being a mean of about 1.5 hours depending on the length treated, source activity, and decay factors. The dose of 15 Gy was chosen upon consideration of single fraction external beam radiation (EBR) to the chest (Hunter R, personal communication, Christie Hospital, Manchester, England).

The use of an HDR Selectron has allowed simplification of this technique with no obvious change in outcome. A standard nasogastric tube is passed under a local anaesthetic and the treatment length determined radiologically. The treatment time is a much more tolerable 10–20 minutes, again depending on source activity and length.[32]

## Results

In our initial study a significant relief of dysphagia was observed at 6 weeks in 70% of squamous cancer and 60% of adenocarcinoma (mainly cardia not extending significantly to the stomach). About 10% survive symptom free at 1 year, which I feel reflects tumor biology and shows how this group, in particular, may bias trials of radical treatment.[28] Questions about assessment of response in these patients (a simple 0–3 scale) continue to be debated.[33]

Toxicities seemed mainly to be related to the placement of the applicator and are much reduced with the nasogastric tube. We observed one fistula (previous radiation for breast cancer with parasternal fields), one perforation (settled with conservative treatment), and two strictures successfully dilated. Other workers describe a higher incidence of side effects,[34] but this often relates to multimodality treatment, and the contribution of each modality remains unclear.

## The China Experience with Brachytherapy—Wei-bo Yin

### Brachytherapy Alone

From May 1970 to August 1974, a mass screening program for esophageal cancer was conducted in the rural area of Linxian County, China. Since external irradiation facilities were not available in that region, 203 patients diagnosed with cancer of the esophagus were treated by brachytherapy alone.[35]

## Clinical Materials

There were 129 male patients (63.5%) and 74 female patients (36.5%). The diagnosis was confirmed in 146 out of 203 (71%) of these patients by histopathology and the other clinical materials shown in Table 3.

## Method

A plastic tube tipped with a condom filled with water or air to increase the treatment distance to 10 mm was used (Fig. 6). Two finer plastic tubes sealed with cobalt-60 wires were introduced one after another into the outer tube with a condom. The specification of the cobalt-60 tubes are given in Table 4. The length of the lesion was marked on the skin of the patient under the fluoroscope. The patient's nose and throat were anesthetized by 1% xylocaine. Guided by the skin markers under fluoroscopy, the outer tube was inserted into the esophagus of the patient and fixed. Then the patient was transferred into the treatment room, and the cobalt-60 tube was introduced

### Table 3
### Distribution of Cases Treated by Brachytherapy Alone

| Tumor site | No. of tumors from a total series of 208 | % |
|---|---|---|
| Neck | 2 | 0.96 |
| Upper third | 34 | 16.30 |
| Middle third | 139 | 67.50 |
| Lower third | 33 | 15.80 |

| Tumor length | No. of tumors from a total series of 207 | % |
|---|---|---|
| Less than 3 cm | 44 | 21.4 |
| 3–5 cm | 92 | 44.4 |
| 5–8 cm | 62 | 30.0 |
| Greater than 8 cm | 9 | 4.4 |

| Difficulty in swallowing | No. of patients | % |
|---|---|---|
| Solid food | 97 | 47.9 |
| Semiliquid food | 76 | 37.4 |
| liquid | 16 | 7.9 |
| liquid in difficulty | 14 | 6.9 |

* 5 patients had two tumors.
** 1 patient had complete obstruction, and the tumor length could not be measured.

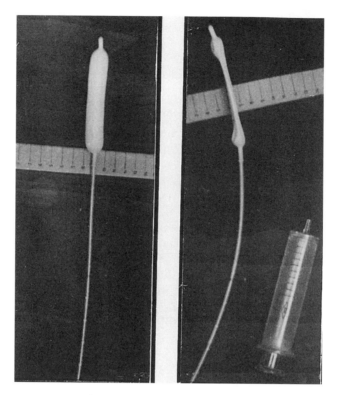

**Fig. 6.** Brachytherapy esophageal tube with balloon dilator.

## Table 4
### Dose Specification for Cobalt 60 Tubes

| Tube length (cm) | Tube activity (mg radium equivalent) | Dose rate at 2.5 cm (cGy/hour) |
|---|---|---|
| 5 | 83 | 750 |
| 7 | 124 | 786 |

into the outer tube. A rubber tube was connected with the outer tube, and the balloon was filled with water or air. The rubber tube was clamped, and treatment started (Fig.7).

## Treatment

Patients were treated for 8 hours per application with an interval of 1 week between the applications. The total number of applications was 2 to 4.

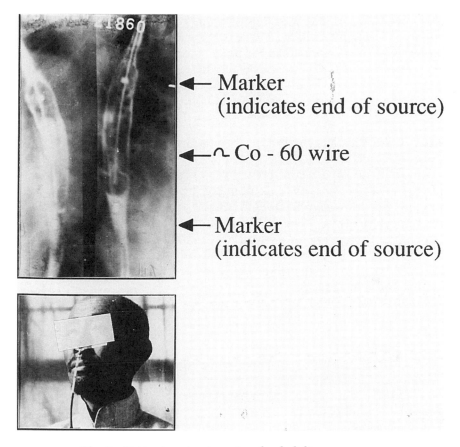

**Fig. 7.** Patient on treatment and cobalt linear source.

## Results

Nine in our series of 203 patients were lost to follow-up. If we assume that these patients have died, we have the following surviving patients: 70, 28, and 17 at 1, 3, and 5 years, respectively. This equates to survival rates of 34.5% (1-year survival), 13.8% (3-year survival), and 8.4% (5-year survival).

## Complications

Acute esophagitis was observed from the third day to 1 month posttreatment. Severe pain on swallowing was experienced by 134 patients (66%) and chest and back pain in 100 patients (49%). Esophagopharyngoscopy was requested in 21 patients, and congestion, erosion, and pseudomembrane were observed in the irradiated area. Sometimes infusion, antibiotics, and steroids were used for relief of their symptoms. Strictures developed in 23 patients as late sequelae to treatment. Local failure was the common cause of death, occurring in 143 patients, which represented 70% of our total series. The survival rates of this series were similar to that of external beam irradiation, but it should be pointed out that this series included some earlier lesions. Owing to the lack of experience, the distance of the reference point was far and dose per fraction and total dose were high, so that complications were severe.

### External Beam Plus Brachytherapy Versus Brachytherapy Alone

A study of external beam therapy plus brachytherapy versus brachytherapy alone for the treatment of carcinoma of the esophagus was conducted from November 1982 to November 1986 in the Department of Radiation Oncology, Shanxi Cancer Hospital.[36] The design of this randomized clinical trial was such that 200 patients were entered, with 100 patients in each group having their tumor confirmed by histopathology or positive cytology. All patients were followed up to 1989; the distribution by sex, age, tumor length, and tumor location is given in Table 5.

### Treatment

The external beam plus brachytherapy group was treated using a 10 MV x-ray isocentric technique with one anterior and two posterior oblique fields. The prescribed tumor dose was 5,000 cGy in 25 fractions over a period of 5 weeks. This was followed by brachytherapy, one application per week with a total of three to four applications, delivering a dose of 1,962 cGy or 2,616 cGy. The brachytherapy equipment was a Gynatron afterloader containing a 150

---

**Table 5**

**Distribution of Patients Treated by a Randomized Trial at the Shanxi Cancer Hospital**

| | Arm of the Clinical Trial | |
| Parameter | External + brachytherapy | External beam alone |
| --- | --- | --- |
| Sex: Male | 63 | 65 |
|     Female | 37 | 35 |
| Age | 37–70 | 37–71 |
| Tumor length: < 3 cm | 31 | 25 |
|     5 cm | 62 | 64 |
|     > 7 cm | 5 | 9 |
| Tumor site: Upper third | 20 | 21 |
|     Middle third | 76 | 74 |
|     Lower third | 4 | 5 |
| Number of patients | 100 | 100 |

MCi source of cesium-137. The external beam alone group was treated by the same 10 MV x-ray technique, delivering a tumor dose of 7,000 cGy in 35 fractions over a period of 7 weeks.

## Results

Numerically, the external beam therapy plus brachytherapy arm gave better survival results at 1, 3, and 5 years (Table 6). However, statistically significant differences were only in 1- and 3-year survival rates, not in the 5-year survival rate. The local control was higher in the group receiving external beam plus brachytherapy (Table 7).

## Brachytherapy for Recurrent Esophageal Carcinoma after External Beam Irradiation

Dr. Yan Zong-yi of the Cancer Hospital at the Chinese Academy of Medical Sciences reported that 28 patients with recurrent carcinoma of the esophagus after radiotherapy were retreated by brachytherapy. HDR was used: 600 cGy per fraction, one fraction per week, 3–4 fractions in total. The average

### Table 6
### Treatment Results and Survival

| Arm of the clinical trial | No. of patients | No. of surviving patients | | | % survival rate | | |
|---|---|---|---|---|---|---|---|
| | | 1 yr | 3 yrs | 5 yrs | 1 yr | 3 yrs | 5 yrs |
| External beam + brachytherapy | 100 | 78 | 31 | 15/88 | 78 | 31 | 17 |
| External beam alone | 100 | 56 | 19 | 9/89 | 56 | 19 | 10 |
| P | | <0.01 | <0.05 | <0.05 | | | |

### Table 7
### Causes of Death

| | External beam + brachytherapy (79 pts) | | External beam alone (88 pts) | |
|---|---|---|---|---|
| Local recurrence | 34 | 43% | 54 | 61.3 |
| Distant metastasis | 17 | 21.5% | 12 | 13.6% |
| Hemorrhage | 5 | 6.3% | 7 | 8.0% |
| Perforation | 5 | 6.3% | 4 | 4.6% |
| Miscellaneous | 18 | 22.6% | 11 | 12.5% |

survival was 7.1 ± 4.2 months as compared with 4.5 ± 4.4 months for the un-treated control group. Retreatment by EBR produced similar results (6.6 ± 4.7 months). Intracavitary irradiation caused radiation ulceration in one patient (confirmed by surgery). Ulceration and perforation of esopharyngeal tissues developed with recurrence. Dr. Fan Ke-cheng of Cancer Hospital, Shanghai Medical University, reported 27 patients with local recurrent carcinoma of the esophagus retreated by intracavitary irradiation. The symptoms improved in 92.5%; esophagograms improved in 40%. Twenty-three patients died: 10 of lo-cal obstruction due to cancer, 3 of fatal hemorrhage, 1 of esophagotracheal fistula, 3 of liver metastasis, 1 of lung metastasis, 3 of lung infection, and 1 of cardiac disease.

## Conclusions

Since most patients who have cancer of the esophagus and cardia have an advanced disease and a very poor prognosis, the main goal of treatment should be an improvement of their quality of life. Unfortunately, of 3,941 recent esophageal papers, only 20 have addressed the quality of life and therapy. Al-though some degree of morbidity is acceptable, it is entirely unjustified to ac-cept a palliative treatment that has the potential risk of mortality. The simplicity of intracavitary irradiation, the convenience of the short treatment time, plus the radiation safety provided by the remote afterloading systems, make this treatment ideal for palliative situations such as cancer of the esophagus.

Our clinical experience over the last 6 years using the combination of in-tracavitary and external irradiation for cancer of the esophagus and cardia has demonstrated to us that this treatment is safe, has low morbidity, and appears to provide an adequate and reasonable palliation for these patients' symptoms. The combination of external radiotherapy and brachytherapy has obvious ad-vantages over conventional external radiotherapy alone. It is also superior to surgery in metastatic or unresectable conditions; and, since it does not increase either the morbidity or the mortality associated with esophagectomy, it pro-vides a better selection of cases for esophagectomy by limiting its use to only potentially curable cases. The anatomical location of the upper esophagus and its closeness to the membranous portion of the trachea with esophagectomy for these lesions may contraindicate surgical management.

In Canada in 1985, it was agreed to use the tracheal bifurcation (carina) to divide the esophagus into two specific sites for the design and development of clinical trials (Fig.8). Patients with tumors above the tracheal bifurcation could be allocated to radiotherapy-based protocols and adjuvant programs that could include chemotherapy, hyperthermia, and/or sensitizers. Patients with tumors below the tracheal bifurcation, however, could be considered for surgically based protocols with an adjuvant program using irradiation preop-eratively, in the form of external radiation and brachytherapy. Since a signifi-cant number of patients also die with metastatic disease, chemotherapy could be added as soon as the ideal combination is found. The advantages of HDR brachytherapy are

# CCABC TRIALS

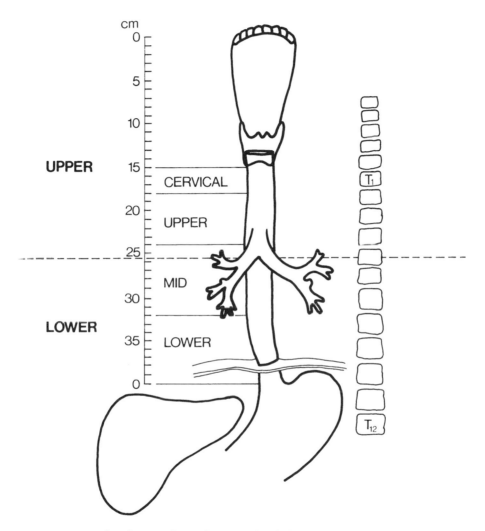

**Fig. 8.** Strategic plan for esophageal protocols. If the center of the tumor is above the carina, radiotherapy-based protocols are proposed. If it is below, then surgical-based protocols will predominate.

(1) short out-patient treatments with minimal supportive care;

(2) a stable and accurately reproducible treatment position;

(3) the tumor is actually treated, not cut or bypassed;

(4) all radiation protection standards are met, particularly for the staff;

(5) cost effectiveness (In Exeter, palliative intubation costs £1,500 as compared to £250 for intracavitary irradiation. The benefit is obvious to health care providers);

(6) the technique is safe for use in general hospitals and not restricted to tertiary referral centers.

Although there are many surgical options for esophagectomy, our preference is to use transhiatal total esophagectomy with extrathoracic anastomosis in the neck for patients receiving preoperative irradiation. This has the advantage of reducing leaks and pulmonary complications; and, because it more adequately removes the remaining proximal esophageal mucosa, it reduces the possibility of local recurrence at the level of the anastomosis. Since there is no difference in the survival rates or local control obtained by the so-called radical en bloc esophagectomy with mediastinal radical dissection versus transhiatal esophagectomy, we feel that this latter procedure should be the preferred choice after irradiation.

Finally, our experience with HDR brachytherapy for cancer of the esophagus and cardia appears to support the following conclusions.

(1) Brachytherapy is an effective palliative treatment for patients with carcinomas of the esophagus and cardia.

(2) The linear quadratic formula can reasonably predict the isoeffects values for different dose rates.

(3) The addition of brachytherapy to external irradiation permits enhancement of local control without increasing operative morbidity nor mortality.

(4) The value of systemic chemotherapy as an adjuvant treatment to external radiotherapy and brachytherapy needs to be explored.

The latest planning systems allow a degree of conformal therapy, providing a higher dose in the tumor volume with a reduced dose in the normal esophagus (the site of anastomotic recurrence). Integration with external beam radiation therapy, hyperthermia, and chemotherapy shows rapid relief of dysphagia (appreciated by the patient) in the 6–8 week period of chemotherapy; normal alimentation; some tumor control in the worrisome delay period before surgery; surgical downstaging; and no increased difficulties in surgical procedure. High dose rate brachytherapy still has much to offer, and its full potential is yet to be exploited.

---

## REFERENCES

1. Blot WJ, Devesa SS, Kneller R, et al. Rising incidence of carcinoma of the esophagus and cardia. JAMA 265:1287-1289, 1991.
2. Earlam R, Cunnha-Melo JR. Esophageal squamous carcinoma: a critical review of radiotherapy. Br J Surg 67:457-461, 1980.
3. Earlam R, Cunnha-Melo JR. Esophageal squamous carcinoma: a critical review of surgery. Br J Surg 67:381-390, 1980.
4. Keane TJ, Harwood AR, et al. Radiation therapy with 5-FU infusion and mitomycin C for esophageal squamous carcinoma. Radiother Oncol 4:205-210, 1985.
5. Seydel H, Leichman K, et al. The Radiation Therapy Oncology Group. Preoperative radiation and chemotherapy for localized squamous cell carcinoma of the esophagus: a RTOG study. Int J Radiat Oncol Biol Phys 14:33-35, 1987.

6. Herskovic A, Martz K, Al-Sarraf M, et al. Intergroup esophageal study: comparison of radiotherapy (RT) to radio-chemotherapy combination: a phase III trial (abstract). Proc. ASCO, 135, 1991.
7. John MJ, Flam MS, Monry PA, et al. Radiotherapy alone and chemoradiation. Cancer 64:2397-2403, 1989.
8. Forrastiere A, Orringer MB, Perez-Tamayo C, et al. Concurrent chemotherapy and radiation therapy followed by transhiatal esophagectomy local-regional cancer of the esophagus. J Clin Onc 8:119-127, 1990.
9. Orringer MB, Forrastiere AA, Perez-Tamayo C, et al. Chemotherapy and radiation therapy before transhiatal esophagectomy for esophageal carcinoma. Am Thorac Surg 49:348-355, 1990.
10. Roth JA, Ajani JA, Rich TA. Multidisciplinary therapy for esophageal cancer. Adv Surg 23:239-260, 1990.
11. Kelsen DP, Bains M, Burt M. Neoadjuvant treatment for cancer of the esophagus. Semin Surg Oncol 6:268-273, 1990.
12. Matthews HR, Waterhouse JA. Cancer of the esophagus: clinical monograph, vol. 1. London, England: The MacMillan Press Ltd, 1987.
13. Muller JM, Erasmi H, Stelzner M, et al. Surgical therapy of esophageal carcinoma. Br J Surg 77:845-857, 1990.
14. Desai PB, Vyas JJ, et al. Current status of surgical treatment of cancer of esophagus. Semin Surg Oncol 5:359-364, 1989.
15. Mantravadi RVP, Lad T, Briele H, et al. Carcinoma of the esophagus: sites of failure. Int J Radiat Oncol Biol Phys 8:1897-1901, 1982.
16. Isono K, Onoda S, Ishikawa T, et al. Studies on the causes of death from esophageal carcinoma. Cancer 39:2173-2179, 1982.
17. Mandard AM, Chasle J, Marnay J, et al. Autopsy findings in 111 cases of esophageal cancer. Cancer 48:329-335, 1981.
18. Ruol F, Segalin A, Castoro C, et al. Patterns of neoplastic recurrence after radical and palliative resection of the esophagus. In: Sievert FDG. Diseases of the Esophagus. Springer-Verlag; 1988, 714-716.
19. Flores A, Nelems B, Evans K, et al. The impact of new radiotherapy modalities on the surgical management of cancer of the esophagus and cardia. Int J Radiat Oncol Biol Phys 17:937-944, 1989.
20. Coia LR, Engstrom PF, Paul AR, et al. Long term results of infusional 5-FU, mitomycin-C and radiation as primary management of esophageal carcinoma. Int J Radiat Oncol Biol Phys 20:29-36, 1991.
21. Kavanagh B, Anscher M, Leopold K, et al. Patterns of failure following combined modality therapy for esophageal cancer, 1984-1990. Int J Radiat Oncol Biol Phys 24:633-642, 1992.
22. Araujo CM, Souhami L, Gil RA, et al. A randomized trial comparing radiation therapy versus concomitant radiation therapy and chemotherapy in carcinoma of the thoracic esophagus. Cancer 67:2258-2261, 1991.
23. Launois B, Delarue D, Campion J, et al. Preoperative radiotherapy for carcinoma of the esophagus. Surg Gynecol Obstet 2:690-692, 1981.
24. Gignoux M, Roussel A, Paillot B, et al. The value of preoperative radiotherapy in esophageal cancer: results of the EORTC. World J Surg 11:426-432, 1987.
25. Huang GJ, Gu X, Wang L, et al. Combined preoperative irradiation and surgery for esophageal carcinoma. In: Wilkins EW, Wong J, eds. International Trends in General Thoracic Surgery: Esophageal Carcinoma. Philadelphia, Pa.: W.B. Saunders; 1988, 315-318.
26. Wang Mei, Gu Xian-zhi, et al. Randomized clinical trial on the combination of preoperative irradiation and surgery in the treatment of esophageal carcinoma; report on 206 patients. Int J Radiat Oncol Biol Phys 16:325-327, 1988.
27. Yin, Wei-bo. Brachytherapy of carcinoma of the esophagus in China. In: Mould RF, ed. Brachytherapy 2nd Proceedings of the 5th International Working Conference. 1989; 139-141.

28. Rowland CG, Pagliero KM. Intracavitary irradiation in palliation of carcinoma of the esophagus and cardia. Lancet 2:981-983, 1985.
29. Dale RG. The application of the linear quadratic dose-effect equation to fractionated and protracted radiotherapy. Br J Radiol 58:515-528, 1985.
30. Mould R. Esophageal applicators before remote afterloading activity. Activity 6(1):44-47, 1992.
31. Lederman M, Jones C, Mould RF. Carcinoma of the esophagus with special reference to the upper third. Br J Radiol 39:193-204, 1966.
32. Burt PA, Notley HM, Stout R. Br J Radiol 62:748-750, 1989.
33. Jager JJ, Pannebaker M, Rijken J, et al. Palliation in esophageal cancer with a single session of intraluminal irradiation. Radiother Oncol 25(2):134, 1992.
34. Hishikawa Y, Kamikonya N, Tanaka S, et al. Radiotherapy or esophageal carcinoma; role of high dose rate intracavitary irradiation. Radiother Oncol 9:13-20, 1987.
35. Yan-jun Miao, Xian-zhi Gu, Wei-bo Yin, et al. Intracavitary irradiation in the treatment of esophageal cancer. Chin J Oncol 4:45-47, 1982.
36. Rui-fen Zhao, et al. Combination of external irradiation and intracavitary cesium-37 radiotherapy for esopharyngeal carcinoma. Chin J Radiat Onc Phys Biol 2:85-87, 1990.

# Chapter 11

# High Dose Rate Brachytherapy for Lung Cancer

*Minesh P. Mehta, Burton L. Speiser, and Hans N. Macha*

## Introduction

With an annual incidence of more than 160,000 cases and a mortality rate of greater than 80%, lung cancer represents our greatest oncologic challenge.[1] Although metastatic disease is not uncommon, failure to obtain local control continues to be a major issue. Local failure rates between 31% to 51% have been reported in several Radiation Therapy Oncology Group (RTOG) studies.[2] In 300 consecutive autopsies from the Veterans' Administration Lung Group (VALG) protocols,[3] residual intrathoracic tumor was responsible for death in 75% of the patients with squamous cell carcinoma and 50% of the patients with adenocarcinoma and large cell carcinoma of the lung.

Endobronchial occlusion is a common and potentially life-threatening complication, not only for patients with recurrent disease, but also at initial diagnosis. According to one estimate, 20–30% of newly diagnosed lung neoplasms will present with atelectasis and pneumonia, due to endobronchial disease.[4]

Symptomatic occlusion often leads to obstructive pneumonitis and hemoptysis followed by slow asphyxiation and a painful death. With a high rate of local failure using conventional therapies, an estimated 50% of patients with lung cancer will develop symptomatic endobronchial involvement.[5] Therefore, management of the endobronchial and peribronchial component of lung cancer takes on the utmost significance in the palliative setting. Additionally, in selected patients, control of endobronchial disease may translate to an improved rate of cure, although properly designed and conducted studies are lacking in this field.

## Strategies for the Management of Endobronchial Disease

Endobronchial tumors may be controlled by a variety of different methods, either used singly or in combination. There are several commonly reported methods that are tabulated in Table 1. In order to better appreciate the role of

From: Nag, S. (ed.): *High Dose Rate Brachytherapy: A Textbook*, Futura Publishing Company, Inc., Armonk, NY, © 1994.

## Table 1
### Techniques for the Management of Endobronchial Disease

1. Biopsy recanalization
2. Electrocoagulation
3. Cryosurgery
4. Laser therapy
5. Photodynamic therapy
6. Endobronchial prosthesis
7. External beam radiotherapy
8. Brachytherapy

high dose rate (HDR) endobronchial brachytherapy, a summary of these complimentary and competing modalities is provided.

### Biopsy Recanalization

Endobronchial recanalization, using forceps biopsy via a rigid bronchoscope under general anesthesia, was reported by Huzly[6] to produce short-term success. However, the many disadvantages of this method include the inability to access lesions beyond the primary bronchi, the necessity for general anesthesia, the inability to control peribronchial tumors, and an unacceptably high hemoptysis rate. For the most part, this method is no longer frequently used, although some "debulking and resection" continues to be performed at the time of bronchoscopy for placement of brachytherapy catheters. Usually, this does not amount to much beyond a biopsy and gentle suction.

### Electrocoagulation

Endoscopic electrosurgery has been extensively used for the removal of colorectal polyps. Limited reports of its application in the airways exist. The cautery probe can readily be passed through the accessory channel of the fiberoptic bronchoscope. Polypoid lesions can be rather readily sectioned out. The alternative approach is to vaporize the lesion, but the risk of fire in the bronchus exists.

### Cryosurgery

The use of extreme variations in heat and temperature represent further physical methods of endobronchial tumor ablation that have now been used for several years. In general, these techniques also require rigid bronchoscopy and hence, general anesthesia. This limits the level of tumor that can be accessed easily. Additionally, these modalities have no impact on peribronchial tumors.

The basic technique of performing endoscopic cryosurgery involves placement of an insulated cannula containing an inner tube into which pressurized liquid nitrogen is fed. The nitrogen, upon contact with the relatively "hot" tip suddenly vaporizes, resulting in the Joule-Thompson effect, that is, rapid cooling secondary to rapid expansion of a gas. The formation of intracellular and extracellular ice crystals results in direct cellular injury as well as indirect injury by affecting the vasculature. Typically, the endobronchial lesion is destroyed and sloughs off over a period of several days, unlike the immediate results from endobronchial laser photocoagulation. Follow-up bronchoscopy is often necessary to remove the tissue slough. Technical problems, such as the necessity for a rigid bronchoscope as well as the short length of the probe, limit its application.

A prospective study was carried out by Walsh et al.[7] to assess the value of bronchoscopic cryotherapy for palliation of malignant airway occlusion. Symptoms, lung function, and radiographic and bronchoscopic findings were recorded serially before and after 81 cryotherapy sessions in 33 consecutive patients. Most patients improved in terms of overall symptoms, such as stridor and hemoptysis, and they had an overall improvement in dyspnea. Objective improvement in lung function was seen in 58% of patients. Bronchoscopic evidence of relief of obstruction was seen in 77% of patients, and 24% showed improvement in the degree of collapse on the radiograph. There were no major complications. These results compared favorably with the results in published series of patients having laser therapy, and it was concluded that bronchoscopic cryotherapy is valuable for the palliation of inoperable bronchial carcinoma.

Considerable interest still exists in utilizing cryosurgery as an adjunct to other therapies in the management of endobronchial tumors. Vergnon et al.[8] performed a trial of cryotherapy followed by irradiation in inoperable non-small cell lung cancer. Thirty-eight patients were treated first by cryotherapy under general anesthesia and then with external irradiation. The success of cryotherapy as assessed bronchoscopically was found to be 26 out of 38 (68%). Seventeen of these 26 patients (65%) had no bronchial residual tumor after irradiation, as contrasted to all of the patients in the nonresponding group (12 out of 38) having residual tumor even after radiotherapy. Survival in the responders (median = 397 days) was significantly higher than the survival of the nonresponders (median = 144 days). Local control was obtained in 65 percent (17 out of 26) of the responders and was never observed in the nonresponders. These results argue for the possible potentiation of irradiation by cryotherapy, raising the intriguing possibility of combining brachytherapy and cryotherapy.

The combined effect of cryotherapy and chemotherapy was studied in 12 patients with bronchial carcinoma.[9] Radiolabeled ($^{57}$Co) Bleomycin (Bristol Myers) was injected intravenously, and detection was carried out with a gamma camera. Plasma half-life and clearance of $^{57}$Co-Bleomycin, as well as the tumor to normal tissue ratios of bleomycin were calculated. The same measurements were repeated 15 days later, immediately after cryotherapy. A mean increase of 30% of radiolabeled Bleomycin was found in the tumor after cryotherapy. Vascular changes following cryotherapy may explain these results, with trapping of the anticancer drug in the tumor and the surrounding area due to vascular stasis. It seems that chemotherapy may be more effective after cryotherapy, and a multicenter study is in progress in France to evaluate this combination of cryochemotherapy.

### Laser Therapy

A comprehensive review of the subject of laser therapy is beyond the scope of this chapter, but because it represents both a competing and a complimentary modality, a brief review is presented. At present, there are three laser systems used for photoablation of endobronchial tumors: the argon laser, the carbon dioxide laser, and the neodymium: yttrium-aluminum-garnet (Nd:YAG) laser, the common features of which are presented in Table 2.

The argon laser light is rapidly and efficiently absorbed by hemoglobin, thus severely limiting the penetration into tissue. When considerable hemorrhage is encountered, this technique can become considerably flawed. The $CO_2$ laser cannot be conducted using quartz monofilament fibers and thus requires rigid bronchoscopy, with all its limitations. The Nd:YAG laser, which can be used both with the rigid as well as the flexible fiberoptic bronchoscope, has a tissue penetration of several millimeters if the dose is increased and has, therefore, become a "favorite" in endobronchial photoresection.[10-19] Although the Nd:YAG laser may be used with the flexible bronchoscope, it has been our experience, as well as the experience reported by others,[20,21] that the best results may be achieved with the rigid bronchoscope because it permits better visualization, ensures safety by allowing for passage of the bronchoscope beyond the tumor and laser resecting only while it is withdrawn, and allows better hemostasis, suction, ventilation, and removal of large pieces of tumor. As a consequence, laser resection is ideally used for tracheal or proximal bronchial lesions[22,23] beyond which the rigid bronchoscope can be passed. Benign tumors, as well as low-grade malignancies, are often well managed by this technique.[24]

The two primary effects of the Nd:YAG laser on tissue are thermal necrosis and photocoagulation. The latter effect provides hemostasis, thereby making it easy to remove relatively large tumor pieces once they have undergone thermal necrosis. However, these effects are also responsible for the possible

### Table 2
### Common Characteristics of the Three Commonly Employed Endobronchial Laser Systems

| Type of laser | Argon | $CO_2$ | YAG |
|---|---|---|---|
| Spectrum | Blue-green | Far infrared | Near infrared |
| Wavelength (nm) | 514 | 10,600 | 1,064 |
| Penetration (mm) | <1 | <1 | 10 |
| Monofilament conduction | Yes | No | Yes |
| Flexible bronchoscopy | Yes | No | Yes |

hazards of laser resection, that is, severe hemorrhage from vascular perforation and the formation of fistulae. Additionally, laser therapy requires that the proportion of oxygen in inhaled air be less than 50%; in compromised patients, this requirement may lead to hypoxemia. Brutinell and colleagues,[25] in an editorial in the journal *Chest*, warn that "The Nd:Yag laser in the treatment of a tracheo-bronchial neoplasm . . . can also be a dangerous one. After a treatment modality becomes accepted in clinical practice, there is a tendency to become complacent about the risks involved in its use." They report a risk of death from hemorrhage of 2%, fire in the tracheobronchial tree, pneumothorax, esophageal fistula, bronchial perforation, and hypoxemia.

Edell et al.[26] have recently suggested the following guidelines when determining whether a patient should be considered for laser resection.

(1) Airway obstruction is unresponsive to other therapies;
(2) Lesion protrudes into the bronchial lumen without evidence of extension beyond the bronchial cartilage;
(3) Axial length of endobronchial lesion is less than 4 cm;
(4) Patent bronchial lumen is visualized beyond the tumor; and
(5) Functional lung tissue is beyond the obstruction.

The major advantage of laser photoresection is almost immediate relief of airway occlusion, resulting in dramatic symptomatic relief in most patients. For example, in a series of 47 patients undergoing laser resection at the Cleveland Clinic,[27] immediate relief was documented in all 47 patients. In fact, in that particular study, a survival advantage was suggested when laser photoresection preceded radiation therapy as compared to radiation only. However, because of the inherent limitations of laser resection, that is, the inability to resect submucosal and peribronchial disease, the dramatic responses are typically quite short-lived, requiring either multiple resections or the addition of endobronchial radiation. A recent study[28] suggested that when compared with external beam radiation, "faster palliation with fewer side effects is probably achieved with laser therapy," but no supporting data were presented. Although this combination is frequently used, it is unclear whether endobronchial radiation might not eventually achieve the same result, and some reports have even suggested that there may be a higher fistualization risk when the combination approach is used.[29]

## Photodynamic Therapy

Photodynamic therapy involves the excitation of a photosensitizer chemical by light, which results in the production of a chemical species capable of interacting with oxygen to produce radicals that cause cellular death and damage.[30-33] The primary targets are believed to be cellular and mitochondrial membranes, but damage to nucleic acids and proteins is also involved.[34-38] Although several chemicals such as methylene blue, eosin, tetracycline, and chlorophylls have been described as possessing these properties, most interest has focused on the hematoporphyrin derivatives[39] that tend to accumulate in neoplastic tissue after intravenous administration. The half-life in neoplastic tissue is on the order of several days,[40] probably as a consequence of hypervascularity and poor lymphatic drainage.

For endobronchial photodynamic therapy, the commonly used photosensitizers include hematoporphyrin derivatives and Photofrin-II. An argon-pumped dye laser producing red light at 630 nm is focused by optical fibers through a fiberoptic bronchoscope to the tumor. More than 300 patients with lung cancer have now been treated with this system, with the largest experience coming from Tokyo Medical College,[26] where in a series of 176 patients, a complete response rate of 78% has been observed. Tumor size less than 1 cm appears to be a positive prognostic factor with 100% complete response rate. At the Mayo Clinic,[26] 65 patients have undergone photodynamic endobronchial therapy with a complete response rate of 55% in patients with radiographically occult disease. For more significant endobronchial disease, the current level of sophistication of photodynamic therapy is unlikely to produce significant tumor resolution.

## Endobronchial Prosthesis

The lumen of the trachea and the major bronchi is kept open by the dynamic properties of the horseshoe-shaped cartilage and the pars membranacea. Destruction of the wall, and especially the cartilage, by tumor growth or thermal destruction secondary to laser coagulation can induce severe airway instability, resulting in severe dyspnea exacerbated by exertion or coughing. An inadequate cough reflex results in substantial retention of secretions. To stabilize the airway and restore patency, a variety of prostheses have been used. These include expandable wire stents,[41] as well as molded silicone stents,[42,43] several models of which can actually be inserted using flexible bronchoscopes. The most comprehensive experience in stent implantation has been gathered by Dumon,[42] who used silicone stents that were implanted using a specially constructed rigid bronchoscope. This procedure required the use of general anesthesia. At least 17 types of stents of different design have since been developed. Most metal wire stents can be implanted under local anesthesia via a flexible bronchoscope. A well-placed stent may be left in place for a year or longer, depending on tumor growth. Additional brachytherapy is feasible.

The ideal indication for stent implantation, after exhaustion of other therapeutic options, is a tumor of the trachea or a main bronchus. Stent implantation requires adequate prior tumor resection by laser and sometimes endobronchial dilatation. An experienced pulmonologist is a must.

Complications after stent implantation include dislocation (often lethal), penetration in the mediastinum (mostly Gianturcostents), and formation of granulation tissue or tumor growth through the network of the wire stents. Because the airflow dynamics and mucociliary clearance are altered or lacking in stents, secretions may be deposited there, which can desiccate and plug the lumen. A newly developed dynamic stent mimics in its construction the trachea with cartilage and the pars membranacea.

### External Beam Radiotherapy

External beam radiation (EBR) alone achieves successful reversal of atelectasis and pneumonitis ranging from 21%[28] to 61%.[44] In the largest reported series, Slawson et al.[45] reported only a 23% rate of improvement in atelectasis following conventional EBR in 330 patients. In the study by Chetty et al.,[28] all of the patients who responded received more than 50 Gy, whereas no patient receiving less than 50 Gy had a favorable response. Even if patients reaerate with EBR, the time required to achieve this is generally longer than with endobronchial radiation. Since a fair number of patients have metastatic disease, an immunocompromised state, or a short median survival, waiting several weeks to achieve a palliative result is not optimal and frequently not feasible.

## Endobronchial Brachytherapy

### Historical Evolution Toward Current Techniques

The earliest reported use of endobronchial brachytherapy is credited to Yankauer[46] from New York who in 1922 reported on the implantation of radon capsules in two patients with bronchial carcinoma via a rigid bronchoscope under local anesthesia with good response. Soon thereafter, Kernan, and later Pancoast, also reported their experiences with endobronchial brachytherapy.[47,48] Unfortunately, this technique suffered from two main disadvantages, that is, the relatively large size of the radon capsules and the low specific activity, requiring long residence times up to 5 days. Consequently, no major clinical series were reported until the 1940s when Ormerod[49] presented his experience in 100 patients, focusing principally on the considerable limitations of radon seed implantation. This led to the abandonment of any major activity in the field of endobronchial brachytherapy for almost two decades.

In the 1960s endobronchial brachytherapy enjoyed a brief resurgence and a sudden demise because of the introduction of Cobalt 60 beads.[50] These beads, with a diameter of 6 to 8 mm, could be attached to an iron wire that could be implanted into the bronchial tree. Compared to the relatively low activity of radon of 30 mCi, these beads were more than twice as active at 80 mCi, permitting a relatively short residence time of 3 to 5 hours. Unfortunately, the lack of afterloading led to considerable personnel exposure, resulting in the abandonment of the technique by the late 1960s.[51]

By 1964 Henschke et al.[52] had already introduced a hand-cranked, remote afterloading device with a cobalt-60 source for use in cervical carcinoma.

Within a few years, the hand crank was replaced by a motor, and the stepwise motion of the source permitted the delivery of tailored brachytherapy. Sauerwein developed computerized control for the device that was named GammaMed I, and this became available for endobronchial treatment in 1979.[53] During this period, experience was being reported not only with this new device,[54,55] but also with Cesium 137[56,57] and with interstitial implantation of gold[58] and iodine. Although this technique reportedly produced excellent palliation in a series of 27 patients,[58] the risks of permanent interstitial implantation included hemorrhage and edema and the potential for seed loss into the pleural space. As a consequence, this technique did not become widespread.

Two developments in the 1980s led to a significant increase in the utilization of endobronchial brachytherapy. First, the advent of fiberoptic bronchoscopy and its widespread dissemination, as well as the simultaneous use of effective local anesthesia, antitussive agents, and intravenous sedation, allowed the insertion of small caliber afterloading catheters in every major branch of the tracheobronchial tree, even in critically ill patients. These flexible catheters could be inserted under direct visual guidance and subsequently afterloaded either manually or with remote afterloaders. The second major development was the availability of high-activity Iridium 192, which could either be obtained as multiple end-to-end seeds simulating a line source[59] or as high-activity seeds driven by a remote afterloader.

The 1980s were characterized by the parallel development of several of these techniques. In 1983 Macha et al.[53] initiated one of the very first endobronchial programs using iridium-192 HDR afterloading with the GammaMed I. The introduction of preimplant Nd:YAG laser photoresection is also credited to Macha. By 1985, when the technique was being introduced in the United States, more than 100 patients had been treated by Macha. In 1985 Schray et al.[60] reported on the use of a blind-end nylon catheter, 2 mm in diameter and 125 cm long, manually afterloaded with iridium seeds and left in situ for 30 to 60 hours. The dose rate at 1 cm was usually 50 to 100 cGy/hour. In 1986 Joyner and Hauskins[61] manually placed iridium seeds into an angiocatheter with an anchoring balloon. The large size precluded the use of the accessory channel on the bronchoscope and, therefore, this angiocatheter was slid over a guide wire that was inserted first at the time of bronchoscopy. Seagren et al.[55] in 1985, used a 3-mm cobalt-60 seed for HDR treatment with a catheter 4 mm in diameter and 46 cm long, which could not be used in the distal airways because of width considerations. In the same year, Korba et al.[62] reported on the use of a 10-Ci iridium-192 source, 1.2 mm in diameter and 1 cm long, attached to a 2-mm thick cable, which was driven by a remote afterloader. The microSelectron HDR was developed in the late 1980s. It uses a high-activity iridium-192 source 1.1 mm in diameter and 6 mm long, attached to a 1.1-mm diameter cable that can be inserted into a 5 French (1.7-mm) catheter. The source position can be programmed in 1 to 48 dwell positions, either in 2.5- or 5-mm increments, thereby allowing coverage of up to 12- or 24-cm lengths.

A tabular summary of the major developments in the evolution of endobronchial brachytherapy is presented in Table 3.

### Table 3
### The History of Endobronchial Brachytherapy

| Year | Event |
| --- | --- |
| 1922 | Yankauer reports first cases treated with radon capsules. |
| 1920s | Kernan and Pancoast report further cases. |
| 1941 | Ormerod's summary of problems of radon implantation leads to a decline in endobronchial brachytherapy. |
| 1962 | Cobalt 60 beads lead to a brief resurgence. |
| 1967 | Personnel exposure leads to an abandonment of this method. |
| 1964 | Henschke introduces remote afterloading. |
| 1979 | GammaMed I remote afterloader for endobronchial remote afterloading brachytherapy becomes available. Interstitial gold and iodine implantation. |
| 1980s | Fiberoptic bronchoscopy, iridium 192, and remote afterloaders lead to widespread use of brachytherapy. |

## Technical Considerations

The prerequisites for an effective endobronchial brachytherapy program based on HDR remote afterloading techniques are

(1) a reliable remote afterloading machine characterized by excellent shielding, small source diameter, high specific activity, availability of multiple channels, and computer control, which allows modulation of source position, dwell spaces, and dwell times;

(2) a good treatment-planning program that allows rapid and accurate calculation of the dose distribution;

(3) suitable endobronchial catheters;

(4) a dedicated team of pulmonologists, radiation oncologists, radiation physicists, and support personnel functioning within a short distance of both the radiation therapy facility as well as the endoscopy suite.

### Remote Afterloaders

The GammaMed II and the microSelectron HDR are the leading afterloading machines currently on the market. Recently, the Omnitron with its ultrasmall source has also become available. A detailed description of these devices is not presented here since this information is contained in Chapter 4. Currently, the manufacturers provide the software for dosimetry.

### Treatment Planning

Most dose-calculation techniques require fast reconstruction of catheter positions. This can be achieved using three different techniques: the semiorthogonal reconstruction, the isocentric method, and the variable angle reconstruction. The semiorthogonal method described by Loeffler et al.[63,64] in 1989 uses a box with cross-wire fiducials on its surfaces, which is placed over the patient prior to obtaining orthogonal radiographs, usually antero-posterior and lateral views. The spatial localization of the x-ray source can be determined by back projecting the fiducials and, therefore, even if the central axes of the two x-ray beams are not perpendicular and even if they are not precisely orthogonal, this determination can be made. In a similar fashion, the position of dummy seeds in the catheters can be determined for dose planning. The isocentric method is suited for isocentric machines, such as a simulator. The two images are obtained by shifting the angle between the central axes of the projecting beams up to 60 degrees such that the two projections of the dummy seeds are still visible on the same radiograph. With a simulator, it is, of course, possible to obtain two different radiographs at different angles, both of which demonstrate the dummy seeds. With orthogonal radiographs, the greatest accuracy in seed placement is achieved. In most commercial systems, catheter localization is expedited by digitizing the dummy seed locations. Van der Laarse[65] has developed an image tracking algorithm that facilitates this process so that only the first image point on both images has to correspond to the same point. Various algorithms to optimize dose distribution based on selected constraints can then be implemented.

Our routine, using the microSelectron HDR (10-Ci initial activity, changed approximately every 3 months at 4.3 Ci) with 6 French catheters, has been to obtain orthogonal radiographs with dummy seeds in place at the "best" angles as determined at the simulator. The seed positions are then digitized from dwell position 1. Although a spacing of 2.5 mm is used to provide 48 dwell positions, this can be varied. In general, the first dummy seed is labeled as the first dwell unless the implant length is expected to exceed 48 dwell positions. Optimization points are then placed at target radii in four cardinal directions, starting from the first active dwell position. As a rough guide, we have found that placing the first active dwell position at approximately half the radial treatment distance from the catheter often produces the desired isodose configuration. When using multiple catheters, it is crucial not to put optimization points closer than the prescription distance. The spinal cord, at several levels, is always entered into. The current treatment planning system, Nucletron Planning System (NPS), runs on a Silicon Graphics Iris Indigo workstation and is compatible with other UNIX workstations, but not DOS.

## Endobronchial Applicators

A variety of different applicators are available for HDR brachytherapy. The major differences between various applicators usually affect the caliber, the composition, the presence of a radio-opaque tip, the presence of an inflatable balloon, and the presence of distance markers. Although various systems including outer sheaths, balloons, and cages have been designed to hold the catheter in a central location in the airway, in order to avoid localized hot spots on the bronchial mucosa, these have generally not been found necessary in the vast majority of patients. The simple procedure of lodging the catheter distal to the obstructed airway is sufficient to hold it in place. Metal-tipped catheters should obviously be avoided if concomitant hyperthermia is contemplated. The most-common calibers used are either 5 (1.7-mm) or 6 (2-mm) French catheters. The 6 French catheter is better at negotiating acute curvature such as the right upper lobe. These catheters are usually quite flexible, but the larger 4-mm catheter is not as flexible. This semirigid catheter has the advantage of keeping its shape during treatment, and dislocation is extremely uncommon. Its introduction requires a ventilation tube that mandates the use of the oral instead of the nasal route. Although extensively used in Europe, it is not commonly utilized in the United States.

## Catheter Placement

Prior to the procedure, a thorough evaluation of the patient, including a full history and physical examination, as well as all pertinent laboratory parameters is essential. It is critical to be aware of the patient's cardiac and pulmonary status. Pretreatment computed tomography (CT) sometimes aids in localizing the obstruction. We do not routinely obtain coagulation studies unless a biopsy is also planned.

Our routine practice involves performance of the procedure in a fully equipped endoscopy suite. Patients are continually monitored in terms of pulse, blood pressure, pulse oxymetry, and ECG at 3-to-5-minute intervals. Continuous oxygen at 3 to 4 liters per minute is provided per nasal cannula. The nasal passages are anesthetized using 10% lidocaine jelly. Fifty to 100 mg of Demerol, given intravenously or intramuscularly, is used for sedation. Either atropine (0.4 to 0.6 mg intravenously) or glycopyrrolate (200–400 mg) is used to minimize secretions. If necessary, 30 to 60 mg of codeine given intramuscularly may be used as an antitussive. To provide adequate sedation, 0.5 to 1 mg of midazolam given intravenously is used and repeated as necessary. Usually, a total dose of 1 to 3 mg is needed, but age is a very important factor in determining total dose. Airway anesthesia is attained with 1% lidocaine in 2 to 3 mL aliquots. In order to ensure adequate anesthesia of the vocal cords, a total of 4 to 5 squirts of 2 to 3 mL each are usually necessary. More lidocaine, as necessary, is used once the bronchoscope has been negotiated past the vocal cords. As a matter of routine practice, we use a video camera head and photographic documentation of the lesion. It is extremely useful to measure the distance between the proximal and, if possible, the distal end of the tumor from a fixed internal landmark such as the tracheal carina. This allows determination of the longitudinal tumor dimension, which can be correlated to a reference point on the simulator radiographs, that is, the carina. After inspecting both sides and determining whether one or more catheters will be necessary, placement is carried out through the accessory port. A radio-opaque internal stiffening cable assists in placing the catheter without kinking, dislodgement, or getting stuck at the obstruction. The goal is to place the catheter at some distance past the obstruction. The distal airways actually hold the catheter in place without the need for fixating devices. The placement is confirmed visually and fluroscopically, and the bronchoscope is withdrawn under continuous fluoroscopy to maintain the catheter position. The catheter is then secured at the nose and marked with indelible ink to provide a visual alert in case of displacement and, as an additional precautionary measure, the external length from the tip of the nostril is documented and verified again prior to actual treatment.

## The Prescription Point

Because various authors have used different prescription points, total doses, and number of fractions, meaningful comparison between different studies is not always possible. Some authors[66] have suggested adopting 1 cm as the standard, but this is not universally accepted.[67] In fact, prescription depths ranging from 0.5 to 2 cm have been used, and these differences reflect the changing caliber of the tracheobronchial tree and the eccentric location of some catheters that are pushed to one side by the endoluminal tumor, as well as the desire to treat some of the peribronchial tumor in order to achieve a sustained response. Of course, toxicity concerns also affect the choice of the prescription point. It is possible to speculate that, with improvements in technology, three-dimensional (3-D) brachytherapy planning may become feasible and cost effective and may then permit tailoring of the dose distribution to the 3-D shape of the tumor. The longitudinal margin is usually 1 to 2 cm and is not the subject of much debate.

## Clinical Results

Endobronchial brachytherapy is most often used for palliative purposes, but is slowly being explored in selected patients as a form of boost with curative intent. No major prospective randomized multiinstitution studies of this modality have been reported, and the lack of uniformity and standardization has remained a major obstacle. The following are the major clinical questions.

- Should brachytherapy be used alone or in combination with laser debulking?
- Is either HDR or low dose rate (LDR) brachytherapy better than the other?
- What is the appropriate dose, fractionation, and prescription point?
- How should palliation be measured?
- Which patients might benefit from the integration of an up-front endobronchial boost as curative therapy?
- What is the toxicity profile?

## Palliative Endobronchial Brachytherapy

This is perhaps the single most common indication of endobronchial brachytherapy. Speiser et al.[68] have described a concise and user-friendly symptom index wherein the four major problems associated with airway occlusion, hemoptysis, pneumonia, dyspnea, and cough are graded on a subjective scale from 0 to 4 (Table 4). They have also described an "obstruction" score for assessment of the degree of endoluminal blockage at the time of endoscopy (Table 5). At the University of Wisconsin, we have utilized a "symptom resolution" data sheet for the determination of response (Table 6). The use of such tools is highly encouraged since it allows for some standardization in this field.

Obviously, the results of any HDR endobronchial brachytherapy clinical trial are likely to be compared to those of low or conventional dose-rate therapy. Several single-institution results of LDR brachytherapy have now been published and are summarized in Table 7. Symptomatic improvement is reported in 50 to 100% of these patients, radiographic improvement in 17 to 78% of patients, and bronchoscopic improvement in 60 to 93%.[60,69-77]

Similar results have been reported in almost 1,000 patients[53,55,68,70,76-84] treated with HDR brachytherapy. A number of different treatment schema have been reported and are summarized in Table 8. The functional, radiographic, and endoscopic improvement following HDR endobronchial brachytherapy is summarized in Table 9. It ranges from 50 to 100% for clinical improvement, 46 to 88% for radiographic reaeration, and 59 to 100% for bronchoscopic response. This variability is explained by several factors, including inhomogenous groups of patients and tumors and variable additional treatments including laser and external radiation, as well as the use of different treatment schema. Therefore, the exact contribution of each of these variables is impossible to tease out. Although some authors[81] have suggested that the addition of the laser improves outcome significantly, this is not borne out in some of the larger series.[68] Similarly, it is difficult to make a case for higher doses since a clear-cut, dose-response relationship does not seem to be apparent. In fact, the only relatively strong data supporting a dose-response relationship come from a LDR study reported by Lo et al.[72] and illustrated in Fig. 1. The palliative response from brachytherapy is therefore excellent, and this modality has now become almost routine at recurrence, when other options have been exhausted and appropriate indications exist. An important aspect of this palliation is its durability. It appears from most studies[70] that almost two-thirds to three-fourths of the remainder of the patients' lifetimes is rendered symptom improved or symptom free.

## Curative Endobronchial Brachytherapy

The logical patient group that could ideally be treated with endobronchial radiation for cure are patients with in situ disease picked up on a screening bronchoscopy. Such patients are not frequently encountered, and in the few small series reported, they have generally been treated with phototherapy.[26]

## Table 4

## Symptom Index

### Hemoptysis

| Score | Definition |
|---|---|
| 0 | None |
| 1 | Less than 2 times/week |
| 2 | Less than daily but greater than 2 times/week. |
| 3 | Daily, bright red blood or clots |
| 4 | Decrease of Hb/Hct. >10%, greater than 150 cc, requiring hospitalization or leading to respiratory distress |

### Pneumonia-elevated Temperature

| Score | Definition |
|---|---|
| 0 | Normal temperature, no infiltrates, WBC <10,000 |
| 1 | Temperature > 38.5 and infiltrate, WBC <10,000 |
| 2 | Temperature > 38.5 and infiltrate and/or WBC >10,000 |
| 3 | Lobar consolidation on radiograph |
| 4 | Pneumonia or elevated temperature requiring hospitalization |

### Dyspnea

| Score | Definition |
|---|---|
| 0 | None |
| 1 | Dyspnea on moderate exertion |
| 2 | Dyspnea with normal activity, walking on level ground |
| 3 | Dyspnea at rest |
| 4 | Requires supplemental oxygen |

### Cough

| Score | Definition |
|---|---|
| 0 | None |
| 1 | Intermittent, no medication necessary |
| 2 | Intermittent, non-narcotic medication |
| 3 | Constant or requiring narcotic medication |
| 4 | Constant, requiring narcotic medication but without relief |

## Table 5

## Obstruction Score Definitions

| | | | |
|---|---|---|---|
| Trachea | >50% is score = 10, but | <50% is score = 6, and | <10% is score = 2 |
| Main Bronchus | >50% is score = 6, but | <50% is score = 3, and | <10% is score = 1 |
| Lobar Bronchus | >50% is score = 2, but | <50% is score = 1 | |
| Atelectasis is score | = 2 per lobe | | |
| Pneumonia is score | = 2 per lobe | | |

## Table 6
### Endobronchial Brachytherapy Data Sheet

Symptom Resolution

Patient name: _____
History number: _____
Date of implant: _____
Date of follow-up: _____

| Symptom | Present | Absent | Improved | Worsened |
|---|---|---|---|---|
| Cough* | | | | |
| Dyspnea* | | | | |
| Pneumonia ⊗ | | | | |
| Hemoptysis° | | | | |
| Chest Pain∅ | | | | |

| * | Grade 0 | Grade 1 | Grade 2 | Grade 3 | Grade 4 |
|---|---|---|---|---|---|
| Cough | None | Mild, dry, no meds. | Persistent, requiring antitussives | Severe, unresponsive to narcotic antitussive | Severe, respiratory |
| Dyspnea | None | Mild dyspnea on exertion | Dyspnea with minimal effort, but not at rest | Dyspnea at rest, intermittent oxygen | Continuous oxygen necessary |

⊗ Pneumonia:
    (a) Clinically obvious findings: antibiotics required.
    (b) Positive sputum cultures with elevated white count (≥1.5 × normal).
    (c) Radiographically obvious pneumonia.
° Hemoptysis: Present or absent
∅ Chest pain: Patient's perception

## Table 7
### Results of LDR Trials

| Author | Patients | Symptoms Improved | X-Ray Improved | Bronch. Improved |
|---|---|---|---|---|
| Schray[60] | 65 | NA | NA | 60% |
| Allen[69] | 15 | 100% | 38% | NA |
| Mehta[70] | 66 | 78% | 78% | 93% |
| Roach[71] | 17 | 53% | 17% | 60% |
| Lo[72] | 87 | 59% | NA | 76% |
| Locken[73] | 18 | 83% | NA | 70% |
| Paradelo[74] | 32 | 66% | 21% | 85% |
| Susnerwala[75] | 14 | 50% | 75% | NA |

## Table 8
### Literature Review of Endobronchial Schema

| Author | Patients | Dose(GY)* | Fractions |
|--------|----------|-----------|-----------|
| Nori[76] | 15 | 60 | 3 |
| Seagren[55] | 20 | 10 | 1 |
| Macha[53] | 56 | 22.5 | 3 |
| Gauwitz[77] | 24 | 18 | 2 |
| Speiser[68] | 144 | 30 | 3 |
| Speiser[68] | 151 | 22.5 | 3 |
| Speiser[68]** | 47 | 15 | 3 |
| Burt[78] | 50 | 15–20 | 1 |
| Fass[79] | 15 | 5–36 | 1–6 |
| Bedwinek[80] | 38 | 18 | 3 |
| Miller[81] | 88 | 30 | 3 |
| Kohek[82] | 81 | 10–21 | 2–3 |
| Stout[83] | 100 | 15–20 | 1 |
| Mehta[70] | 66 | 32 | 4 |
| Sutedja[84] | 31 | 30 | 3 |
| Total | 926 | | |

*Dose at 1 cm
**Intermediate dose rate

## Table 9
### Outcome Data for HDR Endobronchial Brachytherapy

| Author | Clinical Response | Radiographic Response | Bronch. Response |
|--------|-------------------|-----------------------|------------------|
| Nori[76] | 80% | 88% | NA |
| Seagren[55] | 94% | NA | 100% |
| Macha[53] | 74% | 88% | 75% |
| Gauwitz[77] | 88% | 83% | 100% |
| Speiser[68] | 85–99% | NA | 80% |
| Burt[78] | 50–86% | 46% | 88% |
| Fass[79] | 75% | NA | NA |
| Bedwinek[80] | 76% | 64% | 82% |
| Miller[81] | NA | NA | 80% |
| Kohek[82] | 65–77% | 26% | 61% |
| Stout[83] | 51–86% | 46% | NA |
| Mehta[70] | 71–100% | 85% | NA |
| Sutedja[84] | NA | NA | 72% |

There is a small, but increasing, body of data that would suggest that, in selected patients with more advanced disease, endobronchial brachytherapy boost may play a role, in addition to external beam radiotherapy (EBRT). Reddi and Marbach[85] reported on a small study of 32 patients with newly diagnosed, advanced, nonsmall cell lung cancer treated with an initial 60 Gy in

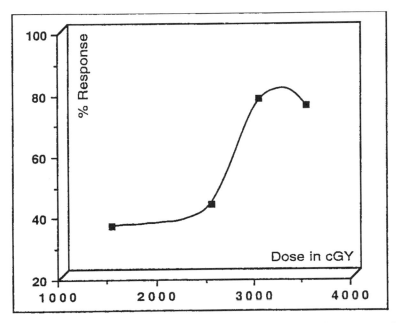

**Fig. 1.** Dose response relationship (clinical improvement). Data from Lo et al.[72] based on LDR dose at 2 cm.

30 fractions followed by HDR boost endobronchial radiation of 7.5 Gy at 1 cm, with an optional second and third brachytherapy boost 2 and 4 weeks later if the residual tumor was found at repeat bronchoscopy. The reaeration response was 100%. In the 8 patients in whom 3-month biopsies were available, none demonstrated residual tumors. The median survival, however, was only 8 months. Aygun and colleagues[86] reported on 62 patients with medically inoperable or surgically unresectable disease who were treated with both EBRT to 50–60 Gy and HDR brachytherapy in 3 to 5 fractions of 5 Gy at 1 cm. The median survival was slightly better at 13 months but probably reflected the fact that some patients had Stage I disease. They noted that median survival for $N_0$ patients was 20 months compared to 9 months for $N_+$ patients. Bastin et al.[87] have previously reported on a group of 22 patients with newly diagnosed Stage IIIA or B nonsmall cell lung cancer who were ineligible for other protocols because of poor KPS, weight loss, significant atelectasis, or other factors and were, therefore, treated with up-front brachytherapy followed by 60 Gy external radiation. A 67% reaeration rate was noted and, using sequential volume integration, we were able to demonstrate 47% and 25% lung volume sparing from external radiation in patients achieving complete and partial reaeration, respectively. Although there was a trend toward improved survival among reaerators, the overall median survival was only 34 weeks. In a case report from Sutedja et al.,[88] a patient with unresectable cancer because of disease extending to the main carina was rendered resectable following brachytherapy.

Such data suggest that, in selected patients, endobronchial boost therapy is likely to produce significant reaeration and, hence, sparing of lung volume from subsequent external radiation. A few cases may even become resectable. Demonstration of a considerable survival advantage will, however, require a larger clinical trial with adequate controls.

Another innovative curative application of this modality is in an adjuvant setting following surgical resection that leaves behind minimal disease at the bronchial stump, either as a positive margin or as positive washings following resection. Macha et al.[89] have recently reported on a series of 17 such patients treated in a pilot study with tumor-free survival times of up to 4 years.

## Complications

### Fatal Hemoptysis

Relatively little has been reported on the long-term tolerance of the tracheobronchial tree to HDR endobronchial brachytherapy. However, more detailed follow-up of patients treated with this modality is beginning to demonstrate that a certain proportion of patients experience fatal hemoptysis. The estimates of the occurrence of this complication is flawed and underreported in most series because only absolute numbers are provided without factoring in patients who were not "at risk."

We have recently analyzed the literature for the reported rates of fatal hemoptysis in patients undergoing either HDR or LDR endobronchial radiotherapy and the data are presented in Tables 10 and 11. Overall, the average fatal hemoptysis rate for LDR, intermediate dose rate (IDR) or HDR do not appear to be significantly different, and the mean values are 5% and 8%. However, the HDR group appears to contain some significant "outliers." The exact causes for this variance have not totally been defined but could include inaccurate re-

### Table 10
### Fatal Hemoptysis Rates (LDR/IDR) Reported in the Literature

| Author | Year | Technique | Patients | No. | % Fatal Hemoptysis |
|---|---|---|---|---|---|
| Schray[60] | 1988 | IDR | 65 | 7 | 11 |
| Locken[73] | 1990 | LDR | 27 | 0 | 0 |
| Roach[71] | 1990 | LDR | 17 | 0 | 0 |
| Lo[72] | 1992 | LDR | 87 | 3 | 3 |
| Mehta[70] | 1992 | LDR | 66 | 4 | 6 |
| Susnerwala[75] | 1992 | LDR | 14 | 0 | 0 |
| Paradelo[74] | 1992 | LDR | 32 | 3 | 9 |
| Speiser[68] | 1993 | IDR | 47 | 2 | 4 |
| Total | 1988–1993 | | 355 | 19 | 5 (average) |

### Table 11
### Fatal Hemoptysis Rates (HDR) Reported in the Literature

| Author | Year | Technique | Patients | No. | % Fatal Hemoptysis |
|--------|------|-----------|----------|-----|--------------------|
| Seagren[55] | 1985 | HDR | 20 | 5 | 25 |
| Macha[53] | 1987 | HDR | 56 | 4 | 7 |
| Nori[76] | 1987 | HDR | 15 | 0 | 0 |
| Burt[78] | 1990 | HDR | 50 | 0 | 0 |
| Miller[81] | 1990 | HDR | 88 | 0 | 0 |
| Stout[83] | 1990 | HDR | 100 | 0 | 0 |
| Kohek[82] | 1990 | HDR | 81 | 3 | 4 |
| Fass[79] | 1990 | HDR | 15 | 0 | 0 |
| Khanavkar[92] | 1991 | HDR | 12 | 6 | 50 |
| Bedwinek[80] | 1992 | HDR | 38 | 12 | 32 |
| Sutedja[84] | 1992 | HDR | 31 | 10 | 32 |
| Gauwitz[77] | 1992 | HDR | 24 | 1 | 4 |
| Aygun[86] | 1992 | HDR | 62 | 9 | 15 |
| Mehta[70] | 1992 | HDR | 31 | 1 | 3 |
| Speiser[68] | 1993 | HDR | 295 | 23 | 8 |
| Total | 1985–1993 | | 918 | 74 | 8 (average) |

porting, variable follow-up, different patient populations, different prior concomitant and sequential therapeutic measures, different rates of follow-up bronchoscopy and biopsy, which could induce trauma, the total length treated, and the total dose as well as fractionation. These issues can only be sorted out in a prospective trial.

When we made the switch from LDR to HDR at our institution, radiobiological modeling was carried out in an attempt to limit this particular complication.[70] In our LDR group, we had routinely prescribed a dose of 20 Gy at 2 cm, which equates to approximately 50 Gy at 1 cm. Using radiobiological modeling, we predicted a 60% increase in late effects if a single equivalent fraction were to be utilized for HDR. We, therefore, opted to pursue a schema using 4 fractions of 4 Gy each at 2 cm delivered over 2 days with the catheter left in place for the duration. We have not found a significant difference in fatal hemoptysis using this approach.

Bedwinek et al.[80] noted a surprisingly high 32% rate of fatal hemoptysis in their series of 38 patients. In an attempt to sort out treatment-related hemoptysis from tumor-related hemoptysis, they constructed a time curve of cumulative probability of hemoptysis, which suggested a greater than 90% risk beyond 25 weeks. However, because a substantial number of these events occurred at such a short point in time following brachytherapy, the role of tumor progression in causing hemoptysis must be seriously evaluated. In fact, 3 of 5 patients undergoing bronchoscopic evaluation prior to hemoptysis were found to have tumors. This may, in fact, suggest that hemoptysis might even represent a failure of therapy rather than a consequence![90] In a further analysis to identify risk factors for hemoptysis, Bedwinek et al.[80] noted that prior laser therapy, prior external radiation, and the size of extrabronchial disease did not influence the rate of hemoptysis. Hemoptysis as a presenting symptom also did not influence the ultimate rate of hemoptysis. Interestingly, 2 of 4 (50%) patients who had two courses of brachytherapy died from hemoptysis compared to a 29% rate for the single-course group. The factor most closely associated with a high risk was location, with the left upper lobe demonstrating a 75% (6 out of 8 patients) risk. Autopsy data on patients dying from lung cancer not treated by brachytherapy reveal that the left upper lobe is, in fact, a "high-risk" site. Miller and McGregor,[91] in an autopsy series of 877 cases, found an overall incidence of fatal hemoptysis of 29 out of 877 patients (3.3%), but the risk in the left upper lobe was 15 out of 120 patients (12.5%). An additional risk factor in this autopsy study was the histologic type with squamous cell carcinoma having a 7.4% (24 out of 326 patients) risk. The authors recreated this situation for dosimetric evaluation and demonstrated that the wall of the pulmonary artery could fall within a "hot spot" of 20 to 30 Gy with a single 6 Gy fraction, implying that the total numeric dose to it, including a prior median external beam dose of 60 Gy, could well be in the order of 150 Gy. Obviously, these data must be taken into consideration when retreating left upper lobar lesions. Bedwinek et al.'s[80] final hypothesis was that the tumor had already created a fistula between the bronchus and the pulmonary artery, and the brachytherapy may simply have "unplugged" the tumor. Autopsy verification of such a phenomenon is lacking.

Another report with an alarmingly high hemoptysis rate is the one by Khanavkar et al.[92] reporting a 50% (6 out of 12 patients) occurrence. Interestingly, squamous histology and left upper lobe location predominated in their fatal hemoptysis group. They noted that, although the total radiation dose did not influence the occurrence of this complication, the length of the irradiated segment of bronchus had some correlation. Patients who developed fatal hemoptysis had an average length of 5.3 cm treated compared to 3.5 cm (a 51% difference) for those not experiencing hemoptysis.

Macha et al. (personal communication), using HDR [192]Ir (GammaMed I) have previously noted a 23% rate of fatal hemoptysis in 73 patients. Their most recent analysis of 221 patients suggests a 21% risk of fatal hemorrhage.

### Radiation Bronchitis

Speiser and Spartling have recently described an entity known as radiation bronchitis and stenosis.[93] This was identified during follow-up bronchoscopy and was graded by severity. Grade 1 is a mild mucosal inflammation with swelling, characterized by a thin, whitish circumferential membrane without endoscopic or clinical evidence of obstruction. Grade 2 is represented by greater exudation from this membrane, causing symptoms that might require endoscopic debridement or medical management consisting of steroid therapy, both oral and aerosol, inhalation of alkalinized (with $NaHCO_3$ to reduce the viscosity of mucous) bronchodilators, oral mucolytic agents, and antitussives. Grade 3 is defined as a severe inflammatory response with a marked membranous exudate. Mehta et al.[94] have previously described this as "chronic mucosal sloughing" and suggested that a combination of factors such as high-dose external radiation, multiple laser treatments, and a high dose to the mucosa from brachytherapy may play a causative role. Such a reaction may require multiple debridements. The most severe, or grade 4, reaction is characterized by significant fibrosis, resulting in circumferential narrowing, which requires management with balloon or bougie dilatation, photoresection, or stent placement.

The overall incidence by grade in the report of Speiser et al.[93] was 29%, 22%, 20%, and 29% for grades 1 through 4. They found that risk factors for this complication included large cell histology, concomitant high-dose EBRT, the addition of laser therapy, male gender, and longer survival. The risk of fatal hemoptysis was slightly higher in this group at 12%, compared to 7% in those who did not develop radiation bronchitis.

## Other Fistulae

The occurrence of fistulae at other locations, such as the mediastinum or esophagus, is less common. In several studies, the incidence of this has been reported to be between 1 to 3%.[94] Although not as acutely fatal as tracheovascular fistulae, these fistulae are also ultimately fatal. Patients with tracheomediastinal fistulae develop lethal mediastinitis over a period of several days to weeks, and patients with tracheoesophageal fistulae develop aspiration pneumonia.

---

## REFERENCES

1. Boring CC, Savires TS, Tong T. Cancer statistics, 1991. Ca-Cancer J Clin 41:19-36, 1991.
2. Perez CA, Stanley K, Grundy G, et al. Impact of irradiation technique and tumor extent in tumor control and survival of patients with unresectable non-oat cell carcinoma of the lung. Cancer 50:1091-1099, 1982.
3. Cox JD, Yesner R, Mietlowski W, et al. Influence of cell type on failure pattern after irradiation for locally advanced carcinoma of the lung: from the Veterans' Administration Group (VALG). Cancer 44:94-98, 1979.
4. Minna JD, Higgins GA, Glatstein EJ. Cancer of the Lung. In: DeVita VT, Hellman S, Rosenberg SA, eds. Cancer Principles and Practice of Oncology, 2nd ed. Philadelphia, Pa.: JB Lippincott Co.; 1985, 518.
5. Moylan D. Overview of endobronchial brachytherapy and review of literature. In Proceedings of AERALTS II; 1987; New Orleans, La.
6. Huzly A. Bronchoskopie in Lokalanasthesie. In: Giesbach R, Muller RW, eds. Bronchoskopische Eingriffe. Berlin, Germany: Springer Verlag; 1974.
7. Walsh DA, Maiwand MO, Nath AR, et al. Bronchoscopic cryotherapy for advanced bronchial carcinoma. Thorax 45:509-513, 1990.
8. Vergnon JM, Schmitt T, Alamartine E, et al. Initial combined cryotherapy and irradiation for unresectable non-small cell lung cancer: preliminary results. Chest 102:1436-1440, 1992.

9. Homasson J, Pecking A, Roden S, et al. Tumor fixation of bleomycin labeled with 57 cobalt before and after cryotherapy of bronchial carcinoma. Cryobiology 29:543-548, 1992.

10. Arabian A, Spagnolo SV. Laser therapy in patients with primary lung cancer. Chest 86:519-523, 1984.

11. Brutinel WM, Cortese DA, McDougall JC, et al. A two year experience with the neodymium-YAG laser in endobronchial obstruction. Chest 91:159-165, 1987.

12. Cavaliere S, Foccoli P, Farina PL. Nd:YAG laser bronchoscopy: a five year experience with 1,396 applications in 1,000 patients. Chest 94:15-21, 1988.

13. Gelb AF, Epstein JD. Nd-YAG laser in lung cancer. West J Med 140:393-397, 1984.

14. Hetzel MR, Millard FJC, Ayesh R, et al. Laser treatment for carcinoma of the bronchus. Br Med J 286:12-16, 1983.

15. McDougall JC, Cortese DA. Neodymium-YAG laser therapy of malignant airway obstruction: a preliminary report. Mayo Clin Proc 58:35-39, 1983.

16. McElvein RB. Laser endoscopy. Ann Thorac Surg 32:463-466, 1981.

17. Personne C, Colchen A, Bonnette P, et al. Laser in bronchology: methods of application. Lung 168(S):1085-1088, 1990.

18. Shapshay SM, Dumon JF, Beamis JF Jr. Endoscopic treatment of tracheobronchial malignancy: experience with Nd-YAG and $CO_2$ lasers in 506 operations. Otolaryngol Head Neck Surg 93:205-210, 1985.

19. Wolfe WG, Cole PH, Sabiston DC Jr. Experimental and clinical use of the YAG laser in the management of pulmonary neoplasms. Ann Surg 199:526-531, 1984.

20. Dumon JF, Reboud E, Garbe L, et al. Treatment of tracheobronchial lesions by laser photoresection. Chest 81:278-284, 1982.

21. Toty L, Personne C, Colchen A, et al. Bronchoscopic management of tracheal lesions using the neodymium yttrium aluminum garnet laser. Thorax 36:175-178, 1981.

22. Kvale PA, Eichenhorn MS, Radke JR, et al. YAG laser photoresection of lesions obstructing the central airways. Chest 87:283-288, 1985.

23. Parr GVS, Unger M, Trout RG, et al. One hundred neodymium-YAG laser ablations of obstructing tracheal neoplasms. Ann Thorac Surg 38:374-379, 1984.

24. Diaz-Jimenez JP, Canela-Cardona M, Maestre-Alcacer J. Nd:YAG laser photoresection of low grade malignant tumors of the tracheobronchial tree. Chest 97:920-922, 1990.

25. Brutinell WM, Cortese DA, Edell ES, et al. Complications of Nd:YAG laser therapy. Chest 94:902-903, 1988.

26. Edell ES, Cortese DA, McDougall JC. Ancillary therapies in the management of lung cancer: photodynamic therapy, laser therapy, and endobronchial prosthetic devices. Mayo Clin Proc 68:685-690, 1993.

27. Desai SJ, Mehta AC, Medendorp SV, et al. Survival experience following Nd:YAG laser photoresection for primary bronchogenic carcinoma. Chest 94:939-944, 1988.

28. Chetty KG, Sassoon CSM, Viravathana T, et al. Effect of radiation therapy on bronchial obstruction due to bronchogenic carcinoma. Chest 95:582-584, 1989.

29. Mehta MP, Shahabi S, Jarjour N, et al. Effect of endobronchial radiation therapy on malignant bronchial obstruction. Chest 97:662-665, 1990.

30. Mitchell JB, McPherson S, DeGraff W, et al. Oxygen dependence of hematoporphyrin derivative-induced photoactivation of Chinese Hamster cells. Cancer Res 45:2008-2011, 1985.

31. Lee See K, Borbes LJ, Betts WH. Oxygen dependency and photocytoxicity with hematoporphyrin derivative. Photochem Photobiol 39:631-634, 1984.

32. Moan J, Sommer S. Oxygen dependence of the photosensitizing effect of hematoporphyrin derivative in NHIK 3025 cells. Cancer Res 45:1608-1610, 1985.

33. Gibson SL, Hilf R. Interdependence of fluence, drug dose and oxygen on hematoporphyrin derivative induced photosensitization of tumor mitochrondria. Photochem Photobiol 42:367-373, 1985.

34. Gibson SL, Hilf R. Photosensitization of mitochondrial cytochrome c oxidase by hematoporphyrin derivative and related porphyrins in vitro and in vivo. Cancer Res 43:4191-4197, 1983.
35. Hilf R, Warne NW, Smail DB, et al. Photodynamic inactivation of selected intracellular enzymes by hematoporphyrin derivative and their relationship to tumor cell viability in vitro. Cancer Lett 24:165-172, 1984.
36. Foote CS. Mechanisms of photooxygenation. In: Doiron DR, Gomer CJ, eds. Porphyrin Localization and Treatment of Tumors. New York, NY: Liss; 1984, 3-18.
37. Fiel RJ, Datta-Gupta N, Mark EH, et al. Induction of DNA damage by porphyrin photosensitizers. Cancer Res 41:3543-3545, 1981.
38. Moan J, Waksvik H, Christensen T. DNA single-strand breaks and sister chromatid exchanges induced by treatment with hematoporphyrin and light or by x-rays in human NHIK 3025 cells. Cancer Res 40:2915-2918, 1980.
39. Doiron DR, Gomer CJ. In: Doiron DR, Gomer CJ, eds. Porphyrin Localization and Treatment of Tumors. New York, NY: Liss; 1984, xxiii.
40. Bugelski PJ, Porter CW, Dougherty TJ, et al. Autoradiographic distribution of hematoporphyrin derivative in normal and tumor tissue of the mouse. Cancer Res 41:4606-4612, 1981.
41. Simonds AK, Irving JD, Clarke SW, et al. Use of expandable metal stents in the treatment of bronchial obstruction. Thorax 44:680-681, 1989.
42. Dumon JF. A dedicated tracheobronchial stent. Chest 97:328-332, 1990.
43. Insall RL, Morritt GN. Palliation of malignant tracheal strictures using silicone T tubes. Thorax 46:168-171, 1991.
44. Majid DA, Lee S, Khushalani S, et al. The response of atelectasis from lung cancer to radiation therapy. Int J Radiat Oncol Biol Phys 17:847-851, 1989.
45. Slawson RG, Scott RM. Radiation therapy in bronchogenic carcinoma. Ther Radiol 132:175-176, 1979.
46. Yankauer S. Two cases of lung tumour treated bronchoscopically. New York Med J (Je 21), 741-742, 1922.
47. Kernan JD. Carcinoma of the lung and bronchus. Treatment with radon implantation and diathermy. Arch Otolaryngol 17:457-475, 1933.
48. Pancoast HK. Superior pulmonary sulcus tumor. JAMA 99:1391-1396, 1932.
49. Ormerod FC. Some notes on the treatment of carcinoma of the bronchus. J Larynx Otol 56:1-10, 1941.
50. Schlungbaum W, Blum H, Brandt HJ. Ergebnisse der endobronchialen strahlentherapie des bronchialkarzinoms. Radiologie Austria XIII/3:201, 1962.
51. Bublitt G, Labitzke R. Ergebnisse endobronchialer kontaktbestrahlung des bronchuskarzinomas mit Co 60 Perlen. Strahlentherapie 134:332, 1967.
52. Henschke UK, Hilaris BS, Mahan GD. Remote afterloading for intracavitary applicators. Radiology 83:344-345, 1964.
53. Macha HN, Koch K, Stadler M, et al. New technique for treating occlusive and stenosing tumours of the trachea and main bronchii: endobronchial irradiation by high dose iridium-192 combined with laser canalization. Thorax 42:511-515, 1987.
54. Rooney SM, Goldnier PL, Bains MS, et al. Anaesthesia for the application of endotracheal and endobronchial radiation therapy. J Thorac Cardiovasc Surg 87:693-697, 1984.
55. Seagren SL, Havvel JH, Havv RA. High dose rate intraluminal irradiation in recurrent endobronchial carcinoma. Chest 88(6):810-814, 1985.
56. George PJM, Hadly JM, Mantell BS, et al. Medium dose rate endobronchial radiotherapy with Cesium 137. Thorax 47:474-477, 1992.
57. Mendiondo OA, Dillon M, Beach LJ. Endobronchial brachytherapy in the treatment of recurrent bronchogenic carcinoma. Int J Radiat Oncol Biol Phys 9:579-582, 1983.
58. Hilaris BS, Martini N, Loumanen RK. Endobronchial interstitial implantation. Clin Bull 9:17-20, 1979.

59. Shahabi S, Mehta MP, Wiley AL, et al. The role of computed tomography in dosimetric evaluation of endobronchial implants. Endocurie/Hypertherm Oncol 4:187-191, 1988.

60. Schray MF, McDougall JC, Martinez A, et al. Management of malignant airway compromise with laser and low dose rate brachytherapy. Chest 93:264-269, 1988.

61. Joyner LR, Hauskins L. Iridium afterloading and Neodymium-YAG laser treatment of segmental and lobar intrabronchial malignant obstructions. Tumor Diagnostik and Therapie 7:183-187, 1986.

62. Korba AL, Spear RK, Howard D, et al. High dose fraction intrabronchial radiation therapy for non-small cell carcinoma of the lung. Presented at Current Endobronchial Therapy: State of the Art; 1987; Phoenix, Ariz.

63. Loeffler EL, van der Laarse R. Technique and individual afterloading treatment planning simulating classic Stockholm brachytherapy for cervix cancer. In: Vahrson H, Rauthe G, eds. High Dose Rate Afterloading in the Treatment of the Uterus, Breast and Rectum. Munich, Germany: Urban and Schwarzenberg; 1988 (suppl.) 82, 83, 89.

64. Loeffler EL. Quality control in brachytherapy. In: Rotte K, Kiffer J, eds. Changes in Brachytherapy, Quality Control in Brachytherapy. Nurenberg, Germany: D.E. Wacholz KG; 1989.

65. van der Laarse R: In: Mould RF, ed. The Selectron Treatment Planning System. Leersum, The Netherlands: Nucletron Corp.; 1985, 176-186.

66. Speiser BL. High dose-rate endobronchial brachytherapy: whither goest thou? Int J Radiat Oncol Biol Phys 23:250, 1992.

67. Mehta MP. Endobronchial brachytherapy: whither prescription point? Int J Radiat Oncol Biol Phys 23:251, 1992.

68. Speiser BL, Spratling L. Remote afterloading brachytherapy for the local control of endobronchial carcinoma. Int J Radiat Oncol Biol Phys 25:579-587, 1993.

69. Allen MD, Baldwin JC, Fish VJ, et al. Combined laser therapy and endobronchial radiotherapy for unresectable lung carcinoma with bronchial obstruction. Am J Surg 150:71-77, 1985.

70. Mehta MP, Petereit DG, Chosy L, et al. Sequential comparison of low dose rate and hyperfractionated high dose rate endobronchial radiation for malignant airway occlusion. Int J Radiat Oncol Biol Phys 23:133-139, 1992.

71. Roach M III, Leidholdt EM Jr, Tatera BS, et al. Endobronchial radiation therapy (EBRT) in the management of lung cancer. Int J Radiat Oncol Biol Phys 18:1449-1454, 1990.

72. Lo TCM, Beamis JF Jr, Weinstein RS, et al. Intraluminal low-dose rate brachytherapy for malignant endobronchial obstruction. Radiother Oncol 23:16-20, 1992.

73. Locken P, Dillon M, Patel P, et al. Palliation of locally recurrent non-small cell lung cancer with low dose rate Iridium-192 endobronchial implant combined with localized external beam irradiation. Endocurie/Hypertherm Oncol 6:217-222, 1990.

74. Paradelo JC, Waxman MJ, Throne BJ, et al. Endobronchial irradiation with 192Ir in the treatment of malignant endobronchial obstruction. Chest 102:1072-1074, 1992.

75. Susnerwala SS, Sharma S, Deshpande DD, et al. Endobronchial brachytherapy: a preliminary experience. J Surg Oncol 50:115-117, 1992.

76. Nori D, Hilaris BS, Martini N. Intraluminal irradiation in bronchogenic carcinoma. Surg Clin North Am 67:1093-1102, 1987.

77. Gauwitz M, Ellerbroek N, Komaki R, et al. High dose endobronchial irradiation in recurrent bronchogenic carcinoma. Int J Radiat Oncol Biol Phys 23:397-400, 1992.

78. Burt PA, O'Driscoll BR, Nortley HM, et al. Intraluminal irradiation for the palliation of lung cancer with the high dose rate micro-Selectron. Thorax 45:765-768, 1990.

79. Fass DE, Armstrong J, Harrison LB. Fractionated high dose rate endobronchial treatment for recurrent lung cancer. Endocurie/Hypertherm Oncol 6:211-215, 1990.

80. Bedwinek J, Petty A, Bruton C, et al. The use of high dose rate endobronchial brachytherapy to palliate symptomatic endobronchial recurrence of previously irradiated bronchogenic carcinoma. Int J Radiat Oncol Biol Phys 22:23-30, 1991.

81. Miller JI Jr, Phillips TW. Neodymium-YAG laser and brachytherapy in the management of inoperable bronchogenic carcinoma. Ann Thorac Surg 50:190-196, 1990.

82. Kohek P, Pakisch B, Rehak P, et al. Nd-YAG laser debulking combined with $^{192}$Ir HDR brachytherapy for obstructing cancer of the central bronchial airways: technique and results. Selectron Brachytherapy Journal S1:45-47, 1990.

83. Stout R, Burt PA, O'Driscoll BR, et al. HDR brachytherapy for palliation and cure in bronchial carcinoma: the Manchester experience using a single dose technique. Selectron Brachytherapy Journal S1:48-50, 1990.

84. Sutedja G, Baris G, Schaake-Koning C, et al. High dose rate brachytherapy in patients with local recurrences after radiotherapy of non-small cell lung cancer. Int J Radiat Oncol Biol Phys 24:551-553, 1992.

85. Reddi RP, Marbach JC. HDR remote afterloading brachytherapy of carcinoma of the lung. Selectron Brachytherapy Journal 6(1):21-23, 1992.

86. Aygun C, Weiner S, Scariato A, et al. Treatment of non-small cell lung cancer with external beam radiotherapy and high dose rate brachytherapy. Int J Radiat Oncol Biol Phys 23:127-132, 1992.

87. Bastin KT, Mehta MP, Kinsella TJ. Thoracic volume radiation sparing following endobronchial brachytherapy: a quantitative analysis. Int J Radiat Oncol Biol Phys 25:703-707, 1993.

88. Sutedja T, Zoetmulder F, Zandwijk N. High dose rate brachytherapy improves resectability in squamous cell lung cancer. Chest 102:308-309, 1992.

89. Macha HN, Wahlers B. Adjuvant endobronchial irradiation with curative intent: a report of 17 patients. Presented at the Eighth International Brachytherapy Conference; April 1993; New York, NY.

90. Speiser B, Spratling L. Fatal hemoptysis: complication or failure of treatment. Int J Radiat Oncol Biol Phys 25:925, 1993.

91. Miller R, McGregor D. Hemorrhage from carcinoma of the lung. Cancer 36:904-913, 1975.

92. Khanavkar B, Stern P, Alberti W, et al. Complications associated with brachytherapy alone or with laser in lung cancer. Chest 99:1062-1065, 1991.

93. Speiser BL, Spartling L. Radiation bronchitis and stenosis secondary to high dose rate endobronchial irradiation. Int J Radiat Oncol Biol Phys 25:589-597, 1993.

94. Mehta MP, Shahabi S, Jarjour NN, et al. Endobronchial irradiation for malignant airway obstruction. Int J Radiat Oncol Biol Phys 17:847-851, 1989.

**Chapter 12**

# High Dose Rate Brachytherapy for Breast Cancer

*Daniel H. Clarke, Frank Vicini, H. Jacobs, Chris G. Rowland, and Robert R. Kuske*

## Introduction

Over the past 20 years, there has been a dramatic shift in the understanding of the role of local therapy in the treatment of early stage breast cancer. Multiple retrospective studies, as well as seven prospective randomized trials, have convincingly shown that lumpectomy, followed by radiation therapy, is equivalent to mastectomy in terms of disease-free and overall survival.[1] The recognition that breast-conserving techniques are as effective as amputation has resulted in a gradual shift away from mastectomy and a declaration by the National Cancer Institute Consensus Development Conference in 1990 that lumpectomy plus radiation therapy should now be considered as the preferred treatment in the management of this disease.[2]

As with any cancer treatment, it is desirable to improve treatment techniques to optimize the end results. With breast conserving therapy (BCT), there are two methods for accomplishing this: (1) refinement of the selection criteria that determine the patients most suitable for BCT and (2) improvements in the techniques of treatment for those patients selected. A considerable body of literature has been published in both these areas. While there is some controversy as to the full effect of various prognostic factors on the success of BCT, published reports have shown that young age, an extensive intraductal component (EIC), mononuclear cell reaction, high grade, tumor necrosis, endolymphatic invasion, and infiltrating lobular histology can be associated with a higher risk of relapse in the breast after BCT.[3,4] What constitutes the most appropriate technique of BCT, however, has yet to be agreed upon.

Most of the debate regarding the optimal technique of BCT centers on two questions: (1) What is the most appropriate extent of surgical resection; and (2) How much radiation should be delivered? Though each of these concepts may, at first, appear to be independent, recent data have convincingly shown that they are both interrelated and complimentary. The surgical options that have been used to treat breast cancer include biopsy, gross local excision, wide excision, and quadrantectomy. In general, the more limited surgeries produce the

From: Nag, S. (ed.): *High Dose Rate Brachytherapy: A Textbook*, Futura Publishing Company, Inc., Armonk, NY, © 1994.

least cosmetic distortion but at a cost of higher risk of local recurrence. Conversely, larger surgeries appear to yield the best local control rates but at the price of less-satisfactory cosmetic results. Recent data from the Joint Center for Radiation Therapy, Boston, Massachusetts, clearly illustrate both of these points. Olivetto et al.[5] demonstrated that the cosmetic outcome was adversely affected when the lumpectomy specimen measured more than 75 cm.[3] Conversely, Vicini et al.,[6] analyzing the same group of patients, showed that the risk of local recurrence decreased as the extent of surgical resection increased. What then represents the optimal extent of tumor excision to provide both good local control and an acceptable cosmetic result? Ideally, wide excision or a re-excision should be performed to achieve pathologically negative surgical margins. However, from a practical point of view, histologic assessment of the adequacy of margins is difficult to perform. Moreover, achieving pathologically negative margins is likely to be most important in cases with an EIC but considerably less so when an EIC is absent. In the analysis above by Vicini et al.[6] (Table 1), the impact of surgical resection on decreasing the risk of local recurrence was most pronounced in patients with an EIC. In patients without an EIC, local control was easily achieved with standard doses of whole breast radiation therapy (supplemented by a carefully designed boost) even in the case of focally positive margins or a small breast resection. In the presence of an EIC, standard doses of radiation did not appear to be adequate to control local disease, and only in those patients with larger surgeries was the local control rate acceptable. Thus, the need for wide surgical margins and for re-excision should be carefully assessed and tailored to the individual case.

With respect to the optimal dose of radiotherapy in BCT, the literature is also controversial. Multiple investigations have shown a "dose response relationship" between the tumor-bed dose and the rate of local control. Nobler et al.[7] reported a better control rate in the breast with doses > 60 Gy. A dose response was also shown by van Limbergen et al.[8] Clarke et al.[9] also reported a dose response relationship; when a nominal standard dose (NSD) of less than 1,840 ret was given to the tumor bed, a higher recurrence rate was noted. Others have not shown this clear-cut dose response relationship. This controversy may, in large part, be explained by the findings published by Holland et al.,[10] who performed a pathological and radiographic study on mastectomy specimens to assess where the residual tumor was located after a simulated tumor excision. They found that 43% of patients would have had a residual tumor remaining in the breast after tumor excisions with a 2-cm margin. Of greater significance, however, was the fact that patients with EIC were more likely to have a prominent amount of residual ductal carcinoma-in-situ (DCIS) remaining in the breast after tumor excision than patients without an EIC (44% vs. 3% $P <$ 0.0001). What these data imply is that much of the risk of tumor recurrence in the breasts after BCT may be related to the volume of disease remaining in the breast after surgery. In patients with an EIC, either an increased breast resection or a higher tumor-bed dose (or both) may be needed to overcome the effect of this risk factor. Thus, with the knowledge of what constitutes a high-risk subgroup, and with an understanding of the extent of surgical resection that

### Table 1

### 5-Year Actuarial Rate of Local Breast Recurrence in Relation to the Extent of Breast Resection and the Presence of EIC

| | | *Extent of Breast Resection* | | | |
|---|---|---|---|---|---|
| | *Tumor Size* | *Smallest* | *Intermediate* | *Largest* | *Probability Value* |
| EIC+ | T1 | 29% | 22% | 10% | 0.07 |
| | T2 | 36% | 26% | 9% | 0.04 |
| EIC− | T1 | 9% | 2% | 0% | 0.02 |
| | T2 | 6% | 2% | 3% | NS |

has been undertaken, the aggressiveness of breast radiation therapy can be appropriately tailored to improve outcome.

On the basis of the above data, the following recommendations can be made regarding treatment to the breast with radiation in patients treated with BCT. After adequate surgery has been performed, whole breast radiation to doses in the range of 45–50 cGy should be delivered. This is followed, in virtually all patients, with a boost to the tumor bed. As noted above, it has been suggested that a dose effect with breast cancer does exist. In all the series where this has been analyzed, it is the tumor bed dose, not the breast dose, that is most important. In patients without adverse histopathological findings, a tumor-bed dose of 60 Gy should be adequate. Patients with significant risk factors for local recurrence (i.e., high grade, an EIC that is inadequately excised, young age, etc.) should be boosted more aggressively. For these patients, an interstitial implant is advised since higher doses can be delivered with good or excellent cosmesis. These boosts should include a generous volume and, in cases with significant DCIS, should probably include the nipple-areolar complex.

Vicini et al.[11] recently analyzed their implant experience in a series of 402 patients treated with BCT at William Beaumont Hospital, Royal Oak, Michigan (Table 2). Patients underwent excisional biopsy and were treated to the tumor bed to at least 60 Gy using either electrons, photons, or an interstitial implant that used either Ir-192 or I-125. With a median follow-up of 60 months, no statistically significant differences were noted among the various boost modalities with regard to local control or cosmesis.[11] However, 72% of patients

### Table 2

### 5-Year Actuarial Rate of Local Breast Recurrence in Relation to the Boost Technique

| *Boost Techniques* | *No. of Pts.* | *Med Follow-up (mos)* | *Distant Failure* | *Local Recurrence* |
|---|---|---|---|---|
| I-125 | 86 | 46.0 | 14.0% | 3.0% |
| Ir-192 | 197 | 75.7 | 13.9% | 3.8% |
| Electrons | 204 | 50.4 | 10.2% | 5.4% |
| Photons | 15 | 54.4 | 0% | 0% |

boosted with an I-125 implant were considered to have significant risk factors for local recurrence (i.e., EIC, high grade, tumor necrosis, inadequate margins). The excellent rate of local control in these patients (97%) suggests that implant boosts may be capable of providing high rates of local control even in subsets of patients considered to be at high risk for recurrence.

Recently, it has been suggested that certain patients with early-stage breast cancer may only need treatment to the tumor bed after breast-conserving surgery. Recent studies appear to indicate that prophylactic treatment of the whole breast may not be required.[12] Most of the logistical problems with BCT relate to the protracted course of external beam radiation directed to the whole breast. As a result, several investigators are assessing the outcome of wide local excision followed by an interstitial implant alone as a definitive local treatment. Early results from pilot trials in Europe suggest that this approach can provide both an acceptable cosmetic outcome and excellent local control in carefully selected patients.[13]

The sections that follow address the use of interstitial implants of the breast both as a method of boost therapy with standard BCT and as the sole method of radiation treatment. The results of several European trials will be presented with an emphasis on the role that high dose rate (HDR) brachytherapy may have in improving both outcome and treatment acceptance.

## Interstitial Implants of the Breast—Boost Therapy

Interstitial implant boosts should be considered in patients treated with BCT if significant risk factors for local recurrence (both clinical and/or histopathological) have been identified or in patients with large breasts not easily suitable to electron-beam teletherapy. In most patients, the implant boost is performed 7–10 days after whole breast irradiation under local or general anesthesia. These implants can also be performed perioperatively (i.e., at the time of axillary dissection) thus avoiding an additional surgical procedure and allowing the surgeon's input into the identification of the tumor bed.

Traditionally, interstitial implants have been performed using low dose rate (LDR) techniques that use the isotopes Ir-192 or I-125 (see previous section). More recently, these techniques have been modified in order to incorporate the advantages of HDR treatment. Various implant techniques can be used, but most employ either a rigid template or a freehand system of needle placement. After the area to be implanted is identified, hollow stainless steel needles are inserted into the breast. These are then replaced with afterloading tubes that accommodate either an LDR or HDR source. Depending upon the implant technique or isotopes chosen, these catheters remain in position from as little as several hours up to 4 days.

### The Winterberg-Krankenhaus Experience

In 1977 breast-conserving therapy (BCT) was introduced at Saarbrücker Winterbergkliniken. Following external beam radiation (EBR) to the breast, an interstitial HDR boost was performed for the majority of patients. The results in patients with a minimum 3-year follow-up are presented.

Tumors 3.5 cm or smaller were included in the protocol. The tumor-node metastasis (TNM) stage distribution of 403 patients is shown in Table 3. The treatment protocol was as follows.

(1) gross tumor excision;
(2) 46 Gy in 23 fractions with 6 MV photons to the breast;
(3) interstitial HDR brachytherapy—a single fraction of 10–15 Gy;or
(4) electron beam boost of 10–15 Gy to the 85% isodose line at 2–2.5 Gy/fraction.

The target volume of the boost field included the surgical bed with additional margin provided in cases of duct cancer in situ or lymphatic space involvement. The target volume did not include the skin; the source-dwell positions did not come closer than 1.0 cm from the skin surface.

Special templates were used to facilitate parallel placement of stainless steel needles. The implant was performed under local or general anesthesia 10 days after EBR. Most patients had two plane implants with a mean treatment volume of 40–45 cc.

The breakdown by stage and type of boost is shown in Table 4. The majority of patients received HDR boosts. The crude local control rate for the entire group was 93%. The risk of local relapse by type of boost is shown in Table 5.

The cosmetic results were good to excellent in most patients (HDR: 81%, electrons: 75%, no boost: 88%). Early in the HDR experience, some patients had skin unintentionally treated because of poor fixation of the template. These

#### Table 3

#### Stage Distribution

| TNM Stage | Number of patients |
|-----------|--------------------|
| T1N0 | 187 |
| T2N0 | 95 |
| T1N1 | 72 |
| T2N1 | 49 |
| T1N0–T2N1 | 403 |

#### Table 4

#### Stage and Type of Boost

| Stage | HDR | Electron | None |
|-------|-----|----------|------|
| T1N0 | 90 | 61 | 36 |
| T2N0 | 59 | 23 | 13 |
| T1N1 | 38 | 34 | 0 |
| T2N1 | 37 | 12 | 0 |
| T1N0–T2N1 | 224 (56%) | 130 (32%) | 49 (12%) |

**Table 5**

**Crude Local Control Rate by Type of Boost**

| | HDR (1982–1988) | Electron (1977–1988) | None (1977–1988) |
|---|---|---|---|
| Overall local control | 210/224 (94%) | 120/130 (92%) | 44/49 (90%) |
| Control in original quadrant | 214/224 (96%) | 122/130 (94%) | 44/49 (90%) |
| Median follow-up | 5.8 yrs | 7.4 yrs | 7.6 yrs |

patients developed circular telangiectasia around the puncture site. Localized breast fibrosis developed in 20–25% of cases.

In summary, HDR boosts were safely and conveniently administered to patients who were candidates for such a boost. As opposed to LDR boosts, no hospitalization or overnight stay was required, thereby reducing costs and inconvenience for the patient. At the last follow-up, HDR implant boosts appeared to result in the same local control and overall cosmetic results as those achieved with conventional LDR boosts.

## Interstitial Implants of the Breast—Implant Alone

Interstitial breast implants can also be used to provide the entire radiation treatment in selected patients with early stage breast cancer. Earlier pilot trials used LDR techniques (i.e., Ir-192).[13] Currently, most investigators have incorporated HDR systems that maximize the advantages of this modality. These advantages include (1) optimized dose distributions within the implanted volume; (2) no need for patient hospitalization to deliver the radiation treatment; and (3) radiation protection to staff and personnel.

### The Ochsner Clinic Experience: Results of a Pilot Trial—Implant Alone

In January 1992, a pilot study opened at the Ochsner Clinic, New Orleans, Louisiana, exploring a technique that shortens the overall radiation therapy treatment course for BCT patients from the usual 6 weeks to 4 days. Patients with in situ T1 or T2 and N0 or N1 disease were eligible, providing that only 1–3 nodes contained metastases and that there was no extracapsular extension. Negative microscopic surgical margins were required.

The study closed in August 1993 after an accrual of 23 patients. The first 11 patients were treated with LDR iridium-192. The last 12 patients were treated with HDR Ir-192 remote afterloading equipment. With HDR alone, patients received 8 fractions of 4 Gy, with at least 6 hours between fractions over 4 elapsed days. The implants were more generous than those typically used when the implant boost was combined with external beam RT. A freehand technique was preferred to a rigid template. A minimum of 2 cm beyond all surgical clips was required for the target volume. This resulted in large-volume implants; for example, a 5-cm excision cavity with a 2-cm target volume beyond the cavity wall would result in a target volume 9 cm long. A typical implant on this protocol included 10 catheters in the deep plane and 9 catheters in the superficial plane. Only one patient required 3 planes to cover the target volume.

The implant dosimetry was performed according to the Paris Dosimetry System (PDS): the basal dose rates were calculated at the intersource position in the transverse plane, and the treatment time was calculated for a reference dose (RD) rate taken to be 85% of the average basal dose rate (ABD).

The implant calculation was done using a Nucletron planning system (NPS) as follows:

(1) The catheters of the implant were aligned along one of the axes of the cartesian coordinates using the interactive graphics.

(2) In order to have a point of reference, an "applicator point" was selected in "Z" axis external to the implant.

(3) With the desired dose specified at this "applicator point," a geometrical optimization was performed and the dwell times for the implant obtained.

(4) The isodose distribution was displayed in a transverse plane cutting through the center of the implant. In the same plane, the basal dose points were selected and the dose values measured with the distance-dose ruler. The ABD was then calculated.

(5) If the isodose line going through the "applicator point" was not within (± 3%) of the 85% value of the ABD, a new "applicator point" was chosen and the optimization process repeated.

(6) Steps 4 and 5 were repeated until the goal was achieved and the final isodose curves were acceptable.

The median follow-up time of 8 months was too short to adequately evaluate tumor control. However, there have been no local recurrences to date. The preliminary toxicity results were encouraging. There was only one grade III and two grade II toxicities. The grade III toxicity occurred in an LDR patient who experienced cellulitis of the breast and an abscess within the tylectomy cavity, requiring a 10-day hospitalization, debridement, and intravenous antibiotics. The two grade II toxicities comprised self-limiting chest wall pain (probably from myositis) and moist desquamation of the skin. Initial cosmetic results demonstrated good symmetry in the shape of the treated breast compared to the contralateral breast and minimal to no skin changes other than transient dark spots at the skin entry and exit points where the buttons come in contact with the skin.

Patients were enthusiastic about participation in the study, particularly those women who lived more than 50 miles from the clinic, the elderly, or busy working women trying to minimize disruption of their lives by repeated trips to the radiation oncology department.

**Royal Devon and Exeter Hospital Experience**

HDR interstitial brachytherapy was recently introduced as the sole treatment following tumor excision at the Royal Devon and Exeter Hospital, Exeter, England. The age range of patients was 30–90 years and represented referrals from a number of surgeons. The implants were performed by one radiation oncologist. Patients selected for this treatment had T1–T2 (less than 4-cm diameter) cancers moderately or well differentiated, with clear or close margins.

A local tumor excision with at least a 1-cm margin was performed. By prior agreement, the skin incision was made directly over the tumor so as to lessen the chance of a geographical miss; most patients were implanted some weeks after lumpectomy. Hematomas necessitated an early implant since "tissue organization" can complicate the procedure. Lymph node assessment was by clinical examination only; only one axillary dissection was performed.

A rigid template and needle system was used to compress the breast into a well-defined and reproducible volume, in some cases approximating a quadrantectomy. This allowed for very accurate placement of iridium sources with delivery of a low dose to the crucial organ, the skin. In addition, the needles split rather than cut the skin, which allowed excellent healing. Often, there was a small amount of reactionary edema in the breast, but this advantageously conforms the breast to the applicator. The implants were performed under local or general anesthesia, according to patient preference, and suitable patients were allowed home with the applicator in situ. Dosimetry was in accordance with the PDS, and 3 fractionation schedules were used with a minimum 4-hr gap between treatments: (a) 20 Gy in 2 fractions (22 patients), (b) 28 Gy in 4 fractions (17 patients), and (c) 32 Gy in 6 fractions (8 patients).

Cosmesis was assessed by both the radiation oncologist (C.G.Rowland) and the patient on a 1 to 3 scale (1 = excellent, 2 = good, and 3 = poor). No cases of wound infection or skin necrosis were recorded.

Forty-five patients (mean age: 63 years; range: 30–90 years) were entered in the study. Ten patients had been started on tamoxifen prior to treatment. The mean follow-up time was 18 months (range 6–36 months).

Local recurrence (within the treated volume) was observed in four cases. Of these, two have had synchronous axillary recurrence. All these have been successfully salvaged locally by EBR (three cases) or radical surgery (one case). Two patients have died of metastases, one is alive with metastases, and one remains disease free at present. Two additional patients have died of metastases with full local control. Three patients developed new primaries (greater than 3 cm from the treatment volume—one with axillary involvement). These were successfully controlled using EBR or mastectomy. Two patients were lost to follow-up but were disease free when last seen.

Cosmetic outcome was excellent in 95% of cases. There were no cases of wound infection or skin necrosis. Cosmesis related to the amount of tissue surgically excised rather than the long-term effects of radiation.

This pilot study showed that HDR radiation to a limited volume was a practical proposition offering excellent cosmesis and may be appropriate for selected patients. The study population represented referrals from a number of surgeons, mainly prior to the instigation of a screening program. Routine axillary dissection was not performed, and in many cases detailed histology was not available. While this was clearly not an ideal or consensus situation, it is likely to be the actual situation in many parts of Britain and other countries in the world. The question is thus raised as to whether quadrantectomy can be replaced by an equivalent implant giving a high dose of radiation in the area of risk without irradiating the whole breast. As further screening (including biological) methods become common, it may become possible to select a group of women suitable for minimal effective local treatment.

## REFERENCES

1. Harris JR, Lippman ME, Veronesi V, et al. Medical progress: breast cancer. N Engl J Med 327(6):390-398, 1992.
2. NIH Consensus Conference. Treatment of early-stage breast cancer. JAMA 265:391, 1991.
3. Kurtz JM, Jaequemier J, Amalric R, et al. Risk factors of breast recurrence in pre and postmenopausal patients with ductal cancers. Cancer 65:1867, 1990.
4. Clarke D, Martinez AA. Identification of patients who are at high risk for locoregional breast cancer recurrence after conservative surgery and radiotherapy: a review article for surgeons, pathologists, and radiation and medical oncologists. J Clin Oncol 10:474-483, 1992.
5. Olivetto IA, Rose MA, Osteen RT, et al. Late cosmetic outcome after conservative surgery and radiotherapy: analysis of causes of cosmetic failure. Int J Radiat Oncol Biol Phys 17:747-753, 1989.
6. Vicini FA, Eberlein TJ, Connolly JL, et al. The optimal extent of resection for patients with stages I and II breast cancer treated with conservative surgery and radiotherapy. Ann Surg 214:200-205, 1991.
7. Nobler MP, Venet L. Prognostic factors in patients undergoing curative irradiation for breast cancer. Int J Radiat Oncol Biol Phys 11:1323-1331, 1985.
8. van Limbergen E, van den Bogaert W, van der Schueren E, et al. Tumor excision and radiotherapy as primary treatment of breast cancer: analysis of patient and treatment parameters and local control. Radiother Oncol 8:1-9, 1987.
9. Clarke DH, Le MG, Sarrazin D, et al. Analysis of local-regional relapses in patients with early breast cancers treated with excision and radiotherapy: experience of the Institut Gustave-Roussy. Int J Radiat Oncol Biol Phys 11: 137-145, 1985.
10. Holland R, Connolly J, Gelman R, et al. Nature and extent of residual cancer in the breast related to the intraductal component in the primary tumour. Int J Radiat Oncol Biol Phys 15:182-183, 1988.
11. Vicini FA, White J, Gustafson G, et al. The use of iodine-125 seeds as a substitute for iridium-192 seeds in temporary interstitial breast implants. Int J Radiat Oncol Biol Phys 27:561-566, 1993.
12. Ribiero GG, Dunn G, Swindell R, et al. Conservation of the breast using two different techniques: interim report of a clinical trial. Clin Oncol (R Coll Radiol) 2:27-34, 1990.
13. Fentiman IS, Poole C, Tong D, et al. Iridium implant treatment without external radiotherapy for operable breast cancer: a pilot study. Eur J Cancer 27:447-450, 1991.

# Chapter 13

# Remote Afterloading High Dose Rate Brachytherapy for Carcinoma of the Bile Duct

*Dattatreyudu Nori, Subir Nag, David Rogers, and Bhadrassain Vikram*

## Introduction

Carcinoma of the extrahepatic bile duct accounts for 0.5% of all cancers in the United States. Reported 5-year survival ranges from 0 to 10%. Surgery, when available, is a treatment of choice; however, 70–80% of these cancers are unresectable.[1,2] Unresectable lesions are best palliated by drainage procedures followed by radiation therapy with or without chemotherapy.[3] Some authors have boosted the external beam radiation therapy (EBRT) dose by adding various doses of transhepatic intraluminal low dose rate (LDR) [192]Ir brachytherapy over 2–4 days on an in-patient basis.[4-19] This combination has the advantage of delivering a high dose to the tumor while sparing the surrounding normal tissues (liver, kidney, and bowel). Such aggressive local regional therapy can substantially improve both the quality and duration of life for patients with cholangiocarcinoma.[4] However, its use involves issues of radiation exposure, patient convenience, and catheter-related sepsis that must be considered. Intraluminal high dose rate (HDR) remote brachytherapy used on an out-patient basis[20-23] addresses these concerns.

## Methods

Whenever possible, megavoltage radiation therapy is combined in patients receiving intraluminal brachytherapy. The brachytherapy can be delivered by a transhepatic cholangiocatheter[20] or by an endoscopic retrograde technique.[21,22]

### External Beam Radiation Therapy

The target area for external beam radiation therapy (EBRT) is determined by adding a 2-cm margin to the tumor volume and the potential lymph node

From: Nag, S. (ed.): *High Dose Rate Brachytherapy: A Textbook*, Futura Publishing Company, Inc., Armonk, NY, © 1994.

drainage areas identified on computed tomography (CT) and a cholangiogram. Patients are then treated by parallel anterior and posterior EBRT or 4-field EBRT to a dose of 45–50 Gy in 25 fractions. Appropriate shielding is used for the liver and kidneys.

## Brachytherapy

Much of the morbidity associated with biliary drainage catheters is secondary to sepsis. With this in mind, the following guidelines should be considered an integral part of the management of these patients.

(1) Antibiotic prophylactics should be given the day before the procedure, the day of the procedure, and the day after the procedure.

(2) The biliary drainage system is a closed system. It is, therefore, of paramount importance to maintain sterile technique when the system is open for insertion of the afterloading catheter into the biliary drainage catheter.

(3) At the completion of the procedure, the biliary drainage system should be flushed early with at least 50 cc of sterile normal saline.

(4) One month after the last treatment, the patient should be evaluated by the interventional radiologist for placement of an internal stent and removal of the biliary drainage catheter.

## Transhepatic Cholangiocatheter Technique

Currently available remote afterloading HDR catheters can be negotiated without difficulty through a 12 French catheter. For this reason, 10 days after the completion of external beam therapy, patients have their standard transhepatic catheter replaced with a 12 French catheter, if necessary. The pretreatment cholangiogram findings are reviewed with the diagnostic radiologist, and the area of obstruction is identified. This information is then reviewed with the planning physicist who determines the active treatment length by adding a 2-cm margin to both the proximal and distal ends of the obstructed segment. With the aid of a computer, the physicist then determines the number of dwell positions, their optimal separations from one another, and the length of time the sources should remain in each of the dwell positions to deliver a dose of 5 Gy to a depth of 1 cm from the catheter.

The biliary drain is opened, and the orifice is cleansed with sterile betadine wipes. The catheter is then flushed with a minimum of 50 cc of sterile normal saline, and the afterloading catheter is inserted to the predetermined length in the larger biliary drainage catheter. Dummy source ribbons are then inserted through the catheter. Orthogonal films are obtained, and the positioning is reviewed. A customized computer treatment plan is prepared, and the dummy ribbons are removed. A sterile technique is maintained throughout these procedures.

The HDR brachytherapy catheter is then connected to the remote afterloader, and treatment is delivered. HDR brachytherapy tubing is disconnected, and the catheter is removed. The biliary drainage catheter is then flushed and reconnected to the drainage bag. The nursing staff then reviews appropriate follow-up care with the patient and his or her family. Antibiotic treatment is also administered during treatment and on the day before and the day after the treatment. The procedure is repeated three more times at weekly intervals. One month after completion of therapy, the patient is evaluated by the interventional radiologist for removal of the biliary drainage tube and placement of an internal stent.

Between September 1990 and September 1993, 15 patients presenting with signs and symptoms of obstructive jaundice were diagnosed radiologically (4 patients) or histologically (11 patients) with unresectable bile duct cancer at the New York Hospital Medical Center of Queens. Initially, all patients underwent a temporary transhepatic drainage using a 12 hepatic catheter to relieve the obstruction. Subsequently, they were started on external beam radiation (EBR), receiving 45 to 50 Gy at 1.8 Gy per fraction over a period of 5 weeks with concomitant 5-Flurouracil (FU) chemotherapy. Two weeks after EBRT, HDR brachytherapy was initiated on an out-patient basis, delivering a total of 15–20 Gy in total in 3–4 fractions of 5 Gy, spaced 1 week apart. These 15 patients underwent a total of 60 out-patient HDR treatments. The brachytherapy treatment volume encompassed the area of original obstruction and 2–3 cm proximal and distal margins as outlined by the pretreatment cholangiogram. Treatment length varied from 5–7 cm. Transhepatic catheters were removed 1 to 2 months after HDR, and a permanent stent was placed.

## *Endoscopic Technique* [21,22]

Before the procedure, the biliary tract is visualized radiographically by cholangiography to define the stricture and the extent of the disease. An endoscopic retrograde cholangiopancreatography (ERCP) is performed by a gastroenterologist, and sphincterotomy is performed to provide access for a large caliber prosthesis. A 0.035-inch (0.089-cm) guide wire is loaded into a 7 French Van Andel catheter, and, after the bile duct is cannulated, this guide wire is advanced through the malignant stricture.

Under fluoroscopy, the Van Andel catheter is removed, leaving the guide wire in place. A 10 French straight nasobiliary tube is threaded over the guide wire and through the channel. The nasobiliary tube is advanced beyond the stricture and into the biliary tree. The endoscope is then slowly withdrawn over the tube. The position of the guide wire and all other stages of the procedure are repeatedly checked with fluoroscopy. Care is taken to avoid forming a redundant loop in the duodenum since additional turns could be more difficult for the HDR remote afterloading source to negotiate. After removal of the endoscope, the proximal end of the tube is rerouted from the mouth to the nose, and the nasobiliary tube is taped to the patient's cheek.

An extra long (130-cm) 6 French afterloading catheter with an inner radio-opaque wire is then passed through a 10 French nasobiliary tube under fluoroscopy and advanced through the lesion. The dummy wire has radio-opaque markers at intervals that simulate the potential placement of iridium-192 seeds. Localization radiographs are taken for dosimetric purposes. On the basis of the location of the catheter, the radiographic cholangiography, and the CT or magnetic resonance imaging (MRI) scans, the tumor volume is identified. Then, after the dose is calculated, the positions to be programmed and the dwell times of the sources in each position are determined.

One significant advantage of this technique is the ability to optimize, that is, to shape the HDR radiation volume to the shape of the tumor. With conventional brachytherapy techniques, it is rarely possible to obtain a shape other than a tapered cylinder; however, by varying the microSelectron-HDR source positions and dwell times, any desired shape can be obtained.

After the source positions and dwell times are determined, a computerized dose distribution is printed out. The dummy source wire is removed, and the microSelectron-HDR is attached to the nasobiliary afterloading catheter. Under audiovisual monitoring, the patient receives the appropriate dose over a few minutes. For patients who are to receive no EBRT, HDR brachytherapy is delivered at a rate of 5 Gy per fraction prescribed at 1 cm from the center of the catheter. Treatments are delivered twice each day to a total of 6 treatments. The total dose is thus 30 Gy in 6 fractions over 3 days. If indicated, this treatment can be repeated between 3 and 6 weeks later.

For patients who are to receive EBRT and brachytherapy, a total of 45 Gy of EBRT is delivered to the target volume, usually by a 4-field technique. Brachytherapy is delivered either before or after (only occasionally concurrently) EBRT, depending on the clinical circumstances. Brachytherapy is delivered at 5 Gy per fraction, prescribed at 1 cm from the center of the catheter, twice each day for a total of 4 treatments (total dose = 20 Gy in 4 fractions over 2 days). Patients receiving concurrent EBRT and brachytherapy may receive as little as 5 Gy of brachytherapy in one fraction, once a week, for 4 weeks.

After the treatment is completed, the nasobiliary tube is removed, and the patient is returned to the endoscopy unit, where an ERCP is performed again, and a large caliber endoprosthesis is positioned for biliary drainage. The patient is placed on intravenous antibiotics and observed for 24–48 hours; then regular diet is resumed.

## Results at the New York Hospital Medical Center of Queens

The multimodality therapy consisting of EBRT, chemotherapy, and HDR brachytherapy was extremely well tolerated. Eight of 15 patients reported mild to moderate gastrointestinal symptoms, nausea, and diarrhea, and all were treated symptomatically. None of the patients suffered serious morbidity requiring hospitalization. One patient developed signs of vertebral body collapse at L1, which was diagnosed to be an *E. coli* infection and responded to antibiotic therapy. One patient developed duodenal bleeding owing to recurrent cancer 10 months after treatment. The follow-up period ranged from 6 months to 24 months (median of 8 months); 8 patients were alive, disease free, and symptom free, with weight gain and good quality of life at 6, 6, 8, 8, 8, 9, 11, and 24 months, respectively. Pavlou et al.[21] reported on eight patients treated with the endoscopic retrograde technique at Beth Israel Medical Center in New York. Few and insignificant immediate complications were reported. However, one problem encountered was that, in some instances, the HDR source was unable to negotiate the curve from the duodenum into the bile duct. These patients required treatment with LDR manually afterloaded [192]Ir sources. Pakisch et al.[23] reported good palliation in 9 patients treated with 50.4 Gy EBRT and 10 Gy hyperfractionated HDR brachytherapy.

## Discussion

At present, surgery is the only curative treatment for extrahepatic bile duct cancer. The preferred surgical treatment involves excising the tumor and involved ductal systems and establishing enteric bile drainage by a Roux-En-Y hepaticojejunostomy.[24] Of the approximately 25% of patients who undergo surgery, about 50% will be found to have microscopically positive margins; about 80% of those will ultimately develop local recurrence.[24]

Local regional failure is a predominant cause of death in both resectable and unresectable cases. This has led to a vigorous search for methods to im prove both local control and possibly survival. In the late 1970s and early 1980s, early attempts to improve local regional control in inoperable cases involved the use of biliary drainage followed by EBRT (typically in the 0.4–0.6 Gy dose range). Patient tolerance was acceptable, and reports of significant palliation in occasional long-term survival supported its use. Encouraged by these results, several authors reported that further improvement in local control and survival could be achieved with local boost brachytherapy treatment and use of chemotherapy.[4,25]

The use of HDR brachytherapy for palliation of malignant biliary obstruction is a relatively simple technique causing very little morbidity and providing a maximum amount of palliation. For the occasional patient with early disease, its use also offers the possibility of a cure. Radiation given via brachytherapy has been found to be well suited to these cases and can be combined with a drainage procedure and EBRT. It has also been shown to result in increased survival, compared with treatment by surgery alone.[17]

The insertion of a 10 or 12 French biliary catheter, which is large enough to accommodate the remote afterloading brachytherapy catheter in the biliary tract, may be accomplished through either a percutaneous transhepatic catherization[20,23] or a retrograde approach through the ampulla of Vater.[21,22]

The transduodenal endoscopic technique is an effective method to relieve biliary obstruction. Internal biliary drainage offers several advantages over percutaneous drainage, for example, fewer complications, no puncture of the liver, less pain, and no need for an external catheter or hardware. However, it requires a longer catheter (130 cm compared to the standard 100-cm catheter), and sometimes the HDR source cannot negotiate the sharp curve from the duodenum to the common bile duct. In these cases, LDR [192]Ir brachytherapy must be used.

An HDR remote afterloading device to treat patients with malignant biliary tract tumors offers significant advantages over other conventional approaches.

(1) Because the intraluminal brachytherapy is delivered through pre-existing transhepatic drainage catheters, there is no need to place special catheters for brachytherapy.

(2) The brachytherapy is delivered on an out-patient basis by using a remote afterloading system. Thus, there is no exposure to the nursing staff, and the quality of care does not suffer because of the concerns of the radiation exposure.

(3) The out-patient treatments are convenient, safe, and cost effective, making fractionation possible. And fractionation allows for the possibility of tumor shrinkage between fractions and the achievement of better dosimetry with succeeding treatments.

(4) The short duration of treatment (a few minutes) should (a) decrease the potential for the development of sepsis because a closed system is maintained and there is no potential for radioactive sources to obstruct the drainage catheters (leading to bile stasis) since the sources are removed in minutes and (b) improve upon the precision of treatment because the position of the sources in the catheter is less likely to shift during the shorter treatment period.

(5) Out-patient treatment improves patient acceptance and decreases costs compared to conventional in-patient treatment.

(6) HDR remote afterloading brachytherapy allows optimization of the treatment volume according to the extent of the disease.

Further advances in the technique include the use of ultrasound to determine tumor volume[26] and the addition of interstitial microwave hyperthermia.[27] Minsky et al.[26] inserted a small diameter endoluminal ultrasound probe into the bile-duct drainage tube to accurately define the proximal, distal, and lateral extent of the biliary tumor and to assess the response to therapy. Coughlin et al.[27] treated 10 patients with single-antenna, interstitial microwave hyperthermia and iridium-192 brachytherapy. The hyperthermia antenna was inserted into the drainage catheter to heat the tumor volume to 45°C for 60 minutes before and after 55–79 Gy (calculated at 0.5-cm) LDR brachytherapy.

Although HDR brachytherapy offers a potentially effective treatment for these tumors, its use has been limited by some disadvantages. Major disadvantages are the lack of standardization of technique and the wide variation in dose prescription point, making it difficult to compare the clinical results. A broad range of dose prescription points have been reported: the surface of the bile duct,[13] at 0.5 cm,[19,20,23,28] at 0.75 cm,[23] at 1 cm,[11,15,21] at 2.25 cm,[14] at 2.5 cm,[26] or unmentioned in the report.[12] For uniformity, it is suggested that the dosage be prescribed at 1 cm from the source.[11]

## Conclusion

The combination of EBRT, chemotherapy, HDR brachytherapy, and out-patient HDR brachytherapy appears to be well tolerated in patients with unre-sectable primary bile duct cancers. Out-patient HDR brachytherapy has the additional advantage of convenience to the patient, elimination of radiation ex-posure to the staff, precision of radiation delivery, and optimization treatment based on the extent of the disease. Both subjective and objective treatment re-sponses have been very encouraging. We believe that this treatment deserves consideration as part of the standard treatment for this cancer.

## REFERENCES

1. Fields JN, Emani B. Carcinoma of the extrahepatic biliary system. Results of pri-mary and adjacent radiation therapy. Int J Radiat Oncol Biol Phys 13:331-338, 1987.
2. Evander A, Freudlund P, Hoevels J, et al. Evaluation of aggressive surgery for car-cinoma of extrahepatic bile ducts. Ann Surg 191:23-29, 1980.
3. Chitwood WR, Myers WC, Heaston DK, et al. Diagnosis and treatment of primary extrahepatic bile duct tumors. Am J Surg 143:99-106, 1982.
4. Minsky BD, Wesson NF, Armstrong JG, et al. Combined modality therapy of extra-hepatic biliary system cancer. Int J Radiat Oncol Biol Phys 18:1157-1163, 1990.
5. Minsky BD, Kemeny N, Armstrong JG, et al. Extrahepatic biliary system cancer: an update of an combined modality approach. Am J Clin Oncol 14:433-437, 1991.
6. Novell JR, Hilson A, Hobbs KE. Therapeutic aspects of radio-isotopes in hepato-biliary malignancy. Br J Surg 78:901-906, 1991.
7. Trodella L, Mantini G, Barina M, et al. External and intracavitary radiotherapy in the management of carcinoma of extrahepatic biliary tract. Rays 16:71-75, 1991.
8. Nunnerly HB, Karani JB. Interventional radiology of the biliary tract. Intraductal radiation. Radiol Clin North Am 28:1237-1240, 1990.
9. Hayes JK, Sapozink MD, Miller FJ. Definitive radiation therapy in bile duct carci-noma. Int J Radiol Oncol Biol Phys 15:735-744, 1988.
10. Son YH, Nori D, Leibel SA, et al. Biliary tree. In: Interstitial Collaborative Working Group, eds. Interstitial Brachytherapy. New York: Raven Press; 1990, 153-156.
11. Nag S, Tai DL, Gold RE. Biliary tract neoplasms: a simple management technique. South Med J 77:593-595, 1984.
12. Siegel JH, Lichtenstein JL, Pullano WE, et al. Treatment of malignant biliary ob-struction by endoscopic implantation of iridium-192 using a new double lumen en-doprosthesis. Gastrointest Endosc 34:301-306, 1988.
13. Herskovic A, Heaston D, Engler MJ, et al. Irradiation of biliary carcinoma. Radiol-ogy 139:219-222, 1981.
14. Kumar PP, Good RR, McCaul GF. Intraluminal endocurietherapy of inoperable Klatskin's Tumor with high-activity $^{192}$Iridium. Radiat Med 4:21-26, 1986.
15. Mornex F, Ardiet JM, Bret P, et al. Radiotherapy of high bile duct carcinoma using intracatheter iridium-192 wire. Cancer 54:2069-2073, 1984.
16. Fogel T, Weissberg JB. The role of radiation therapy in carcinoma of the extrahe-patic bile duct. Int J Radiat Oncol Biol Phys 10:2251-2258, 1984.
17. Karani J, Fletcher M, Brinkley D, et al. Internal biliary drainage and local radio-therapy with iridium-192 wire in treatment of hilar cholangiocarcinoma. Clin Ra-diol 36:603-606, 1985.

18. Molt P, Hopfan S, Watson RC, et al. Intraluminal radiation therapy in the management of malignant biliary obstruction. Cancer 57:536-544, 1986.
19. Fletcher MS, Brinkley D, Dawson JL, et al. Treatment of hilar carcinoma by bile drainage combined with internal radiotherapy using [192]iridium wire. Br J Surg 70:733-735, 1983.
20. Haffty BG, Mate TP, Greenwood LH, et al. Malignant biliary obstruction: intracavitary treatment with a high-dose-rate remote afterloading device. Radiology 164:574-576, 1987.
21. Pavlou WJ, Vikram B, Urban MS, et al. The use of high dose rate remote brachytherapy in the treatment of malignant biliary obstruction. Activity-Selectron Brachytherapy Journal 5:13-16, 1991.
22. Urban MS, Siegel JH, Pavlou W, et al. Treatment of malignant biliary obstruction with a high-dose rate remote afterloading device using a 10F nasobiliary tube. Gastrointest Endosc 36:292-296, 1990.
23. Pakisch B, Klein GE, Stucklschwieger G, et al. Metallic mesh endoprostheses and intraluminal high dose rate [192]Ir brachytherapy in the palliative treatment of malignant bile duct obstruction: initial results. Rofo Fortschr Geb Rontgenstr Neuen Bildgcb Vergahr 156:592-595, 1992. (In German)
24. Kopelson G, Galdabina J, Warshaw AL, et al. Patterns of failure after curative surgery for extrahepatic biliary carcinoma: implications for adjuvant therapy. Int J Radiat Oncol Biol Phys 7:413-417, 1981.
25. Harvey JH, Smith FP, Schein PS. 5 FU—Fluorouracil, mitomycin, doxorubicin, (FAM) carcinoma of the biliary tract. J Clin Oncol 11 (suppl.):1245-1248, 1984.
26. Minsky B, Botet J, Derdes H, et al. Ultrasound directed extrahepatic bile duct intraluminal brachytherapy. Int J Radiat Oncol Biol Phys 23:165-167, 1992.
27. Coughlin CT, Wong TZ, Ryan TP, et al. Interstitial microwave-induced hyperthermia and iridium brachytherapy for the treatment of obstructing biliary carcinomas. Int J Hyperthermia 8:57-171, 1992.
28. Wong JYC, Vora NL, Chou CK, et al. Intracatheter hyperthermia and iridium-192 radiotherapy in the treatment of bile duct carcinoma. Int J Radiat Oncol Biol Phys 14:353-359, 1988.

# Chapter 14

# Interstitial High Dose Rate Irradiation for Hepatic Tumors

*David S. Thomas and Anatoly Dritschilo*

## Introduction

Isolated hepatic metastases frequently occur in patients with colorectal carcinoma. An estimated 15,000 patients a year will have the liver only as the site of the initial metastatic disease when it is discovered.[1] Since surgical resection of the tumor is possible in only one-third of patients undergoing exploration, approximately 5,000 patients have hepatic metastases suitable for resection.[1] Upwards of 30% of patients who undergo partial hepatectomy will remain disease free at 5 years.[2,3] However, another 31% of explored patients have liver-confined but unresectable metastases.[2] If these lesions could be nonsurgically ablated, a survival rate similar to that seen with surgical resection may be potentially achieved.

Traditional radiotherapeutic efforts have shown either limited success or applicability in only very specific situations. External photon beam irradiation can encompass larger target volumes but is limited by the inability to deliver a tumorcidal dose within hepatic tolerance. Interstitial iodine seed implantation may be effective but cannot encompass large volumes.[4] Newer methods, such as radionuclide-tagged antibodies, apply only to certain tumor types (hepatoma). Nonsurgical and nonradiotherapeutic ablative techniques have been investigated. Although cryosurgery may treat somewhat larger tumors, it may cause bleeding from the hepatic surface and may thrombose hepatic vessels. Intra-arterial embolization may relieve pain but tends to be a palliative therapy since revascularization usually occurs.

Intraoperative electron beam irradiation for extrahepatic tumors can be curative.[5] Thus, a single, large dose of irradiation delivered within the tumor and sparing the surrounding tissues is potentially tumorcidal.[6] Such a therapeutic approach does not take advantage of radiation fractionation and repair and may be termed ablative radiation therapy. Intraoperative interstitial high dose rate (HDR) radiation therapy (IIRT) offers such radiation ablation for tumors inaccessible to intraoperative electron beam and thus is particularly suitable for hepatic tumors, such as colorectal metastases.[6,7]

From: Nag, S. (ed.): *High Dose Rate Brachytherapy: A Textbook*, Futura Publishing Company, Inc., Armonk, NY, © 1994.

Patients with tumors of other histologic types secondarily involving the liver may be candidates for interstitial irradiation. Such an approach is supported by extrapolation from surgical metastasectomy data.[8] Similarly, patients with primary hepatic tumors may also be considered candidates for ablative radiation since cure rates may approach 30% in patients with hepatoma treated by resection.[9]

## Methods

In a Phase I-II trial at Georgetown University Hospital, Washington, D.C., patients with unresectable or medically inoperable colorectal metastases were treated with HDR interstitial irradiation.[6,10] Initially, the procedure was performed in a standard linear accelerator room in the radiation oncology department. One or several 2.1-mm closed-end, beveled-tip needles were percutaneously placed through an intercostal space into the liver tumor. Ultrasound guidance confirmed proper placement.[11] A single fraction of 3.75 to 20 Gy was delivered with the GammaMed IIi afterloader (Mick Radio-Nuclear Instruments, Inc., Bronx, New York) and 10 Ci Ir-192 source. Needles remained in place for up to 30 minutes, and no bleeding was encountered in the six patients. The approach subsequently evolved to an intraoperative technique to better localize the tumor and to improve tumor control. An operative room was shielded with lead for the use of the interstitial intraoperative program.[6]

Eligibility criteria for HDR IIRT included the following:

(1) primary or secondary hepatic malignant tumor confined to the liver; alternately, coexistent minimal extrahepatic disease (either the primary site or other metastatic disease) that is amenable to radical surgery or radiation therapy;

(2) evidence of unresectability, such as involvement of both right and left hepatic lobes or close proximity to the vena cava; surgically resectable disease in the setting of medical inoperability (e.g., significant cardiac disease);

(3) medical condition permitting exploratory laparotomy;

(4) normal coagulation parameters;

(5) residual unirradiated liver parenchyma providing sufficient hepatic function.

(6) ability to encompass all disease within interstitial radiation volumes at laparotomy and thus radical intent;

(7) ability to limit dose to critical structures, such as major biliary ducts, to no more than 20 Gy.

Ineligibility criteria for IIRT included the following:

(1) untreatable extrahepatic primary tumor or metastases;

(2) ability to resect all known disease at the time of surgery;

(3) medical condition prohibiting exploratory laparotomy such as severe pulmonary or cardiac disease;

(4) recent myelosuppressive chemotherapy;

(5) abnormal, uncorrectable coagulation parameters or evidence of moderate to severe cirrhosis;

(6) unirradiated liver parenchyma insufficient for hepatic function;

(7) inability to encompass all known disease within interstitial radiation volumes at laparotomy because of excessive tumor volume, number of lesions, or miliary spread pattern.

## Preoperative Phase

A history and physical examination were performed with emphasis on prior hepatic disease, comorbid cardiopulmonary disease, stigmata of cirrhosis, and performance status. Proctosigmoidoscopy was typically done to ensure no recurrence of the rectal primary tumor. In addition to the usual parameters, laboratory determinations included prothrombin time, partial thromboplastin time, hepatic enzymes, and carcinoembryonic antigen (CEA). Radiographic studies included a chest x-ray (and chest computed tomography [CT] scan if the chest x-ray is abnormal), barium enema, and CT scan of the abdomen and pelvis. Some patients were also studied with magnetic resonance imaging (MRI) as part of the evaluation of MRI for identifying hepatic disease. Patients considered for resection usually underwent angiography. In the early phase of the study, dosimetric preplanning was performed using the Theraplan V05 planning system (Theratronics International Ltd., Kanata, Ontario, Canada). Subsequently, a personal computer-based software developed at Georgetown University was employed. A quality assurance checklist on the afterloader was completed before each session.

## Operative Phase

Exploratory laparotomy was accomplished through a subcostal or median vertical incision. Careful examination of the abdomen and the pelvis was done before any hepatic dissection to ensure that no untreatable extrahepatic disease was present. Ultrasound of the liver was used for disease that could not be palpated. After determination of the extent of hepatic involvement, a biopsy was performed to confirm metastatic disease if not done preoperatively, and the falciform ligament was bisected to allow the liver to drop into the abdomen to improve access to the diaphragmatic recesses. Patients with disease conforming to usual surgical criteria for resection (four or fewer lesions in one lobe or amenable to trisegmentectomy) underwent partial hepatectomy. Patients with unresectable disease underwent interstitial insertion of closed-end needles as the sole therapy.

Needles were inserted in either a planar or volumetric (Quimby) distribution. Spacing between the parallel needles was 1.0 to 1.5 cm, and the distal ends of the needles extended approximately 0.3 cm beyond the lesion to allow for the dead space at the tip of the needle. When protrusion of the needle was not feasible (e.g., at the vena cava or heart), longer dwell times were employed at the distal end. Needles were supported and separated with laparotomy packing, which also displaced uninvolved organs such as the bowel, kidney, and lung from the radiation volume. Needles were connected by cables to the afterloading device, and sterility of the cables was maintained near the point of insertion on the afterloading device.

Treatment was delivered with personnel outside the room, and the patient was monitored remotely with two television and anesthestic monitors. Spacing between stops was 0.8 to 1.0 cm along the needle. The dose-to-tumor periphery was escalated from 20 Gy to 30 Gy in this study. After irradiation, the needles were removed, the bleeding was controlled with pressure or cautery, and the surgical procedure was completed. If the gallbladder was in the radiation field, cholecystectomy was performed, usually at the start of the procedure.

### Postoperative Phase

Initially, patients were monitored for 24 hours in the surgical intensive care unit, but, subsquently, patients were cared for on a standard surgical ward. Serial CEA determinations and chemistries were obtained at 1 to 4 weeks. CT or MRI was performed every 4 months. Progression was defined as greater than a 25% increase in the product of bidimensional measurements; otherwise, the disease was considered stable. Parameters of follow-up included the status at irradiated hepatic sites, unirradiated hepatic sites, and nonhepatic sites and survival.

# Results

### Colorectal Hepatic Metastases

Six patients received 3.75 to 20 Gy to single colorectal hepatic metastases with the percutaneous technique. Although there were no complications, early progression of the disease was seen in most of these patients and marginal miss was considered likely. Thus, the technique was changed, and the next 33 patients with colorectal hepatic metastases were treated with the intraoperative approach. Confirming the experience with percutaneous approach, 14 of the first 15 intraoperative patients had disease underestimated by CT scan in either number or volume. Typically, the CT scan missed lesions less than 2 cm, and either underestimated or overestimated tumor size as determined by measurements at laparotomy. Clinical characteristics of the 33 patients with colorectal hepatic metastases are described in Table 1. Although the median age was 60 years, 8 patients were 70 years or older, and 3 were 76 years or older. The average size of the largest lesion in each patient was 6 cm, and the range was 3 to 13 cm. Nearly all patients had received systemic chemotherapy and had progressive disease.

## Table 1

**Clinical Characteristics of 33 Patients with Hepatic Metastases from Colorectal Carcinoma Undergoing 35 IIRT Procedures**

|  |  | *Range* |
|---|---|---|
| Age, median (yrs) | 60 | 39–82 |
| Male : female | 26:7 |  |
| Lesions, median (n) | 3 | 1–11 |
| Lesions, modal | 1 |  |
| Largest Diameter, average (cm) | 6 |  |
| Largest Diameter, median | 5 | 3–13 |
| Total Volume, average (cc) | 174 | 14–696 |

## Table 2

**Number of IIRT Procedures at Each Dose Level for Patients with Hepatic Metastases from Colorectal Carcinoma**

| *Median No. Lesions (range)* | *Average Volume (cc) (range)* | *20 Gy* | *Procedures Per Dose* *25 Gy* | *30 Gy* |
|---|---|---|---|---|
| 3 (1–11) | 174 (14–696) | 13 | 9 | 13 |

The number of procedures at each dose level in the 33 patients with colorectal carcinoma is described in Table 2. Two patients developed other colorectal hepatic metastases and underwent a second interstitial irradiation procedure. In one patient, no tumor was found on a biopsy of the prior site. In the second patient, no tumor was found at two sites, but a tumor was histologically confirmed at the third site in a distribution suggesting a marginal miss. Thus, pathological confirmation of tumorcidal response to IIRT was established.

The median follow-up is 12 months (range: 2–39 months). Seven patients remained alive, 6 of them with stable disease at IIRT sites at 4, 5, 5, 6, 36, and 39 months. Five patients have died but had stable disease at IIRT sites. The time to death in this group was 5, 9, 14, 25, and 26 months. Thus, considering both alive and deceased patients, disease control at IIRT sites for greater than 1 year was seen in 5 patients (14, 25, 26, 36, and 39 months). The actuarial analysis method shows a 25% local control at 26 months. The median time to progression at IIRT sites was 8 months. In 87% of patients, new sites of disease developed in the remainder of the liver. Systemic disease progression was seen in 42% at a median time of 8 months.

No significant radiation toxicity was seen. In three patients, minimal, transient elevations of hepatic enzymes appeared. One patient with cirrhosis experienced ascites postoperatively and required prolonged diuresis and hospitalization for 23 days. However, the median hospitalization was 8 days (range 3–23), and older patients fared as well as younger patients. Postoperative pneumonia was seen in two patients and wound infection in two patients. These were considered unrelated to irradiation. All patients responded to conservative medical management.

## Hepatic Noncolorectal Metastases and Hepatoma

Eight additional patients with hepatic metastases from noncolorectal tumors also underwent irradiation (Table 3). There were two patients each with breast carcinoma, leiomyosarcoma, ovarian carcinoma, and one each with lung and prostate carcinoma. One patient with ovarian carcinoma underwent two procedures, with disease controlled at the original site of irradiation as demonstrated by biopsy at the second laparotomy. IIRT doses ranged from 15 to 30 Gy in these eight patients. Two patients, one each with ovarian and prostatic carcinoma, also underwent planned external beam irradiation to the hepatic disease; the dose was 41.4 and 40 Gy, respectively (Table 4). In five of seven evaluable patients, the disease remained controlled at IIRT sites. However, only three of these seven patients remained alive at the last follow-up (Table 5). One patient, a 63-year-old woman with an isolated hepatic metastasis from breast carcinoma measuring 8 cm, was treated with 20 Gy IIRT. At a follow-up 5 years later, the single lesion had gradually regressed before a small, new lesion developed elsewhere in the liver.

Disease in two patients was inevaluable. One patient with prostate cancer developed rapidly progressive intrahepatic and extrahepatic disease. One patient with hepatoma and moderate to severe cirrhosis died within 1 month of surgery and IIRT. Death was due to hepatorenal syndrome secondary to hypotension from self-administered narcotic analgesia. Although IIRT was not

## Table 3

### Number of Treated Lesions and Delivered Dose for Patients with Hepatic Metastases from Noncolorectal Origin and for a Single Patient with Hepatoma

| Primary | Number of Lesions | IIRT Dose (Gy) |
|---|---|---|
| Breast | 1 | 20 |
| Breast | 3 | 25 |
| Ovary | 1/1 | 25/25 |
| Ovary | 1 | 15 |
| Sarcoma | 8 | 25 |
| Sarcoma | 1 | 25 |
| Lung | 1 | 30 |
| Prostate | 1 | 25 |
| Hepatoma | 1 | 30 |

**Table 4**

**Clinical and Treatment Characteristics of Eight Patients with Hepatic Metastases from Noncolorectal Origin and for a Single Patient with Hepatoma**

| Primary | Age (Yrs) | Number of Lesions | Largest Diameter (cm) | Total Volume (cc) | XRT (Gy) |
|---|---|---|---|---|---|
| Breast | 63 | 1 | 8 | 288 | |
| Breast | 33 | 3 | 5 | 118 | |
| Ovary | 54 | 1/1 | 3/3 | 14/14 | |
| Ovary | 52 | 1 | 1.5 | 2 | 41.4 |
| Sarcoma | 57 | 8 | 4 | 56 | |
| Sarcoma | 55 | 1 | 2.5 | 13 | |
| Lung | 72 | 1 | 7 | 140 | |
| Prostate | 54 | ? | 8 | 216 | 40 |
| Hepatoma | 62 | 1 | 7 | 178 | |
| Median | 55 | 1 | 5 | 118 | |

**Table 5**

**Treatment Results of Eight Patients with Hepatic Metastases from Noncolorectal Origin and for a Single Patient with Hepatoma**

| Primary | Follow-up Mos | Status | Control IIRT Sites | Other Liver | Systemic Sites |
|---|---|---|---|---|---|
| Breast | 63 | A | Yes | P | |
| Breast | 6.5 | D | No | P | P |
| Ovary | 36/29 | D | Yes/Yes | P/P | P |
| Ovary | 34 | A | Yes | ?P | |
| Sarcoma | 19 | D | P, 13 mos. | P | |
| Sarcoma | 3 | A | Yes | NED | |
| Lung | 10 | D | Yes | NED | P |
| Prostate | 8 | D | Not evaluated | P | P |
| Hepatoma | 1 | D | Not evaluated | | |

considered causative, the precaution remains that intraoperative hepatic irradiation in patients with significant cirrhosis may lead to radiation hepatitis. Increased postoperative morbidity and mortality may be anticipated in patients with significant cirrhosis.

## Conclusions

Hepatic IIRT of 15 to 30 Gy has been demonstrated to be well tolerated in a Phase I-II trial. Tumor control has been shown not only radiographically but also pathologically in some patients. Although it is technically feasible with a percutaneous approach, the intraoperative method has better-defined tumor extent and reduced the chance of "marginal miss." No region of the liver proved inaccessible at operation after dissection of the falciform ligament. Hepatic IIRT offers the potential for long-term disease control in patients with involvement of both lobes or otherwise unresectable metastatic or primary liver cancer. As hepatic resection increases from simple wedge resection to lobectomy, the operative mortality increases from 3% to 9%[3]. IIRT provides an alternative to major resection for "at risk" patients. Further work is indicated to optimize IIRT dose and to ascertain the risk of late radiation hepatitis, biliary sclerosis, or other unknown major complications, as well as to better define efficacy. Possible areas of research include combined modality therapy with conformational external beam, chemotherapy, or surgery.

## REFERENCES

1. Cady B, Stone MD. The role of surgical resection of liver metastases in colorectal carcinoma. Semin Oncol 18:399-406, 1991.
2. Daly JM, Kemeny N. Therapy of colorectal hepatic metastases. In: De Vita VT, Hellman S, Rosenberg SA, eds. Important Advances in Oncology 1986. Philadelphia, Pa.: JB Lippincott; 1986, 251-268.
3. Foster JH. Survival after liver resection for secondary tumors. Am J Surg 135:389-394, 1978.
4. Donath D, Nori D, Turnbull A, et al. Brachytherapy in the treatment of solitary colorectal metastases to the liver. J Surg Oncol 44:55-61, 1990.
5. Abe M. Intraoperative radiation therapy for gastric cancer. In: Dobelbower RR, Abe M, eds. Intraoperative Radiation Therapy. Boca Raton, FL: CRC Press, Inc.; 1989, 165-179.
6. Dritschilo A, Harter KW, Thomas D, et al. Intraoperative radiation therapy of hepatic metastases: technical aspects and report of a pilot study. Int J Radiat Oncol Biol Phys 14:1007-1011, 1988.
7. Thomas DS, Nauta RJ, Rodgers JE, et al. Intraoperative high-dose rate interstitial irradiation of hepatic metastases from colorectal carcinoma: results of a phase I-II trial. Cancer 71:1977-1981, 1993.
8. Rosenberg SA. Principles of surgical oncology. In: De Vita VT, Hellman S, Rosenberg SA, eds. Cancer, Principles and Practice. 3rd ed. Philadelphia, Pa.: JB Lippincott; 1989, 244.
9. Wanebo HJ, Falkson G, Order SE. Cancer of the hepatobiliary system. In: De Vita VT, Hellman S, Rosenberg SA, eds. Cancer, Principles and Practice. 3rd ed. Philadelphia, Pa.: JB Lippincott; 1989, 846.
10. Schildberg FW, Willich N, Krämling H-J, eds. Intraoperative Radiation Therapy. Proceedings of the Fourth International Symposium IORT. Munich, Germany: Essen: Verlag Die Blaue Eule; 1993, 483-489.
11. Dritschilo A, Grant EG, Harter KW, et al. Interstitial radiation therapy for hepatic metastases: sonographic guidance for applicator placement. Am J Roentgenol 146:275-278, 1986.

## Chapter 15

# The Role of High Dose Rate Brachytherapy in Rectal Cancer

*Dattatreyudu Nori and Lincoln Pao*

## Introduction

Radiation therapy has performed a vital role in the treatment of cancer of the rectum during the past 25 years. External beam radiation therapy (EBRT) has become the conventional adjuvant treatment in potentially curable surgical cases, and it is used as the primary therapy in unresectable or medically inoperable patients and in the treatment of recurrent disease. Intraoperative techniques using electrons and brachytherapy have demonstrated improved local control. Interstitial and intracavitary brachytherapy (IBT) has been recently introduced with success in the treatment of early, accessible lesions in carefully selected patients. These patients constitute 3%–5% of all rectal cases, and the tumors are small, exophytic, mobile, and without adverse pathological factors.

The selection of tumors for local therapy is based on clinical and pathological factors. During physical examination, the tumor size, mobility, location, and circumference must be carefully assessed. The pathological information must be obtained from a full-thickness, local excision to determine the depth of invasion.

Adverse clinical features include tumors that are circumferential, fixed, ulcerated, or larger than 3–5 cm in diameter. Ominous pathological factors include high grade, blood vessel and lymphatic invasion, and penetration of tumor into or through the muscularis propria. Intracavitary brachytherapy using either low dose rate (LDR) or high dose rate (HDR) brachytherapy techniques may be used to treat these tumors.

Memorial Sloan-Kettering Cancer Center, New York, New York, reported on a series of patients treated between January 1981 and April 1986. Twenty-eight patients were treated with remote afterloading intracavity HDR for rectal, rectosigmoid, and anal cancers, either for persistence, recurrence, or as an adjunct to current therapy. Twenty-seven cases were evaluable (one patient was lost to follow-up after the treatment): 14 (52%) had rectal cancer; 10 (37%) had rectosigmoid cancer; and 3 (11%) had anal cancer. There were 16 males and 11 females. Patient ages ranged from 27 to 88 years (median: 66 years). Indications for HDR brachytherapy were as follows: 13 patients were treated for

From: Nag, S. (ed.): *High Dose Rate Brachytherapy: A Textbook*, Futura Publishing Company, Inc., Armonk, NY, © 1994.

347

recurrent disease; 12 patients were treated postoperatively (4 for gross residual disease, and 8 following suboptimal surgery but without gross residual disease); and 3 patients were treated with HDR brachytherapy as a boost to primary EBRT.

Prior treatment consisted of surgery plus EBRT in 18 patients, surgery alone in 6 patients, and EBRT alone in 3 patients. Of the 21 patients who received prior EBRT, conventional fractionation of 200 cGy/fraction was used in 12 patients, and 9 had unconventional fractionation (7 patients receiving 300 cGy/fraction; 2 patients receiving 250 cGy/fraction). Total EBRT doses ranged from 2,700 cGy to 6,000 cGy. Almost all patients were treated with 3 or 4 fields. A variety of surgical procedures were performed in these patients, including low anterior resection, abdominoperineal resection (1 patient was treated with HDR brachytherapy for a fistulous tract recurrence), total and subtotal excisions, and fulguration.

## Treatment Technique

All patients were treated with a remote afterloader. The treatment was delivered via a single, cable-mounted, high-activity $^{192}$Ir source. This device was driven from the safe by a stepping-motor guided by a microcomputer. Standard applicator cylinders were used; in some cases, these were custom-made to accommodate the anatomical location and extent of the target volume. Cylinders 2 cm in diameter were used in all patients for HDR brachytherapy, with doses prescribed to 0.5 cm from the surface of the applicator. Treatment lengths varied from 3 to 10 cm. Appropriate shielding was added in selected cases. The dose rate ranged from 100 to 200 cGy/minute, and the dose per fraction ranged from 440 cGy to 840 cGy. The number of fractions ranged from 1 to 5 and were given at weekly intervals. These treatments were delivered on an outpatient basis, using topical anesthesia.

## Results

Patients were followed at regular intervals with a physical exam and appropriate radiological and endoscopic studies. Follow-up ranged from 1 to 74 months (median: 12 months). Actuarial survival and local disease-free survival were determined using the life-table method. Statistical significance was determined using the G-statistic test for independence.

The overall actuarial 5-year survival was 50%, and the overall local, disease-free 5-year survival was 36%. The actuarial, local, disease-free survivals for the 2 groups at 5 years was 43% for Group I and 30% for Group II. The median local disease-free survival was 24 months for Group I and 12 months for Group II. In absolute terms, 71% (10 of 14) of Group I achieved local control; 39% (5 of 13) of Group II achieved local control. Of the 10 patients in Group I achieving local control, 2 were among the 4 patients who presented postoperatively with gross residual disease; 8 had undergone suboptimal surgery but with no gross residual disease. Seven of these 8 patients maintained local control at follow-up ranging from 5 to 60 months. Overall, there were 15 completed responses (56%), 10 partial responses (37%), and 2 (7%) minimal responses.

Four patients have achieved long-term, disease-free survival. Three of these were Group I patients, and one was in Group II. Patient 1, who had an anal carcinoma, achieved a complete response after 3,000 cGy of pelvic EBRT and concomitant 5-Flurouracil (FU) plus mitomycin C and, therefore, received adjuvant IBT instead of previously planned abdominoperineal resection. She had persistent refractory proctitis that ultimately resolved 5 years after IBT. Nine of 10 patients with evaluable symptoms in Group II experienced palliation of those symptoms (median duration: 8 months).

## Complications

Patients were followed at regular intervals to monitor the development of complications, as well as to determine local control. Complications were carefully analyzed for all patients. Overall, 13 patients (48%) had no complications; 3 (11%) had transient treatment-related symptoms not requiring any treatment ($G_1$ complication); 8 (30%) had chronic symptoms requiring conservative treatment ($G_2$ complications), and 3 patients (11%) had complications requiring surgical intervention ($G_3$ complication). Complications included bleeding, pain, diarrhea, proctitis, ulcer, tenesmus, and stricture. Subsequent discussion of complications refers to $G_2$ and $G_3$ complications.

Analysis of complications yielded the following relevant parameters (Table 1): IBT fractionation, total cumulative IBT plus EBRT dose, EBRT fractionation, IBT treatment length, and anatomical location. The total dose

### Table 1

**Intraluminal Brachytherapy in Rectosigmoid, Rectal, and Anal Cancer:
Factors Influencing Complications**

|  | Category | No. of Patients | No. of Patients with Complications | % Complications |
|---|---|---|---|---|
| Fractionation |  |  |  |  |
| IBT | ≤2Fx | 15 | 7 | 47.5 |
|  | >2Fx | 12 | 4 | 33 |
| EBRT | conventional Fx | 12 | 3 | 25 |
|  | unconventional Fx | 9 | 8 | 89 |
| Treatment length | 3–7 cm | 8 | 0 | 0 |
|  | 8–10 cm | 19 | 11 | 58 |
| Total cumulative dose | ≤4000 cGy | 9 | 1 | 11 |
|  | 4,000–7,000 cGy | 18 | 10 | 55 |
| Anatomical site | Rectal | 14 | 7 | 50 |
|  | Rectosigmoid | 10 | 1 | 10 |
|  | Anal | 3 | 3 | 100 |

and number of fields used for EBRT, type of previous surgery, and treatment with systemic chemotherapy had no apparent relation to the development of complications.

Seven of 15 (48%) patients receiving less than 3 IBT fractions had complications, and 4 of 12 (33%) patients receiving more than 2 fractions had complications. Ten of 17 (59%) patients receiving a cumulative dose greater than 4,000 cGy had complications. One of 10 (10%) patients receiving a cumulative dose of 4,000 cGy or less had complications. Three of 12 (25%) patients who received conventional EBRT developed complications, compared with 8 of 9 (89%) patients who received unconventional EBRT and developed complications. None of the 6 patients who had only postoperative IBT (i.e., no EBRT) developed complications.

IBT treatment length seemed to have a significant effect on complication rate. None of the patients treated with a treatment length of less than 7 cm had complications; 48% of those treated with a treatment length greater than 7 cm developed complications.

Anatomical location of the tumor site appeared to contribute to complications. All three patients treated for anal cancer had complications. In the one patient with a rectal carcinoma 0.3 cm from the anal verge, a $G_2$ complication developed as well.

## Discussion

For a long time, it was believed that colorectal cancer was minimally radiosensitive. Among the reasons for this opinion were that there were technical limitations of radiotherapy in past years and that the majority of the experience was with advanced, residual, or recurrent cancer.[1-3] Management of colorectal cancer in patients with persistent or recurrent disease remains a difficult problem. Although palliation is achieved in a great majority of patients treated with radiation therapy and IBT, local control rates have been unsatisfactory, and cures have been infrequent.[4] Wang and Schultz[5] treated 111 patients with persistent or recurrent disease with EBRT, achieving palliation in 84%. Williams[6] reported an 85% rate of pain relief and a 5.8% 5-year survival. The experience reported in this review (90% palliation) also corroborates the experience described in the literature. Results for recurrence are often poorer than for persistent disease, possibly because most recurrences occur in tissue whose vasculature has been compromised by previous surgery.[7] The differences between our Group I and Group II are in keeping with these observations. Although the number of patients is small, the 30% actuarial 5-year disease-free survival for our Group II (recurrent cancer) compares very favorably with that reported for EBRT alone in the treatment of recurrent colorectal cancer.[2,5-7]

Rich et al.[8] used local excision of fulguration and EBRT to treat 26 patients with small cancers limited to the lower two-thirds of the rectum. The indications for this treatment were similar to those for our Group I patients. EBRT after surgery, leaving no gross residual disease, resulted in a 94% local control rate. EBRT after a surgical procedure, leaving gross residual disease, resulted in a 56% local control rate. Although the data of Rich et al.[8] are almost identical to those in this report, many of the patients presented in the IBT review had advanced disease at presentation and, therefore, are not exactly comparable.

Primary radiation therapy is not the treatment of choice in the great majority of colorectal cancers.[6,8-10] However, in carefully selected early rectal and anal cancers, Syed et al.,[11] Jackson,[12] (using combined EBRT and interstitial brachytherapy), Papillon,[13,14] and Sischy[15] (using intracavitary contact radiotherapy) have reported excellent local control rates with minimal side effects and complications. Remote afterloading techniques, such as those used in this report, have an obvious advantage over brachytherapy afterloading techniques in that staff radiation exposure is completely eliminated.[16] Other advanatages include short treatment times, outpatient treatments, use of small sources (which allows intraluminal radiation in otherwise inaccessible sites), an ability to tailor treatment and dose distribution to accommodate the site and extent of disease, a relative ease and convenience of administration of treatment, and a high acceptance rate by the patients.

The biological effects of sparsely ionizing radiation are significantly affected by dose rate.[17,18] The radiobiological manifestations of dose rate are related to SLD repair, cell proliferation, and reassortment in the cell cycle. Both laboratory and clinical studies of HDR effects are not conclusive.[18] Although it may be assumed that qualitative differences in effects on both tumors and normal tissues are incurred with different fractionating schedules, there are no conclusive experimental data to confirm this assumption. The nominal single dose concept has been useful, and Orton[19] and Liversage[20] have observed that total prescribed doses should be reduced by 20% to 50% in going from LDR to HDR treatments. Our previous experience has shown that increased fractionation plays a significant role in reducing treatment-related effects.[10]

We use as standard treatment parameters a dose per fraction of 500 cGy prescribed to 0.5 cm from the surface of the applicator. With a 2-cm cylinder, this yields a 909-cGy surface dose, and, with a 3-cm diameter cylinder, it yields a 700-cGy surface dose. With 2-cm diameter cylinders, the dose rates at a 0.5 cm depth vary from 100 to 200 cGy/minute. Before beginning a treatment course with IBT, depth dose and surface dose must be thoroughly considered.

In analyzing the data from this study, it is instructive to compare them to those of an analogous technique established by Papillon[14] and reported on by Sischy.[21] The treatment was via proctoscopy using a contact 50-KeV orthovoltage unit. The dose rate was 1,000 to 2,000 cGy/minute prescribed to the surface. Three to 4 fractions were administered at intervals of 2 to 3 weeks with total doses of 10,000 to 15,000 cGy. Only lesions up to 5 cm by 3 cm could be treated, with 5-cm lesions requiring 2 overlapping fields. For primary therapy, lesions were required to be low grade, exophytic, and no more than 11 to 12 cm from the anal verge. Sischy[21] reported local control in 95% of 94 patients, and Papillon[14] reported a 78% 5-year disease-free survival in patients meeting these requirements. Although none of our patients could be described as being in a favorable risk category, 71% of the Group I patients did achieve local control. Sischy[21] treated 73 patients whose lesions did not meet the size, circumferential extent, or thick ulcerative morphology criteria; he reported 31 (42%) of these patients as achieving local control. Papillon[14] reported 35% local control in 16 patients who had ulcerative lesions located near the sphincter; for these patients, he recommended EBRT plus brachytherapy. In 39% of our patients in Group II, local control was achieved. There are high rates of complications with both techniques when treating lesions near the anal sphincter. Apparently the transitional mucosa is quite sensitive to radiation, and the underlying sphincter muscle is susceptible to necrosis.

## Other Institutional Experience

Doss et al.[22] treated eight patients with the microSelectron HDR afterloading machine; three of these had received previous EBRT for persistent disease. Two of the eight patients were treated preoperatively because of obstruction and bleeding. Five of the eight were treated to palliate pain and severe bleeding. Commercially available 180° internal tungsten shielding was used. One patient was treated with an interstitial implant using Nucletron rigid 14 gauge needles. Tumor regression was noted in all patients. Complete response was seen in two of the patients. Bleeding and pain resolved in all patients, and they reported no acute or long-term toxity.

## Summary and Conclusions

Between 1981 and 1986, 28 patients who had previously undergone surgery and/or EBRT received IBT with remote afterloading technique. Local control was achieved in 71% of Group I and 39% of Group II patients, and 7 of the 8 patients who were treated adjunctively maintained local control. The factors identified as related to increased complications were EBRT fractionation, total cumulative EBRT plus IBT dose, IBT fractionation, IBT treatment length, and anatomical location.

The rationale for treating colorectal cancer with remote afterloading IBT is explained principally by the favorable characteristics of the technique itself. It is simpler and more convenient than interstitial brachytherapy or intraoperative EBRT and does not require the strict selection criteria of the Papillon technique. The experience is limited, but it appears that IBT is a feasible form of treatment, either alone or in combination with EBRT. Combined with standard EBRT, IBT using multiple fractions and treatment lengths no greater than 7 cm appears to result in satisfactory local control and acceptable morbidity in the treatment of colorectal cancer.

---

## REFERENCES

1. Gunderson LL, Cohen AM, Dosoretz D, et al. Residual, unresectable or recurrent colorectal cancer: external beam irradiation and intraoperative electron beam boost + resection. Int J Radiat Oncol Biol Phys 9:1597, 1983.

2. Sidorchenkov VO. Intracavitary brachytherapy for rectal cancer. Selectron Brachytherapy Journal 5:137-139, 1991.
3. Tepper JE, Cohen AM, Wood WC, et al. Intraoperative electron beam radiotherapy in the treatment of unresectable rectal cancer. Arch Surg 121:421-423, 1986.
4. Fourquet A, Enker WE, Shank B, et al. The value of interstitial radiation in advanced and recurrent colorectal cancer. Endocurie/Hypertherm Oncol 1:113-117, 1985.
5. Wang CC, Schulz MD. The role of radiation therapy in the management of carcinoma of the sigmoid, rectosigmoid and rectum. Radiology 79:1-5, 1962.
6. Williams IG. Radiotherapy of Carcinoma of the Rectum. Edinburgh, Scotland: Churchill-Livingstone; 1960, 210-219.
7. Rao AR, Kagan AR, Chan PYM, et al. Effectiveness of local radiotherapy in colorectal carcinoma. Cancer 42:1082-1086, 1978.
8. Rich TA, Weiss DA, Mies C, et al. Sphincter preservation in patients with low rectal cancer treated with radiation therapy with or without local excision or fulguration. Radiology 156:527-531, 1985.
9. Cummings BJ, Rider WD, Howard AR, et al. External beam radiation therapy for adenocarcinoma of the rectum. Dis Colon Rectum 26:30, 1983.
10. Nori D, Hilaris BS, Chadha M, et al. Clinical applications of a remote afterloader. Endocurie/Hypertherm Oncol 1:193-200, 1985.
11. Syed AMN, Puthawala A, Neblett D, et al. Primary treatment of carcinoma of the lower rectum and anal canal by a combination of external irradiation and interstitial implant. Radiology 128:199-203, 1978.
12. Jackson BR. Iridium implants in treatment of anorectal carcinoma. Dis Colon Rect 23:145-150, 1980.
13. Papillon J. Intracavitary irradiation of early rectal cancer for cure: a series of 186 cases. Cancer 36:696-701, 1975.
14. Papillon J. Rectal and anal cancers: conservative treatment by irradiation—an alternative to radical surgery. New York: Springer-Verlag; 1982.
15. Sischy B. Endocavitary irradiation for adenocarcinoma of the rectum. Cancer 34:333-339, 1984.
16. Henschke UK, Hilaris BS, Mahan GD. Remote afterloading with intracavitary applicators. Radiology 83: 344-345, 1964.
17. Hall, EJ. Time-dose relationships in brachytherapy. In: Hilaris B, ed. Afterloading: Twenty Years of Experience, 1955-1975. New York: Memorial Sloan-Kettering Cancer Center; 1975, 35-40.
18. Hall EJ. The biological basis of endocurietherapy: the Henschke Memorial Lecture, 1984. Endocurie/Hypertherm Oncol 1:141-151, 1985.
19. Orton CG. Radiobiological dose rate considerations with remote afterloading. In: Shearer DR, ed. Recent Advances in Brachytherapy Physics. New York: American Institute of Physics; 1981, 190-200.
20. Liversage WA. Comparison of the predictions of the CRS, TDF, and Liversage formula with clinical experience. Br J Radiol No. 17(special report), 1981.
21. Sischy B. The place of radiotherapy in the management of rectal adenocarcinoma. Cancer 50:2631-2637, 1982.
22. Doss LL, Schaffner SJ, Lange BJ, et al. Remote afterloading brachytherapy in rectal and anorectal carcinoma. Selectron Brachytherapy Journal 6:58-62, 1992.

# Chapter 16

# High Dose Rate Brachytherapy of the Prostate

*Timothy P. Mate, György Kovács, and Alvaro A. Martinez*

## Introduction

Prostate carcinoma, which is diagnosed annually in tens of thousands of men, represents the most common male genitourinary malignancy. Over the years, interstitial radioactive implants have been employed in the management of these carcinomas to enhance local tumor control rates. Treatment schemes employing brachytherapy have the added benefit of minimizing adverse effects on adjacent radiosensitive organs, resulting in improved quality of life for these patients. Demographically, with an aging population and wider application of prostate cancer screening, improved brachytherapy techniques will be in increased demand.

Various radioisotope techniques have been used in prostate brachytherapy tasks. Long-term results have been reported with suprapubically placed I-125 and gold seeds.[1] Likewise, several institutions have described the perineal application of temporary low dose rate (LDR) iridium-192 as a boost either before or after pelvic external beam radiotherapy (EBRT).[2-4] This combination has yielded excellent local control rates. In particular, for bulkier stages B and C and high-grade lesions, results appear to be superior to what can be achieved with external beam alone or permanently placed I-125 seeds. Favorable dose rates, photon penetration, and fixed implant geometry provided by the template may be the explanation. Because of the proven efficacy of iridium-192, this isotope will continue to play a major role in interstitial brachytherapy prostate applications.

With the advent of transrectal ultrasound (TRUS) technology, there has been a resurgence in prostate brachytherapy. Holm et al.[5] first described the use of transrectal ultrasonography to guide the insertion of I-125 seeds into the prostate. There is an overwhelming consensus that ultrasound-guided template implants result in more accurate seed placement.

Furthermore, the development of high dose rate (HDR) iridium-192 remote afterloaders has provided new avenues for genitourinary brachytherapy tasks. Based upon the experience with cervical and endometrial cancers and

From: Nag, S. (ed.): *High Dose Rate Brachytherapy: A Textbook*, Futura Publishing Company, Inc., Armonk, NY, © 1994.

guided by the predictions that the linear quadratic equation provides, dose fractionated schedules have been devised that allow substitution of HDR iridium-192 for LDR iridium-192 procedures.[6]

High dose rate iridium-192 has the added appeal of complete radiation safety and potential for dose optimization. This chapter describes the work in progress at three centers: Kiel, Germany; Seattle, Washington; and Royal Oak, Michigan.

## The Kiel Experience

HDR brachytherapy for prostate carcinoma was first introduced at Kiel University in March 1986. The Kiel rationale for using HDR Iridium-192 brachytherapy for the treatment of prostate carcinoma was as follows:

- HDR iridium-192 treatment has the advantages of dose optimization, shorter treatment time, and better quality control;
- The ultrasound guided method developed by Holm et al.[5] improves the accuracy of needle application and provides an opportunity for in vivo dosimetry.

The Kiel treatment scheme combined conventional fractionated external beam radiation (EBR) with two HDR iridium-192 boosts given during the course of EBR so as not to increase the overall treatment time.

### Materials and Methods

From March 1986 to December 1992, 150 patients with histologically confirmed carcinoma of the prostate were selected for treatment. The majority were clinically staged, though, in some instances, a patient underwent staging lymphadenectomy. TRUS technology was used to assist staging. The patients were staged according to a tumor node metastasis (TNM) system with some modifications. Stage T3 was assigned to a patient who had evidence (by TRUS) of capsular invasion by a tumor greater than 5 mm, ejaculatory duct tumor invasion, or asymmetry of the seminal vesicles. Invasion of the rectal wall, levator muscles, or base of the bladder was classified as stage T4. The distribution by stage was $T_1$,-1, $T_{2a}$,-22, $T_{2b}$,-38, $T_3$, and 38. The histological stage according to the criteria of Helpap et al.[7] is as follows: Grade $G_1$-20, $G_2$-42, and $G_3$-37.

Patients were not eligible for interstitial needle implantation if on TRUS there was less than 0.5 cm between the tumor and rectal mucosa. Furthermore, if patients were found to have a prostate ultrasound volume greater than 50 cc, patients were first surgically and hormonally debulked by an androgen blockade using a luteinizing hormone-releasing hormone (LHRH)-analog plus flutamide. In these situations, radiation therapy was deferred for 3 months. At the onset of radiation, the androgen blockade was discontinued.

According to the general treatment scheme, a total of 50 cGy via conventional fractionated EBR therapy was given (5 times/week, 200 cGy/fraction) and 2 separate HDR-Ir[192] boosts of 15 Gy each were incorporated. The Kiel treatment regimen is seen in Table 1 and in Figs. 1a, 1b, and 1c. The total dose and treatment blocks are shown in Table 2.

The HDR iridium-192 boost was preplanned using TRUS imaging. Transverse ultrasound images from the bladder neck to the apex was obtained at 5-mm intervals. On each ultrasound image, the outer capsule of the prostate was marked as the target volume (Fig. 2.) Some general guidelines were followed. To avoid the urethra, no needles were placed in the midline. Needles were placed at positions where the tumor penetrated the prostate capsule.

On the days of HDR iridium-192 treatment, EBR treatment was not given. The patient was given a regional or general anesthetic and placed in the lithotomy position. A three-way transurethral balloon catheter was placed in the bladder. One channel was used for prostatic in vitro dosimetry, and one channel was used to fill the bladder with contrast. The transrectal ultrasound probe was placed in the rectum, and a needle template guide, which was fixed to the probe, pushed the perineum. The template has a 3.33-m spaced grid of 1.7-mm holes with a thickness of 20 mm. This grid corresponded to an electronically generated grid overlying the video ultrasound image. Generally, 6 to 12 needles were inserted. In vivo rectal dosimetry was also used.

If needles deviated more than 3 mm from their intended preplanned position at implantation, the plan was corrected. This was done by adjusting dwell times or by entering the correct needle positions.

Once there was an acceptable plan, the transducer water balloon was deflated to relax the compression of the rectal mucosa against the prostate. With

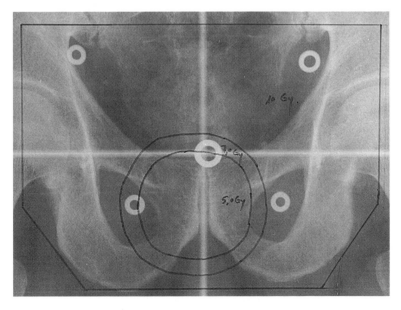

**Fig. 1a.** AP/PA portal simulation image for the individual dose modification absorption body.

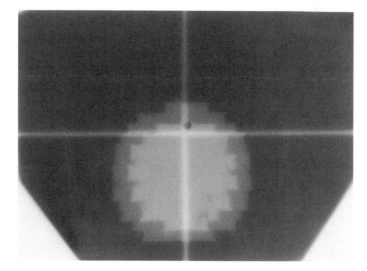

**Fig. 1b.** Dose modification absorption body field control image with the therapy beam.

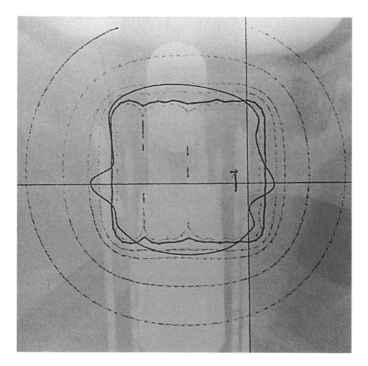

**Fig. 1c.** Subtraction of isodose plan and AP HDR-brachytherapy control image. Note the geometry of the needles and the head of ultrasound probe: the last cranial cross-section image is the control image for the needle implantation.

**Table 1**

**Kiel Treatment Regimen**

| | |
|---|---|
| 1st therapy block: | AP/PA opposing portals (inferior margin on the bottom of the ischial tuberosities, lateral margin 2 cm lateral from bony pelvis, upper margin at $L_5$. |
| 1st day of the 2nd therapy block: | First 15 Gy-Ir$^{192}$ application dose defined at the prostate capsule. Treatment planning for the dose-modification absorption body. |
| 3rd day of the 2nd therapy block: | Beginning of AP/PA opposing portals with a special dose-modification absorption body for the prostate (conventional fractionated). The dose modification is as follows: 100% for the subclinical disease, 70% or a security area according to the 3 Gy isodose of the implant, and 50% for the prostate, according to the 5 Gy isodose of the implant (Fig. 1a, 1b, and 1c). |
| 3rd therapy block: | Reduced EB volume. Margins of the field: inferior on the bottom of the ischial tuberosities, lateral the middle of the foramina obturator, and the upper margin at the top of the linea terminalis. |
| 1st day of the 4th therapy block: | Second 15 Gy HDR-Ir$^{192}$ application dose deferred at the prostate capsule. |
| 3rd day of the 4th therapy block: | Beginning of the $5\times2$ Gy EB with the dose modification absorption body. |

**Table 2**

**Dose and Treatment Blocks of the Kiel Treatment Regimen**

| Treatment Block | Dose (Gy) To | |
|---|---|---|
| | *Prostate Capsule* | *Subclinical Disease* |
| 1st | 20 Gy via EB | 20 Gy via EB |
| 2nd | 15 Gy via HDR +5 Gy via EB | 10 Gy via EB |
| 3rd | 10 Gy via EB | 10 Gy via EB |
| 4th | 15 Gy via HDR +5 Gy via EB | 10 Gy via EB |
| Total | Prostate | Subclinical Disease |
| 6 weeks | 70 Gy Total | 50 Gy Total |

the patient remaining in the lithotomy position, treatment was rendered with a GammaMed II HDR Ir$^{192}$ afterloading device. The overall elapsed time for implantation and treatment was approximately 50–80 minutes.

Following the HDR iridium-192 treatment, the needles were removed. Several radio-opaque small metallic coils were then ultrasonically placed into the

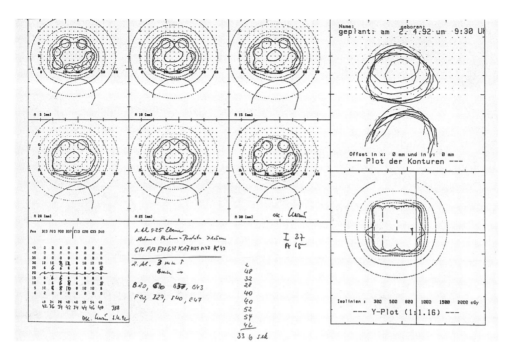

**Fig. 2.** 3D TRUS reconstruction of the prostate and rectal wall. The planning of the dwell times was done in 5-mm steps, according to the steps of the TRUS probe.

prostate to help localize the prostate for eventual EBR field size reductions (Block numbers 3 and 4).

## Results

Ninety-nine patients are available for analysis with a minimum follow-up of 18 months and a mean follow-up of 38 months. Of these 99 patients, 14 had a high risk $UT_{2b}G_3$, and 20 patients had a $UT_3G_3$ tumor. Thirty-six patients had preirradiation surgical and hormonal debulking. Twenty-nine of these patients had transurethral resection of the prostate (TURP), and seven had open prostate adenectomies.

Sixty-eight patients had pretreatment prostate specific antigens (PSAs), of which 53 were greater than normal (4.0 ng/ml). There was no significant correlation found between initial PSA, UT, and G stages. At 12 months following radiation therapy, PSAs fell to a normal range (0–4 ng/ml) in 62 patients. As follow-up continued, all the patients with posttreatment PSAs ≥ 20 ng/ml in the first year exhibited a disease progression. Most patients had abnormal pretreatment digital rectal examinations (DREs), but following treatment there were only 6 abnormal DREs evident. However, follow-up TRUS imaging revealed 35 patients to have persistent abnormal prostates.

Follow-up TRUS-guided biopsy showed tumor regression in 60% of patients with high-risk Grade III and IV lesions. In 18% of patients, the tumor was evident, and the balance had indeterminate biopsies. Local disease progression was observed in three patients. Two of these had $UT_3G_3$ tumors, and one had a $UT_{2b}G_3$. The median interval to local progression was 37.3 months with a range of 18–58 months. Systemic progression was found in 10 patients as follows by stage: $UT_3G_3$—6 patients; $UT_3G_2$—1 patient; $UT_{2b}G_3$—1 patient; $UT_{2b}G_2$—2 patients. The median interval to system progression was 15.5 months, with a range of 9–29 months.

**Side Effects and Complications**

Eight patients developed urethral stricture and were managed by an internal urethrotomy. Seven of these 8 patients had previous adenectomies or TURPs. Seven patients developed advanced cystitis 4–18 months after treatment, of which 6 required electrocoagulation or TURP. All seven had previous TURPs or adenectomies. Moderate incontinence was found in four patients, all of whom had operations because of posttreatment cystitis. Twenty-two of 73 patients (30%) developed dysuria. In 22 patients, it was described as moderate, but in 4 patients severe dysuria occurred. Proctitis lasting greater than 12 months was described in 17 of 73 patients. Ten of these described mild to moderate symptoms, and 7 (23%) had severe symptoms. Three of 99 patients developed rectal ulceration 6–12 months after radiation treatment. All the patients healed conservatively over 24 months, and no operations were required. Thirty of 73 patients developed erectile dysfunction after treatment. Eleven of these patients had pretreatment androgen blockade. One case of osteoradionecrosis occurred 6 months following radiation treatment. This fracture healed with conservation therapy. Scrotal edema occurred in three patients.

# The Seattle Experience

Encouraged by the early Kiel results, Mate and coworkers in 1989 began integrating HDR iridium-192 afterloading technology into the management of prostate carcinoma. The approach at the Swedish Medical Center Tumor Institute, Seattle, Washington, was to develop a treatment scheme consisting of initial external beam pelvic radiotherapy to be followed by single interstitial prostate implant using fractionated HDR iridium-192 to deliver the boost. This approach was designed to mimic traditional North American practices of an initial external beam to the target volume, followed by an interstitial boost as is commonly used in the management of cervix, breast, head, and neck tumors.

In the Seattle scheme of using a single prostate implant following EBR, the number of HDR fractions used in the dose per fraction were selected to be approximately equivalent to the standard LDR iridium-192 boost in terms of tumoricidal effects. The linear quadratic equation was used to estimate the number of HDR fractions and the mean peripheral dose required. It was also predicted that the use of fractionated HDR as a boost with the equivalence of 1,500–2,000 cGy LDR would not lead to a significant increase in adverse late tissue effects.

It was also anticipated that dose optimization capabilities inherent to HDR iridium-192 technology could be used to great advantage in prostate brachytherapy. Stamey et al.[8] in the analysis of radical prostatectomy specimens reported that the bulkier portions of the prostate carcinomas clinically lie in peripheral regions of the prostate. The Seattle approach, therefore, was to differentially increase the implant dose to medial lateral and posterior-lateral aspects of the prostate relative to those prostatic areas immediately adjacent to the anterior rectal wall and superior urethra. Such differential dosing might lead to improved local control rates compared to plans with relatively uniformly dosing across the whole prostate.

The same dose optimizing functions could also be utilized to tailor the maximal permissible dose (MPD) to the prostate's irregular shape, thereby minimizing the dose to adjacent radiosensitive tissues. In the midsagittal plane, the prostate has a pear-shaped configuration from apex to base. The prostate's posterior surface is at different distances from the anterior rectal wall. Furthermore, the base of the prostate joins the bladder at an oblique angle. These anatomical relationships provide an opportunity to specify an MPD isodose curve that conforms to the prostate's shape by minimizing the dose to the adjacent radiosensitive rectum and bladder. The above differential and conformal dosing considerations played a major factor in the design of the implant portion of this treatment scheme.

## Materials and Methods

Patients with biopsy-proven localized prostate adenocarcinoma were eligible for treatment consisting of initial external beam pelvic radiotherapy, followed by a single interstitial prostate implant for fractionated HDR iridium-192. More recently, the implant is being done prior to EBR treatment. This greatly simplifies logistics and is especially useful if coupled with a staging laparoscopic node dissection.

All patients underwent complete clinical staging, including physical examination, pelvic computed tomography (CT) or magnetic resonance imaging, bone scan, serum PSA and prostatic acid phosphatase (PAP). Some patients underwent preimplant laparoscopic pelvic lymph node dissection. Patients were categorized according to a modified American Joint Committee (AJC) staging system as follows:

- A1: Nonpalpable; diagnosis by TURP or transrectal ultrasound; less than 5% malignancy; Gleason pattern score < 4/10.
- A2: Nonpalpable; diagnosis by TURP or transrectal ultrasound; greater than 5% malignancy and/or Gleason pattern score > 4/10.
- B1: Unilobar nodule less than 2 cm in diameter.
- B2: Unilobar nodule equal to or greater than 2 cm in diameter.
- B3: Bilobar; intracapsular.
- C: Clinical extracapsular extension.

Initial therapy consisted of EBRT. Patients received either prostate irradiation alone by a bilateral 120° arc technique or limited pelvic radiotherapy, using the isocentric four-field technique. Field sizes were generally 8 × 8 cm for the arc technique and 10 × 10 cm for the limited four-field pelvic techniques. Radiation was delivered at a dose rate of 180–200 cGy daily, 5 days per week. Total external beam doses ranged from 5,000–5,400 cGy.

Two to 3 weeks after the completion of EBRT, patients then underwent a closed transperineal prostate needle implant with ultrasound guidance as described by Holm et al.[5] but modified for temporary implants. A Bruel and Kjaer ultrasound machine was used with an axial transducer. A volume ultrasound from base to apex at 5-mm intervals was obtained. Two to three metallic markers (dummy I-125 seeds) were first inserted under ultrasound guidance into the prostate apex as radiographic markers of this area. At implantation, a specifically designed template with a detachable perineal portion was used (Real Word Design, Seattle, Washington). Closed-end 20-cm trochar point needles, 1.9 mm in diameter, were inserted into the prostate according to a predetermined pattern. Generally, 10–14 needles were implanted. After all the steel needles were inserted, they were then replaced with 15-gauge Flexiguide needles (Best Industries. Springfield, Virginia). Following needle insertion, the detachable portion of the template was sutured to the perineum to hold the template and needles in position (Fig. 3.)

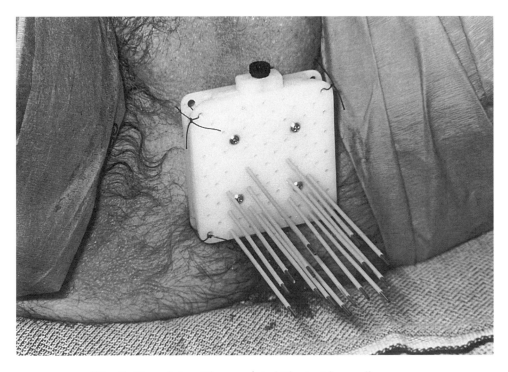

**Fig. 3.** Template with completed Flexiguide needle array.

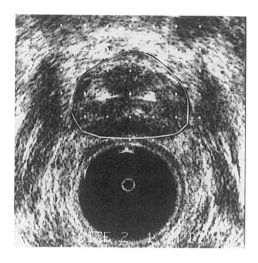

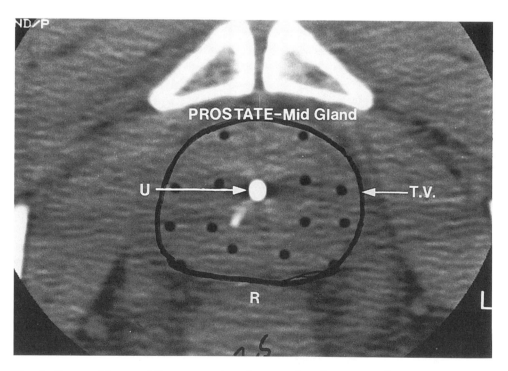

**Fig. 4.** (top and bottom) Intraoperative ultrasound and a postimplant CT are used to determine the target volume, which is 0.0 to 0.5 mm from the visible prostate capsule. Note that no additional margin is specified at the anterior rectal wall. U, R, and TV denote urethra, rectum, and target volume, respectively.

Flexible cystoscopy was then performed following the implant under direct cystoscopic vision. The tips of the Flexiguide needles were advanced to a submucosal position in the bladder base. This was performed with the patient in the operative dorsal lithotomy position and repeated with the patient in the resting supine position.

After a satisfactory recovery, a CT scan of the prostate with bladder and rectal contrast was obtained perpendicular to the long axis of the implant. CT images were taken at 5-mm slice intervals from bone to apex. This procedure radiographically verified and recorded the actual needle position. On each CT image, the prostate's capsule was outlined to be the target volume (Fig. 4). The intraoperative ultrasound was also used to assist identification of the prostate's margin on CT. Treatment planning was done with the Nucletron Treatment Planning system.

For prophylaxis against infection and deep vein thrombosis, patients were placed on prophylactic antibiotics and fitted for sequential pneumatic stockings. Adequate pain control was achieved by utilizing nonsteroidal steroids and patient-controlled analgesia. A catheter was left in the bladder.

Four afterloading treatments were given during this single interstitial implant. The first HDR fraction was given on the afternoon of the procedure; two fractions were given on the next day with a minimum of 6 hours between HDR[192] fractions, and the fourth and final fraction was given on the morning of the second postoperative day. There was a minimum of 6 hours between HDR-IR[192] fractions. The overall Seattle treatment scheme is seen in Table 3.

Initially, each HDR fraction delivered 300 cGy for a total of 1,200 cGy in the 4 fractions. Later, the dose per fraction to the target points was increased to 400 cGy while slightly reducing the dose over the posterior midline portion of the prostate closest to the rectum to 350–400 cGy per fraction. A target mean peripheral isodose curve was designed to conform to the varying shape of the prostate from base to apex. As seen in Fig. 5, significantly higher doses of 600–700 cGy/fraction occurred just within the margins, especially at the posterior lateral portions where carcinomas frequently lie. Urethral doses are in the range of 500 cGy per fraction.

### Table 3
### Seattle Fractionation Scheme

| Week (Day) | Treatment | Fractionation | Dose |
|---|---|---|---|
| 1-5 (1–37) | External Beam | 180 cGy/fx 5 fx/week | 5,040 cGy |
| 7 (50–53) | HDR-IR[192] (single implant) | 400 cGy/fx Day 50—pm Day 51—am/pm* Day 52—am | 1,600 cGy |

* 6 hours between fx

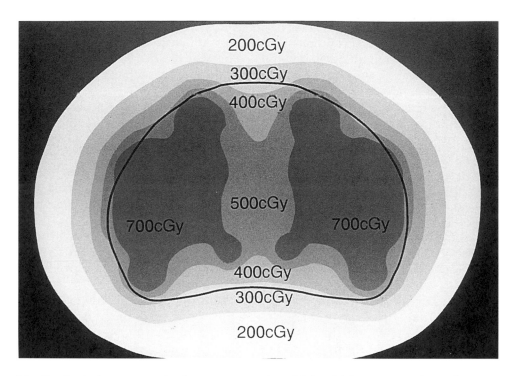

**Fig. 5.** Typical transverse isodose curves at the midgland. The target MPD conforms to the prostate's shape in the sagittal planes as well. Differential loading achieves relatively higher posterior lateral doses.

## Results

Between October 1989 and April 1993, 75 patients were entered in the study. The patients' ages range from 53 to 77 years of age, with a mean age of 68. Eight patients had prior TURPs, and seven patients had pretreatment laparoscopic node dissections. Following complete staging, the distribution by stage were A-9, B1-22, B2-25, B3-15, and C-4.

No significant intraoperative complications were encountered in the 75 procedures performed. No serious perioperative complications such as interstitial bleeding, infection, moderate to severe pain, or deep vein thrombosis have occurred. Some patients had brisk, but temporary, urethral bleeding upon needle removal. All but one patient were discharged immediately following implant removal. Most patients had urinary frequency and mild hematuria for 1–7 days following the procedure. Two patients developed acute postoperative urethral obstruction, one due to prostate edema and one due to an obstructing blood clot. Mild diarrhea and rectal irritation usually occurred but required no specific therapy. Postimplantation pain was minimal, and most patients returned to full activities within 1 week of the procedure.

Acute radiation morbidity defined as symptoms occurring within 90 days of the procedure was principally related to mild urethritis and proctitis. These symptoms generally required no treatment. Acute Grade 3-4 Radiation Therapy Oncology Group (RTOG)-defined rectal or genitourinary morbidity has not been observed.

In 55 patients with a minimum of 1 year follow-up and a mean follow-up of 22 months, no clinically significant late-developing radiation proctitis, cystitis, or urethritis has been observed. Three patients have developed urethral stricture and were subsequently dilated and corrected. Two episodes of acute urinary retention have been encountered with no apparent etiology. One patient developed mild rectal bleeding with sigmoidoscopy findings consistent with proctitis. No incontinence has been observed.

In 55 patients with a minimum of 1 year follow-up, 48 of these patients have had their PSAs return to normal levels of $\leq 4.0$ ng/ml. All of these patients' posttreatment digital examinations were normal. In seven patients, the serum PSAs fell to a nadir and then subsequently rose. Pretreatment PSAs in this group ranged from 11 to 43. One patient after treatment had a persistently abnormal DRE, and the other six had normal posttreatment DREs. One patient was found to have metastatic disease, and another was presumed to have metastatic disease because the PSA continued to increase following treatment. Three of five remaining patients have been rebiopsied, including the one patient with the grossly abnormal DRE. The other two have had negative biopsies.

In the six individuals whose implant were performed simultaneously with laparoscopic pelvic lymph-node dissection, there was no apparent difference in the tolerance of the procedures and EBR, as compared to the rest.

## The Royal Oak Experience

A phase II nonrandomized study of combined EBR and escalating iridium-192 HDR brachytherapy for locally advanced adenocarcinoma of the prostate was started in November 1991 at William Beaumont Hospital, Royal Oak, Michigan. The rationale for developing the HDR technique were as follows:

- A requirement of 1 week of hospitalization for LDR implants.
- The highly selected nature of the patient group that is eligible for general anesthesia.
- Moderately severe toxicity associated with LDR implants.

In order to find a biological equivalent between an external beam boost and an interstitial implant boost, the linear-quadratic model was used. If the assumption that the alpha/beta ratio is equal to 4 Gy for late damage of the rectal wall and is equal to 10 Gy for prostatic carcinoma cells is made, an HDR fraction of 550 cGy $\times$ 3 will increase the rectal mucosa dose by 2.6% and underdose the tumor by 5%. A dose of 570 cGy $\times$ 3 will increase the rectal mucosa by 4.8% and underdose the tumor by 3.3%. A dose of 614 cGy $\times$ 3 will achieve tumor control equal to EBR but might increase normal tissue injury (rectal) by 10%.

This model appears to overstate rectal injury because it makes the assumption that treated volumes and dose distributions with the two techniques are equivalent. In fact, the implanted volume is much smaller than the external boost volume, and the dose gradient is much sharper with the implant. However, this model is probably the best approximation of biological equivalence. On the basis of this formulation, they began a program based on the fractionation scheme described in Table 4.

**Materials and Methods**

Between November 1991 and May 1993, 117 implants have been performed on 38 patients, 31 protocol and 7 nonprotocol, with newly diagnosed $B_2/C$ prostatic adenocarcinoma. The mean age was 67 years, and the mean Gleason score was 6.7. Those with prior TURPs were not excluded. Patients were treated with (a) 4,560 cGy whole pelvis 4-field irradiation and (b) 3 HDR fractions of 550 cGy each (29 patients) or 600 cGy each (9 patients) to the prostate. Under spinal anesthesia, transperineal needle implants utilizing real-time ultrasound guidance with on-line isodose distributions as described by Edmundsen.[9] These were performed weekly on an outpatient basis during weeks 1, 2, and 3 of external irradiation. The brachytherapy target volume included the entire prostate gland and the medial aspects of the seminal vesicles. An average of 14 needles were required to adequately cover this volume. Rectal dose calculations and thermoluminescent dosimetry (TLD) measurements were performed. Acute toxicity was recorded weekly during treatment and at 1.5, 3, and 6 months following treatment using modified RTOG/European Organization for the Research and Treatment of Cancer grading criteria.

**Results**

The mean follow-up from treatment completion is 6 months. No significant intraoperative or perioperative complications occurred. Grade 3 toxicity was encountered in three patients, two with dysuria and one with diarrhea. All toxicities were otherwise grades 1 or 2 and were, as expected, from pelvic external irradiation. Implant-related toxicities included urinary retention (41%),

**Table 4**

**William Beaumont/Royal Oak Fractionation Scheme**

| Week | Pelvis External Fractionation | Prostate HDR Fractionation | Pelvis Dose To Date | Prostate Dose To Date |
|------|---------|---------|---------|---------|
| Week 1 | 200 cGy × 4 | 550 cGy × 1 | 800 cGy | 1,350 cGy |
| Week 2 | 200 cGy × 4 | 550 cGy × 1 | 1,600 cGy | 2,700 cGy |
| Week 3 | 200 cGy × 4 | 550 cGy × 1 | 2,400 cGy | 4,050 cGy |
| Week 4–6 | 180 cGy × 12 | 0 cGy | 4,560 cGy | 6,210 cGy |

hemorrhagic cystitis (18%), bladder spasms (5%), hematospermia (18%), and perineal pain (27%). Southwest Oncology Group performance status changed from 0 to 1 in 2 patients (7%). The mean calculated rectal dose per fraction was 58% of the HDR dose with acceptable agreement demonstrated by TLD measurements within the limitations of iridium-192 TLD dosimetry. PSA levels obtained at 3 months showed $\geq$ 50% reduction in 83% of patients.

## Discussion

Over 200 patients at three institutions have undergone HDR-Ir[192] prostate brachytherapy. All three institutions used a transperineal implant approach assisted by transrectal ultrasound to guide needle placement into the prostate. There were no reported technical difficulties either with the needle application or the HDR-Ir[192] treatment. All patients tolerated implantation well with no significant intraoperative or perioperative morbidity.

Different implant dose and fractionation schedules were employed among the three institutions as seen in Tables 1, 2, and 3. Two institutions (University of Keil and William Beaumont Hospital) performed separate multiple HDR iridium-192 applications on an outpatient basis during the course of EBR. The Keil group used two HDR-Ir[192] implants delivering 15 Gy each, and the Beaumont group used 500 cGy per fraction for each of its three implants. In contrast, the Seattle group chose to perform only a single prostate implant with a 2-day hospital stay either before or after EBR. During this single application, 4 fractions of 300–400 cGy each were delivered with a minimum of 6 hours between fractions on those days when 2 fractions were given.

All three institutions are reporting early encouraging results with regard to PSA responses and clinical local tumor control. In the Keil group, which has the longest follow-up, only 3% of the patients have been observed to have locally progressed. Only 1 of the Seattle patients has shown clinical local disease progression. The majority of the Beaumont-treated patients have shown a significant reduction in posttreatment PSAs. On the basis of these observations, HDR-Ir[192] brachytherapy in combination with EBR appears as effective as LDR-Ir[192] or permanent seed implants.

With regard to late tissue effects, there appear to be differences between the dose fractionation schedules. The Keil group reported the highest number of posttreatment rectal, bladder, and urethral complications. This can be partially explained by the fact that the Keil group has the largest experience and longest follow-up of the three institutions. Symptomatic proctitis occurred in approximately 23% of the Keil-treated patients, and three patients developed rectal ulceration. All patients, however, healed with conservative management. In contrast, the Seattle group has reported no significant rectal complications in a group of 55 patients with at least a 1 year follow-up. Likewise, only one of the 38 Beaumont-treated patients has developed posttreatment rectal difficulties. In an attempt to reduce future complications, the Keil group has modified its technique of EBRT. The group is presently using a four-field external-beam boosting technique with individual shielding of the anterior rectal wall on the lateral portals. Its impression is that the acute side effects have been lessened, but follow-up is too short to report on late effects.

With regard to late GU effects, 30% of the Keil-treated patients reported dysuria following treatment. Most of the cases are reported as mild to moderate, and in four instances it was described as severe. Seven patients developed advanced cystitis 4–18 months after treatment. Incontinence was reported in 4% of the patients. It appears that a prior TURP or adenectomy was a predisposing condition for both cystitis and incontinence. Eight of 99 Keil patients developed urethral stricture. The Seattle group reported 3 minor urethral strictures. One patient developed moderate posttreatment dysuria, and this patient had a prior TURP; otherwise, there were no reported instances of cystitis or incontinence.

The incidence of adverse late GI and GU effects reported herein can be compared to those observed in two large series in which patients with prostate carcinoma were treated by transperineal LDR Ir[192] and EBR. Khan et al.[4] reported a 0.6% to 6.5% rate of Grade 2 GU and GI complications. In this report, Grade 2 symptoms were defined as those that persisted 1 month but responded to simple outpatient management without life-style changes. Two of their 321 patients developed urethral strictures. No other serious complications were reported. Puthawala et al.[10] reported moderate to severe cystourethritis in 3.7% of their treated patients, incontinence in 3.2%, and urethral strictures in 1%. Severe proctitis was reported in 7%, but most of these cases occurred early in their experience. Subsequent treatment modifications have reduced this proctitis rate considerably.

In summary, HDR-Ir[192] prostate brachytherapy, when used as a boost in conjunction with EBR, can be substituted for LDR-Ir[192]. The potential for dose optimization and differential weighting are particular advantages in addition to radiation safety concerns. With the HDR-Ir[192] reported herein, there appears to be no apparent decrease in local tumor control when compared to LDR-Ir[192] and other isotopes.

Treatment schedules employing 3–4 HDR fractions of 400–500 cGy per fraction appear to be better tolerated in terms of late tissue effects when compared to fewer HDR fractions of greater dose per fraction. Further follow-up is awaited from these institutions before the optimal dose-fraction schedule can be determined.

---

## REFERENCES

1. DeBlasio DS, Hilaris BS, Nori D, et al. Permanent interstitial implantation of prostatic cancer in the 1980's. Endocurie/Hypertherm Oncol 4:193-201, 1988.
2. Brindle JS, Martinez A, Schray M, et al. Pelvic lymphadenopathy and transperineal interstitial implantation of Ir[192] combined with external beam radiotherapy for bulky stage C prostatic carcinoma. Int J Rad Onc Biol Phys 17:1063-1066, 1989.

3. Marinelli D, Shanberg AM, Tansey LA, et al. Follow-up prostate biopsy in patients with carcinoma of the prostate treated by [192] Iridium template irradiation plus supplemental external beam radiation. J Urol 147:922-925, 1992.
4. Khan K, Thompson W, Bush S, et al. Transperineal percutaneous iridium-192 interstitial template implant of the prostate: results and complications in 321 patients. Int J Rad Onc Biol Phys 22:935-939, 1992.
5. Holm HH, et al. Transperineal 125-iodine seed implantation in prostatic cancer guided by transrectal ultrasonography. J Urol 130:283, 1983.
6. Martinez AA, Orton CG, Mould RF. Brachytherapy HDR and LDR. In Proceedings of Brachytherapy Remote Afterloading: State of the Art Meeting; May 4–6, 1989; Dearborn, Mich.;121-137.
7. Helpap B, Bocking A, Dhom G, et al. Klassifikation, histologisches und zytologisches grading sowie regressionsgrading des prostatakarzinoms (ger). Urologe A 24:156-159, 1985.
8. Stamey TA, McNeal JE, Freiha FS, et al. Morphometric and clinical studies on 68 consecutive radical prostatectomies. J Urol 139:1235-1241, 1989.
9. Edmundson GK. Ultrasound in treatment planning: a prototype real-time planning system. Presented at the Seventh International Brachytherapy Working Conference; 1992; Baltimore, Md.
10. Puthawala A, Syed AMN, Austin P, et al. Temporary iridium-192 implant in the management of carcinoma of the prostate. Presented at the Fourth Annual Symposium on Prostate Cancer: The Role of Interstitial Implantation; June 1993; Seattle, Wash.

# Chapter 17

# High Dose Rate Brachytherapy for Carcinoma of the Cervix

*André A. Abitbol, Judith A. Stitt, James G. Schwade, and Alan A. Lewin*

## Introduction

Although the standard radiotherapeutic management for carcinoma of the cervix in the United States combines external beam pelvic radiation therapy (EBRT) and low dose rate (LDR) brachytherapy, there is increasing interest in high dose rate (HDR) brachytherapy. High dose rate brachytherapy has been increasingly utilized in Europe, Asia, and some third world countries. The impetus for considering HDR brachytherapy includes the ability to deliver the treatment expeditiously in an outpatient setting, thereby avoiding prolonged bed rest with its attendant risks of thrombophlebitis, pulmonary embolism, pulmonary atelectasis, cardiac decompensation, and urinary sepsis.[1] The miniaturization of the radiation source and applicator allows a more facile placement, frequently obviating the need for endocervical canal dilatation and general anesthesia. The rapid delivery of the radiation assures a more constant source placement and may allow for normal tissue sparing by retraction of the adjacent rectum and bladder. Moreover, dose distribution may be enhanced and optimized using computer dosimetry.[2,3] By integrating HDR brachytherapy earlier in the treatment program while continuing EBRT to the parametria and pelvic sidewalls, a greater emphasis is given to the brachytherapy component.

Despite the above advantages, the enthusiasm for this approach has been tempered by the need for an initial capital expenditure for the purchase of an HDR unit and the building of a dedicated shielded procedure room. Moreover, the lack of standardization of the treatment protocols and treatment-related morbidity scoring between various institutions has made comparisons of clinical results difficult.[4] The paucity of randomized trials comparing LDR brachytherapy and HDR brachytherapy has added to this difficulty. Despite the relatively large body of published results, the lack of a well-established and optimal regimen of HDR brachytherapy has created concern to some investigators.[5] Increasing attention to quality control issues has underscored the need for developing a cohesive and consistent therapeutic approach within each institution that initiates a program of gynecologic HDR brachytherapy. More-

From: Nag, S. (ed.): *High Dose Rate Brachytherapy: A Textbook*, Futura Publishing Company, Inc., Armonk, NY, © 1994.

over, increasing focus by radiobiologists on the issue of dose fractionation in converting from an LDR brachytherapy program to an HDR brachytherapy program has provided a useful framework from which the clinical researcher may begin devising a therapeutic plan.[6-8]

It is not within the scope of this paper to analyze clinical results. The reader is referred to the comprehensive analysis of the literature by Fu and Phillips.[4] Instead, this chapter will concentrate on the methodology adopted by two different institutions and focus on the technical aspects necessary to achieve a successful program. A brachytherapy "system" defines a specific type of gynecologic applicator, the isotope, the strength and distribution of sources in the applicator, dose specification points for normal or diseased tissues, and the total dose and time course to deliver this dose. With the development of HDR remote afterloading units, all the components that define a traditional brachytherapy system have been modified. Emphasis will be placed on developing fractionation schedules that make sense radiobiologically and that are clinically usable. Individualization of treatment planning will be discussed with specific reference to computerized dose optimization for each insertion. Lastly, resource utilization for HDR gynecologic brachytherapy will be discussed.

## University of Miami Protocol

### Overview

Patients entered on protocol are treated with a combination of pelvic EBRT and HDR brachytherapy. Every effort is made to administer HDR brachytherapy after a dose of 19.80 Gy EBRT (four field box technique; 1.80 Gy/fraction). In the situation where it is not possible to insert a tandem after a baseline dose of 19.80 Gy, EBRT continues to 39.60 Gy, and a second attempt at HDR brachytherapy is initiated. In the former situation, which prevails most of the time, six HDR brachytherapy procedures are given on a weekly basis, whereas in the latter situation only four HDR brachytherapy procedures are given on a weekly basis. In both cases, each application delivers 6.00 Gy to point A. Using a progressively enlarging midline block encompassing the 6.00 Gy isodose line, EBRT (1.8–2.0Gy/fraction) continues concurrently to the parametria and pelvic sidewalls 4 days each week to a baseline dose of 45.80 Gy for nonbulky tumors (stage I or II < 4 cm) and 50.40 Gy for bulky tumors (stage II > 4 cm or stage III or IV A). Patients having pelvic sidewall fixation and/or parametrial involvement receive additional booster doses to the involved side(s) between 5.40 and 9.0 Gy with attention given to excluding the small bowel. The program described above is consonant with the consensus guidelines for HDR brachytherapy of the cervix by the Clinical Research Committee of the American Endocurietherapy Society.[9]

## Technique

A commercially available miniaturized fixed-ring ovoid and tandem applicator with a built-in fixed rectal retractor is currently utilized (Fig. 1 and Fig. 2).[10] The salient features of this applicator are contrasted to a Fletcher-Suit

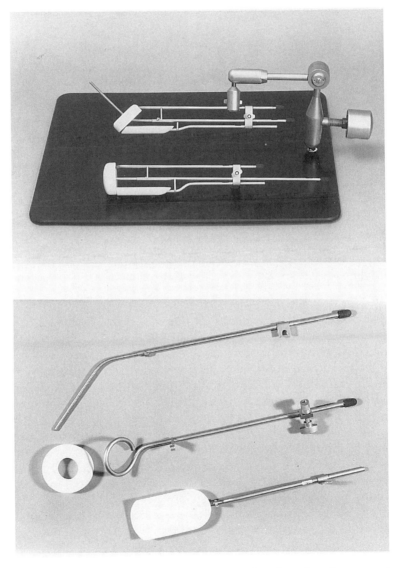

**Fig. 1.** Ring applicator. (Top) Standard applicator (in clamp) and transvaginal applicator. (Bottom) Applicator components (left to right): intrauterine tube, ring tube with plastic cap removed, rectal retractor.

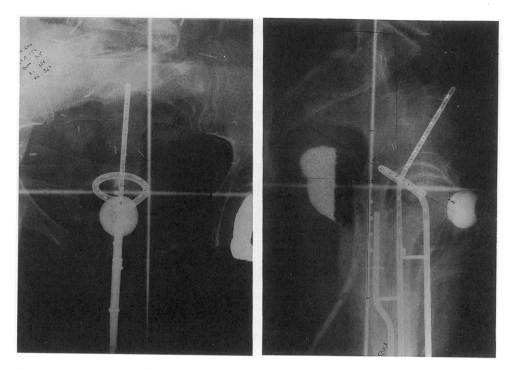

**Fig. 2.** HDR cervix brachytherapy with ring applicator and orthogonal x-ray films. Left: AP view. Right: lateral view.

LDR applicator as well as a modified Fletcher-Suit HDR applicator (as described below in the Madison System) in Table 1. The radiation oncologist has the option of suturing to the cervix an indwelling intrauterine plastic sleeve at the time of the initial exam under anesthesia or first HDR brachytherapy application. This facilitates subsequent placement of the weekly insertion and obviates the need for anesthesia. Alternatively, the radiation oncologist, using sedation, introduces weekly the tandem and ring ovoid. The applicator is secured to an external immobilizing device that facilitates adjustments of adverse anatomical positions of the uterus (i.e., a markedly retroverted fundus or a markedly anteverted uterus, thereby avoiding an excessive dose to the rectosigmoid and bladder, respectively). The use of the external immobilizing device obviates the need for vaginal packing. It has the added advantage of preventing cephalad displacement of the applicator by the vaginal packing technique, thereby potentially decreasing the dose to the adjacent organs, including the small bowel.

## Dose Prescription and Monitoring

Orthogonal films of the application are obtained and a point A identified by calculating a point 2 cm cephalad from the epicenter of the ring ovoid, plus

**Table 1**

**Comparison of Low Dose Rate and High Dose Rate Uterovaginal Applications**

| | Fletcher-Suit (LDR) | Ring (HDR) | Fletcher-Suit Modified (HDR) |
|---|---|---|---|
| Size | Standard | Miniature | Miniature |
| Tandem position | Dependent on uterine anatomical position and vaginal packing. | Adjustable AP/PA external fixation; caudal displacement possible. | Adjustable AP/PA with external fixation. |
| Colpostat size | Variable, with addition of plastic caps. | 2.6 cm, 3.0 cm, 3.4 cm diameter with plastic caps (3–4 mm thick). | 1 cm to vaginal surface |
| Colpostat position | Variable AP/PA; dependent on anatomy and packing. | Fixed; tandem is at epicenter of of ring. | Fixed; external fixation causes tandem to bisect colpostats. |
| Cervical lateral spread | Possible | Fixed (Ring-size dependent) | Possible |
| Cervical dilatation | Required | Minimal | Minimal |
| Optimization of dose distribution | Limited | Possible | Possible |
| Rectal retraction | No | Yes | Yes |

an allowance for the thickness of the ring and plastic cap (arbitrarily 5 mm) along the axis of the tandem and 2 cm laterally on either side perpendicular to the tandem.

Bladder and rectal dose monitoring are illustrated in Fig. 3 and follow the International Commission on Radiation Units (ICRU) Report No. 38.[11] For the usual situation where 6 HDR brachytherapy procedures are performed, the maximum allowable rectal or bladder dose per HDR brachytherapy should not exceed 75% of the point A, and the cumulative rectal or bladder dose integrating EBRT and HDR brachytherapy should not exceed 50.00 Gy. In the atypical case of the patient receiving 39.60 Gy EBRT and 4 HDR brachytherapy applications, the above rules are modified to allow a maximum total cumulative rectal or bladder dose of 60.00 Gy.

# The Madison System of Dose Specification, Fractionation, and Techniques

## Overview

The Department of Radiation Oncology at the University of Wisconsin, Madison, considered a number of parameters when developing the gynecologic

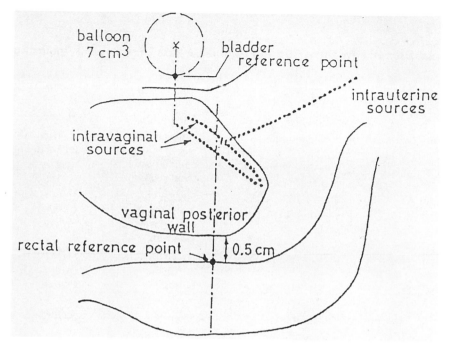

**Fig. 3.** Bladder and rectal dose monitoring. (ICRU report no. 38).

HDR brachytherapy program in 1989. The Madison system of HDR gynecologic brachytherapy describes the technique for intracavitary insertion, applicator type, dose specification points, external beam and HDR brachytherapy doses, and the integration of external and intracavitary doses using high-activity iridium-192.[12,13]

Based on practical considerations and the clinical experience of European and Japanese institutions, the Madison system prescribes five intracavitary insertions using a uterine tandem and vaginal ovoids or a tandem and cylinders. EBRT for carcinoma of the cervix is given at 1.7 Gy per fraction with four external fractions per week and one HDR brachytherapy fraction per week for five fractions. The HDR dose per fraction, integration of EBRT and HDR brachytherapy, and the use of central blocking is tailored to the tumor stage, volume, and distribution of local and regional disease (see Table 2).

**Dose Specification**

Dose specification in the Madison system defines a central tumor reference point M and a lateral pelvic lymph node point E. Point M lies 2 cm lateral to the center of the uterine canal and 2 cm cephalad from a line joining the center dwell position of the vaginal colpostat sources. Point E is a point on the pelvic wall at the intersection of a horizontal line tangential to the most cephalad portion of the acetabula and a line perpendicular to that passing through the medial aspect of the acetabula (Fig. 4).

<None>Table 2

**Treatment Protocols for Cervical Carcinoma: Madison System**

| Stage | HDR @ M Gy/fx | No. fx | HDR @ M | External beam:1.7 Gy/fx, 4 fx/wk | Total Dose (Gy) M | E |
|---|---|---|---|---|---|---|
| IA and IB | 9.1 or 9.9 | 5 | 45.5 49.5 | 60 Gy parametrial (with central area blocked) | 45.5 49.5 | 60 60 |
| IB bulky and IIA | 7.2 or 8.2 | 5 | 36.0 41.0 | 20–30 Gy whole pelvis prior to HDR and parametrial boost to "E" if needed. | 56–66 61–71 | 60 60 |
| IIB | 3.7 or 4.9 | 5 | 18.5 24.5 | 51 Gy whole pelvis | 69.5 75.5 | 60 60 |
| IIIA, IIIB, IVA | 3.7 or 4.3 | 5 | 18.5 21.5 | 60 Gy whole pelvis | 78.5 81.5 | 60 60 |

Note: If unable to perform intracavitary insertion, use 65–70 Gy whole pelvis or interstitial HDR.

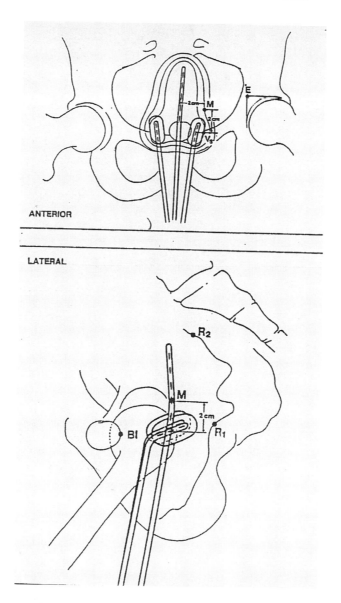

**Fig. 4.** Treatment planning for cervical carcinoma. The Madison system defines dose specification points for cervical carcinoma that include M as the central reference dose point and E for the pelvic wall contribution. Bladder (B1) and rectal $R_1$, $R_2$) dose points are also illustrated. $V_s$ = vaginal surface.

## Technique

Techniques of applicator insertion, fluoroscopy, and radiography for treatment planning films have been developed over time. High dose rate procedures are performed in the department in a shielded procedure suite. Modification of radiographic equipment and the procedure table allows performance of insertions, evaluation of the position under fluoroscopy, and delivery of the HDR treatment without moving the patient from the dorsal lithotomy position or out of the procedure room. Nursing personnel monitor the patient's vital signs and oximetry during the procedure. Sedation is utilized with intravenous doses of versed and midazolam. Initial doses of 50 mcg fentanyl and 2 mg midazolam are administered intravenously with additional doses titrated to achieve patient comfort during the procedure. Insertion of the intrauterine tandem and placement of the vaginal ovoids is accomplished by using the same techniques as for LDR procedures.

Several methods of decreasing the dose to critical normal structures are employed to protect the bladder and rectum. Doses to these critical structures are kept to approximately 80% of the prescription point M dose. Treatment planning optimization enhances the ability to customize therapy and to avoid delivering high doses to normal structures. Procedural manipulations also serve to protect critical structures. A posterior retractor is always used underneath the colpostat to move the anterior rectal wall further from the ovoids. Saline-soaked packing is placed anterior to the applicator to raise the bladder trigone region away from the applicator. Seven milliliters of contrast is used in the bladder catheter balloon and very dilute barium is placed in the rectum to identify critical dose regions of these normal structures. A biplane fluoroscopic and radiographic system allows imaging in anterior-posterior (AP) and lateral projections without moving the patient or x-ray equipment. Evaluation of the applicator position by fluoroscopy determines if adjustments should be made before taking dosimetry films. If the patient is moved to take dosimetry films and returned to the room for treatment, the applicator position and location of normal tissues may be altered enough to invalidate the accuracy of treatment planning.

## Resource Utilization for HDR Gynecologic Brachytherapy

High dose rate gynecologic brachytherapy done as an outpatient procedure in the radiation oncology department causes a cost-shift in reimbursement by increasing radiotherapy department billings and reducing billings by the hospital. A cost comparison for LDR brachytherapy versus HDR brachytherapy for carcinoma of the cervix was performed at the University of Wisconsin, Madison. Low dose rate therapy consisted of two intracavitary applications with three hospital days per application, operating and recovery room use, spinal anesthesia, and radiotherapy and physics charges. High dose rate treatment included five outpatient applications in the radiation oncology department, intravenous sedation without an anesthesiologist, and radiotherapy and physics charges. An overall 244% higher charge for LDR therapy was found primarily because of hospital and operating room expenses.[14]

The initial capital investment, maintenance requirements of the source and computer software, and the depreciation cost for HDR brachytherapy must be included in a decision to move to HDR brachytherapy. A 7-year total expenditure may approach $800,000, excluding hospital overhead, with the afterloader and treatment planning system representing the largest capital expenditure. A dedicated treatment room and radiographic verification system are needed for HDR procedures. Using linear accelerator rooms for treatment and therapy simulators for dosimetry films can reduce the initial cost but may reduce the efficacy of treatment or contribute to complications because of moving the patient from one location to another.

High dose rate programs are disproportionately sensitive to yearly capital depreciation and maintenance costs and are financially more risky than LDR programs. To reach economy parity between LDR and HDR at the University of Wisconsin nearly 200 gynecologic insertions must be performed annually. With ongoing restrictions in reimbursement policies by third-party carriers, the ratio of HDR cost to revenue will probably narrow.

## Conclusion

The initiation of an HDR brachytherapy gynecologic program for the treatment of carcinoma of the cervix involves a complex undertaking and requires a thorough understanding of radiobiological concepts, clinical trial results, and financial cost analysis. We have attempted to outline the methodology necessary to initiate such a program. It is incumbent upon the individual investigators to develop a consistent approach that will ultimately allow end results to be analyzed in a meaningful way.

*Acknowledgment*

The authors express their appreciation for the advice and guidance provided by Professor Charles Joslin in the development of the gynecologic HDR program at the University of Miami.

---

## REFERENCES

1. Dusenbery KE, Carson LF, Potish RA. Perioperative morbidity and mortality of gynecologic brachytherapy. Cancer 67:2786-2790, 1991.
2. Houdek PV, Schwade JG, Abitbol AA, et al. Optimization of high dose-rate cervix brachytherapy; part 1: dose distribution. Int J Radiat Oncol Biol Phys 21:1621-1625, 1991.
3. Houdek PV, Schwade JG, Wu X, et al. Dose determination in high dose rate brachytherapy. Int J Radiat Oncol Biol Phys 24:795-801, 1992.
4. Fu K, Phillips T. High-dose-rate versus low-dose-rate intracavitary brachytherapy for carcinoma of the cervix. Int J Radiat Oncol Biol Phys 19:791-796, 1990.
5. Eifel P. High-dose-rate brachytherapy for carcinoma of the cervix: High tech or high risk? Int J Radiat Oncol Biol Phys 24:383-386, 1992.
6. Dale RG. The use of small fraction numbers in high dose-rate gynecologic afterloading: some radiobiological considerations. Br J Radiol 63:290-294, 1990.

7. Brenner DJ, Huang Y, Hall EJ. Fractionated high dose rate versus low dose rate regimen for intracavitary brachytherapy of the cervix: equivalent regimen for combined brachytherapy and external irradiation. Int J Radiat Oncol Biol Phys 21:1415-1423, 1992.
8. Fowler JF, Stitt JA. High dose rate afterloading: how many fractions for gynecological treatments? Activity 5:135-136, 1991.
9. Nag S, Abitbol AA, Anderson LL, et al. Consensus guidelines for high dose rate remote brachytherapy (HDR) in cervical, endometrial, and endobronchial tumors. Int J Radiat Oncol Biol Phys 27:1241-1244, 1993.
10. Abitbol AA, Houdek PV, Schwade JG, et al. Ring applicator with rectal retractor: applicability to high dose rate brachytherapy of cervical cancer. Activity 4:68-69, 1990.
11. International Commission on Radiation Units and Measurements. ICRU report no. 38: dose and volume specification for reporting intracavitary therapy for gynecology. Bethesda, Md.; Mar. 1985.
12. Stitt JA, Fowler JF, Thomadsen BR. High-dose-rate intracavitary brachytherapy for carcinoma of the cervix: the Madison system: I: Clinical and radiobiological considerations. Int J Radiat Oncol Biol Phys 24:335-348, 1992.
13. Thomadsen BR, Shahabi S, Stitt JA. High-dose-rate intracavitary brachytherapy for carcinoma of the cervix: the Madison System: II: procedural and physical considerations. Int J Radiat Oncol Biol Phys 24:349-357, 1992.
14. Bastin K, Buchler D, Stitt J, et al. Resource utilization: High dose rate versus low dose-rate brachytherapy for gynecological cancer. Am J Clin Oncol 16(3):256-263, 1993.

# Chapter 18

# The Role of High Dose Rate Brachytherapy in Carcinoma of the Endometrium

*Dattatreyudu Nori, Judith A. Stitt, and Lincoln Pao*

## Introduction

Since the discovery of radium in 1896, the techniques of brachytherapy in carcinoma of the endometrium have evolved from Heymans capsules to high dose rate (HDR) applications. Total abdominal hysterectomy and bilateral salpingo-oophorectomy (TAH-BSO) is the traditional surgical procedure accepted as the standard treatment for patients with endometrial cancer. Following surgery alone, there is a 2%–15% reported incidence of vaginal recurrence in surgical stage I disease.[1] The use of adjuvant vaginal irradiation reduces the vaginal recurrence rate to 1%–3%.[1,2] Debate over adjuvant irradiation centers on the indications for therapy, particularly whether preoperative or postoperative irradiation is preferable and whether vaginal apex irradiation is of any value for patients with well-differentiated and superficially penetrating tumors.

## HDR Brachytherapy-Adjuvant Vaginal Treatment

### New York Medical Center of Queens and Memorial Sloan-Kettering Cancer Center Experience—Dattatreyudu Nori

At the New York Medical Center of Queens, stage I endometrial tumors of the International Federation of Gynecology and Obstetrics (FIGO) grade 2 and 3 and those with greater than one-third myometrium invasion are considered to be at high risk for recurrence, and these patients receive adjuvant whole-pelvis external radiation and intravaginal brachytherapy. Since vaginal recurrence can occur in low-grade tumors treated with surgery alone, intravaginal radiation is given to all FIGO grade 1 patients. For patients treated in this fashion by us at Memorial Sloan-Kettering Cancer Center (MSKCC), New York, New York, the 5-year survival rate for stage I disease increased from 70% to 92% and for stage II disease from 46% to 82%.[3] A striking decrease in pelvic

From: Nag, S. (ed.): *High Dose Rate Brachytherapy: A Textbook*, Futura Publishing Company, Inc., Armonk, NY, © 1994.

and/or vaginal recurrences from 22% (119 out of 538 patients) in the stage I historical control group to 2.7% in the combined stages I and II in the current series is notable (Table 1).

Increased dose fractionation had been shown to be a major factor in lowering radiation-related complications with the HDR remote afterloading technique. A submucosal dose of 21 Gy vaginal radiation delivered in 3 fractions spaced 2 weeks apart provides excellent tumor control, and when combined with pelvic external radiation treatment of 40 Gy in 4 weeks for patients with poor prognosis risk factors, it is well tolerated with minimal complications.[2]

*Technical Considerations*

At both the New York Medical Center of Queens and MSKCC, HDR adjuvant vaginal treatment is delivered using an applicator that provides good surface contact throughout the vaginal mucosa for uniform dose distribution. Caution must be taken when using small (2-cm diameter) cylinders because the surface dose is relatively high. Radiographic studies are performed to ascertain the position of the applicator in the vagina. The treatment duration is dependent on the diameter of the applicator and the linear length of the moving source. Patients are treated supine in the dorso-lithotomy position to accommodate applicator placement. No sedation is required either before or during treatment, and all applications are performed on an outpatient basis. The treatment room is heavily shielded and monitored with safety door lock devices to ensure complete radiation protection for medical personnel. Patients are observed during the treatment with closed circuit television to monitor proper treatment position.

Posttreatment observations relative to any abnormal vaginal signs and symptoms are recorded with photomicrographs of the vagina in selected cases. All mucosal changes are documented. Follow-up examinations are performed every 3 months during the first year, every 6 months during the second year, and once yearly thereafter.

**Table 1**

**Comparative Survival and Recurrences:**
**Memorial Sloan-Kettering Cancer Center Experience**

| Review Period | Stage | Type of Treatment | Total No. | 5-yr NED Survival | Pelvic Recurrences |
|---|---|---|---|---|---|
| 1949–1965 | I | S | 536 | 70% | |
| | II | S | 24 | 46% | 22% |
| 1969–1979 | I | S+RT | 278 | 91% | |
| | II | S+RT | 22 | 77% | 2.5% |

NED: no evidence of disease.

*Results*

Long-term evaluation of 300 patients with follow-up ranging from 11–15 years is reported here. Eleven patients (4%) developed a recurrence, and 8 out of 11 patients have died of the disease. One patient with local recurrence was subsequently treated with further radiation and is currently alive and free of disease. Four patients died of nonmalignant causes, and 12 died of a second primary cancer including cancer of the colon, bladder, or breast, and lymphoma. The 5- and 10-year disease-free survivals in stage IA are 96% and 91%; in stage IB they are 83% and 75%.

Nine percent of patients experienced mild to moderate complications. Complications include cystitis (4.5%), vaginal stenosis (2.5%), proctitis (1.5%), vaginal vault necrosis (0.5%), and partial bowel obstruction (0.5%). All complications were managed successfully with conservative treatment without the necessity for surgical intervention.

This analysis has identified three categories of patients with markedly improved survival at 10 years or beyond. These categories are

(1) grade 1 tumors compared with grade 2 and 3 tumors (90% vs 60% 10-year survival);

(2) microscopic extension outside the uterus compared with those patients who have gross involvement of the pelvic structures at the time of hysterectomy (90% vs. 80% 10-year survival);

(3) patients younger than 55 years of age compared to those older than 55 years (92% vs.75% 10-year survival).

In the subsequent series from May 1980 to June 1985, 174 patients at MSKCC, New York, New York, were evaluated as high-risk stage I and stage II endometrial carcinoma because of grade 2 or 3 tumors and/or more than one-third myometrial invasion. Patients were treated with adjuvant preoperative or postoperative radiation therapy, including external pelvic irradiation to 40 Gy over 4 weeks and postoperative intravaginal cuff irradiation with HDR iridium-192 remote afterloading techniques using 2-cm, 2.5-cm, or 3-cm diameter vaginal cylinders at a dose rate of 100–140 cGy/min.

Patients were treated with two different fractionation schedules. Those treated from May 1980 to February 1984 received 21 Gy in 3 fractions at 2-week intervals with the dose prescribed 0.5 cm from the applicator surface (Group 1). From March 1984 to June 1985, the dose per fraction was decreased to 5 Gy for 3 fractions for a total dose of 15 Gy (Group 2). This change in fractionation was made to investigate whether a lower dose per fraction would result in acceptable local control rates and further reduce complications from the previous dose schedule.

In Group 1, 6 of 118 patients are dead of disease, giving a 5-year actuarial disease-free survival rate of 86%. In group 2, 8 of 56 patients are dead of disease with a 5-year actuarial disease-free rate of 86%. There was no significant difference in disease-free survival when the results were compared by stage of disease. (Table 2)

**Table 2**

**Remote Afterloading Treatments: Comparative 5-Year Survival in High Risk Endometrial Cancer (Patients Treated with 2 Different IVRT Regimes after 40 Gy External Pelvic Radiation Therapy)**

| Category | Group I 700 × 3 | Group II 500 × 3 |
|---|---|---|
| Stage I | 88.7% | 88.5% |
| Stage II | 82% | 82% |
| Complication Rate | 6% | 2% |
| Local Failure Rate | 6% | 6% |

Two hundred patients were reviewed for this analysis.

The median time to local recurrence was 13 months in Group 1 and 16 months in Group 2. The difference between local recurrence rates in the two groups was not statistically significant ($P = 0.78$). The actuarial 5-year local recurrence rate was 6% for both groups. All recurrences occurred within 2 years of treatment.

Grade I complications were difficult to quantify retrospectively and, therefore, were not analyzed. Grade 2 complications that were resolved without treatment intervention developed in 29 out of 118 Group 1 patients and in 7 out of 56 of Group 2 patients. Vaginal stenosis resulting in dyspareunia was analyzed separately. Seven patients in Group 1 (6% at 5 years) developed dyspareunia, but no patient in Group 2 had this complaint.

## Madison Experience—Judith A. Stitt

At the University of Wisconsin Comprehensive Cancer Center in Madison, Wisconsin, patients with stage IA grade 1 or 2 cancers receive no further therapy if their tumors are smaller than 2 cm.[4,5] For early stage disease with tumors larger than 2 cm and those with stage IB grade 1 or 2 disease, vaginal cuff irradiation is recommended. Whole pelvis irradiation is indicated for stage IB grade 3, stage IC grade 1, 2, and 3 and stage IIA and IIB. Vaginal cuff irradiation may be added to the whole pelvis depending on the tumor volume, location in the uterus, and degree of cervical involvement (Table 3).

The Madison system of HDR gynecologic brachytherapy for adjuvant cuff irradiation prescribes just two HDR fractions of 16.2 Gy per fraction to the

**Table 3**

**Adjuvant Therapy for Surgically Staged Endometrial Cancer**

| Stage IA; Grade 1, 2 | Stage IA; Grade 3 Stage IB; Grade 1, 2* | Stage IB; Grade 3 Stage IC; Grade 1, 2, 3 Stage IIA, B; Grade 1, 2, 3 |
|---|---|---|
| No Further Therapy | Vaginal Cuff Irradiation | Whole Pelvis Irradiation + Cuff XRT |

*Treat Stage IB, Grade 2 > 2 cm with whole pelvis XRT.

vaginal apex using vaginal colpostats. The decision to use so few fractions was based upon patient convenience in accordance with reasonable radiobiological principles. Vaginal colpostats rather than cylinders are used to avoid treating too long a segment of the vagina. Additionally, because of the anisotropy of iridium-192 when used in cylinders, the dose at the vaginal apex is less than at the cylinder sides and could theoretically cause an overdose to this region. When colpostats are used, source anisotrophy serves to lower the dose to the bladder trigone and to the anterior rectal wall.[4,5]

## Technical Considerations

Techniques of applicator insertion, fluoroscopy, and radiography for treatment-planning films have been developed over time. Ovoid insertions are performed in the department in a shielded procedure suite. Nursing personnel monitor the patients' vital signs and oximetry during intravenous sedation using intermittent doses of fentanyl and midazolam. Modifications in radiographic equipment and the procedure table allow the staff to perform the insertion, evaluate the applicator position with fluoroscopy, take dosimetry films, and give HDR treatment without moving the patient from the dorsolithotomy position or out of the procedure room.

Several methods of decreasing the dose to critical normal structures are employed to protect the bladder and rectum. A posterior retractor is always used underneath the colpostats to move the anterior rectal wall away from the ovoids. Saline-soaked packing is placed anterior to the applicator to raise the bladder base away from the applicator. Seven cc of contrast is used in the bladder catheter balloon, and very dilute barium is placed in the rectum to identify critical dose regions of these normal structures. A biplane fluoroscopic and radiographic system permits obtaining AP and lateral images without moving the patient or x-ray equipment. Evaluation of the applicator position by fluoroscopy determines if adjustments should be made before taking dosimetry films. If the patient is moved from the room to take dosimetry films and returned for treatment, the applicator position and location of normal tissues may be altered enough to invalidate the accuracy of treatment.

Treatment is specified to the vaginal surface. Because 16.2 Gy is being given for each fraction, it is mandatory to achieve technically meticulous insertions and perform optimized dosimetry for each of the two treatments. The bladder and rectal dose calculation points can be kept to approximately 80% of the prescription dose via these means. Treatment-planning optimization enhances the ability to customize therapy and to avoid delivering high doses to normal structures.

## Other Institutional Experience

In the late 1960s, various institutions in Europe introduced HDR brachytherapy for vaginal cuff irradiation in endometrial carcinoma. Sorbe et al.[6] at the Orebro Medical Center Hospital in Sweden treated 404 women with endometrial carcinoma stage I with a $^{60}$Co HDR afterloading technique. Cylindrical vaginal applications were used to treat the proximal two-thirds of the vaginal wall, sparing the distal one-third and introitus. The prescribed dose depth was 1 cm from the surface of the applicator. Four different fractionation schedules were used: 4 × 900cGy, 5 × 600 cGy, 6 × 500 cGy, 6 × 450 cGy. The rate of vaginal recurrence was 0.7%. It was noted that vaginal shortening increased from 31% to 79% as the dose escalated from 450 cGy to 900 cGy. Applicator diameter, dose per fraction, and the vaginal length treated all contributed to the degree of vaginal shortening.

## Discussion

An overview of the international experience in the treatment of postoperative endometrial cancer reveals that cuff irradiation commonly begins 4 to 5 weeks after TAH-BSO. The largest possible diameter vaginal cylinder or colpostat is used at the vaginal apex. Fraction size, dose per fraction, and interval between fractions are variable among institutions. Dose specification is commonly defined at 0.5 cm from the cylinder surface. Minimal acute toxicity results from vaginal cuff irradiation. The most common late effect is vaginal fibrosis and shortening, with the incidence ranging from 5%–37%. Factors increasing vaginal fibrosis include using 2-cm diameter vaginal cylinders, higher dose per fraction, addition of pelvic external beam radiation, and treatment-dose specification beyond 0.5 cm.

# HDR Brachytherapy-Recurrent Vaginal Disease

The prognosis for patients with vaginal recurrence is poor. Recently, the view that vaginal recurrence is often a solitary metastasis is supported by improved 5-year survival rates of 33% to 50%.[3] Factors influencing a prognosis of vaginal recurrence of endometrial cancer include site of recurrence and type of primary therapy. Apical recurrences are associated with better survival compared to lesions of the anterior, suburethra, and lower vaginal walls. Late recurrences have a better prognosis than disease that develops soon after primary therapy.[3] Papillary-type adenocarcinoma has a less favorable outcome than nonpapillary cell types. It tends to relapse outside of the pelvis with a pattern of spread similar to papillary adenocarcinoma of the ovary and is less amenable to regional or systemic therapy.

Twenty patients with vaginal recurrence of endometrial carcinoma treated with HDR brachytherapy and external pelvic irradiation were reported from MSKCC.[3] For most patients, 21 Gy was delivered at 0.5 cm from the mucosal surface over 3 fractions spaced 2 weeks apart over 4 weeks. Radiation was combined with surgical resection in 6 patients. Each patient's treatment was individualized to account for tumor site, resectability, prior radiation therapy and/or surgery. The overall response rate after aggressive treatment was 85% (17 patients). The treatment-related complication rate was 15% (3 patients). Small bowel obstruction occurred in two patients and was resolved with conservative management. Mild vaginal vault necrosis developed in the third patient and healed within 2 months with conservative management. A minimum follow-up of 4 years is available for 18 patients. Actuarial 4-year and no evidence of disease survival rates were 50% and 40%, respectively. The median survival is 39 months.

## HDR Brachytherapy-Inoperable Endometrial Carcinoma

There is a subset of patients with carcinoma of the endometrium who are not candidates for general anesthesia and total abdominal hysterectomy because of severe medical problems, either due to gross obesity, significant cardiovascular disease, diabetes, hypertension, or life-threatening respiratory compromise. Curative radiation therapy, either using intracavitary brachytherapy alone or in combination with external beam radiation, is the treatment of choice in these patients. The same contraindications to surgery are also relative contraindications to whole pelvic external beam radiation and increase the risk of bowel toxicity. These patients are also at increased risk for thromboembolic events due to the prolonged bed rest required for low dose rate (LDR) brachytherapy. High dose rate brachytherapy plays a vital role in the treatment of inoperable carcinoma of the endometrium.

Standard intrauterine radiation techniques require using a uterine tandem or packing the uterine cavity with multiple radioactive sources. The original Heymans capsules used radium that contributed to excessive exposures to the radiation oncologist and operating room personnel. MSKCC developed an endometrial applicator that permitted afterloading of isotopes and improved dose distribution in the uterus by adjusting the number of radioactive sources and their position within the uterus. The same applicator can be used for HDR or LDR brachytherapy.[7]

The current recommendation at Madison for inoperable cases is to deliver a dose of 20 Gy in 2 fractions at 2 cm from the central axis of the uterus with HDR brachytherapy. This is supplemented with 40 Gy whole pelvis external beam therapy over 4 weeks.

A dose specification system to define critical dose points was developed to reflect the structures of interest for endometrial cancer.[5] The paracervical region is designated as point M and lies 2 cm lateral to the center of the uterine canal and 2 cm cephalad from the center dwell position of the vaginal colpostat. The myometrium is represented by point W laterally and point S superiorly. Point W lies 2 cm caudal from the midline of the uterine cavity apex and 3 cm lateral to the uterine tandem in uteri sounding less than 10 cm and 4 cm lateral to the tandem for uteri greater than 10 cm. The Madison system recommends using a single tandem for uteri sounding greater than 10 cm, two 15° tandems for 10–12-cm uteri, and a triple tandem (two 30°, one 15°) for uteri greater than 12 cm. When using multiple tandems, point W is redefined on the basis of anatomical observation of the myometrial location. Optimization of treatment planning using these dose specification points insures adequate coverage of the myometrium. Rotte[7] has used the Heyman packing technique for HDR brachytherapy. The treatment volume is prescribed to a distance of 1.5–2 cm lateral to each of the capsules.

---

# REFERENCES

1. Joslin CA, Smith CW. Postoperative radiotherapy in the management of uterine corpus cancer. Clin Radiol 22:118-124, 1971.
2. Nori D, Hilaris BS, Tome M, et al. Combined surgery and radiation in endometrial carcinoma: an analysis of prognostic factors. Int J Radiat Oncol Biol Phys 13:489-497, 1987.
3. Mandell LM, Nori D, Anderson LL, et al. Postoperative vaginal radiation in endometrial cancer using a remote afterloading technique. Int J Radiat Oncol Biol Phys 11:473-478, 1985.
4. Stitt JA. High-dose-rate intracavitary brachytherapy for gynecologic malignancies. Oncology 6:59–79, 1992.
5. Stitt, JA. Dose specification for inoperable endometrial carcinoma: the Madison System. Activity/International Selectron Brachytherapy Journal (suppl. 2):32-34, 1991.
6. Sorbe BG, Smeds AC. Postoperative vaginal irradiation with high dose rate afterloading technique in endometrial carcinoma stage I. Int J Radiat Oncol Biol Phys 18:305-314, 1990.
7. Rotte K. Technique and results of HDR afterloading in cancer of the endometrium. In: Martinez AA, Orton CG, Mould RF, eds. Brachytherapy HDR and LDR. Columbia, Md.: Nucletron; 1990, 68-79.

## Chapter 19

# The Role of High Dose Rate Brachytherapy in the Management of Adult Soft Tissue Sarcomas

*Subir Nag, Arthur T. Porter, and David Donath*

## Introduction

Soft tissue sarcomas tend to invade locally along anatomical planes. Excisional biopsy, therefore, is inadequate as the sole therapy, and over 90 percent of these patients will have local recurrences. In an American College of Surgeons survey, treatment failures occurred in 37% of patients without metastasis at initial diagnosis and with gross resection of soft tissue.[1] Approximately 80% of all lesions that recur after surgery do so within 2 years.[2] Twenty to 25% of patients undergoing amputation or radical local excision have local recurrences,[2,3] compared to 60%–75% rate of local recurrences for patients undergoing conservative excision.[2-4]

Recently there has been a strong interest in evaluating conservative surgery with adjuvant radiation therapy. A National Institute of Health Consensus Conference review of limb-sparing surgery plus adjuvant radiation or chemotherapy for the management of high-grade extremity sarcoma indicates that the results of the conservative approach with radiation therapy were equivalent to those obtained by more radical surgical procedures in selected patients with reservation of function.[5]

Radiation therapy alone using doses of 60 to 80 Gy can control a small percentage of unresectable soft tissue sarcomas.[6,7] The inverse relation between tumor size and ability to obtain local control is illustrated by control rates of 88%, 53%, and 33% with tumors less than 5 cm, 5 to 10 cm, and greater than 10 cm, respectively.[8] Thus, radiation therapy is generally used as adjuvant therapy to treat the microscopic residual after surgery, or it is given preoperatively to decrease the risk of tumor implantation in the surgical wound and to produce tumor regression that facilitates resection.[9,10]

A few centers have combined surgery with low dose rate (LDR) brachytherapy.[11-18] The advantages of tumor bed brachytherapy include more accurate demarcation of the tumor site and delivery of a high tumor dose with a low dose to the surrounding normal tissues. The loading of radioactive sources is usually performed 5 to 7 days after surgery to allow adequate wound healing, and

From: Nag, S. (ed.): *High Dose Rate Brachytherapy: A Textbook*, Futura Publishing Company, Inc., Armonk, NY, © 1994.

the radiation is usually performed over a period of 4 to 7 days. Thus, there is a very short delay between surgery and the start of radiation therapy. If a high dose (40–45 Gy) of brachytherapy is delivered, no postimplant external beam radiation therapy (EBRT) is employed. If lower doses of brachytherapy (15–25 Gy) are used as a boost, it is followed by external radiation therapy of 45–50 Gy to a larger volume. Memorial Sloan-Kettering Cancer Center, New York, New York, conducted a prospective randomized trial on 126 patients with soft tissue sarcoma of the extremity or superficial trunk between July 1982 and July 1987.[17] Patients were randomized to receive limb-sparing surgery or limb-sparing surgery with LDR brachytherapy using Ir-192 to deliver 4,200 to 4,500 cGy over 4–6 days. At 5 years, the local control was 80% in the brachytherapy group and 62% in the group not receiving brachytherapy ($P = .029$). For high-grade tumors, local control was 88% with brachytherapy and 58% without brachytherapy ($P = .007$). There was no difference in local control in the low-grade patients in either arm of the study. There was no statistical difference in the disease-specific survival at 5 years.

Intraoperative brachytherapy requires a very close cooperation between the surgeon and the radiation oncologist and requires expertise in brachytherapy techniques. Brachytherapy for soft tissue sarcoma requires implantation of large volumes, which results in high radiation exposure to the medical staff. Although use of removable iodine-125 seeds can reduce the radiation exposure problem, this is both more time consuming and more expensive.[11] The use of remote afterloading high dose rate (HDR) brachytherapy would eliminate the radiation exposure and would also allow dose optimization. It seems logical to combine the advantages of EBRT (homogenous dose to a large volume), and HDR brachytherapy (high localized tumor dose, sparing of surrounding normal tissues, elimination of radiation exposure to personnel, short treatment times, and optimized dose distribution). Very few authors have reported on the use of HDR brachytherapy for soft tissue sarcoma.[19,20] Certainly more investigation is required in this field.

## Methods

The patient selection criteria, pretreatment evaluation, surgical procedure, and implantation of the brachytherapy catheters are very similar to those used with LDR brachytherapy[11-16] and will, therefore, be described only briefly.

### Biopsy

The nature of the biopsy is an important aspect of overall management of patients with soft tissue sarcomas. The biopsy site must be removed in any resection; hence care should be taken in placing the biopsy incision at a location and orientation that will not compromise subsequent surgical excision. The biopsy should be an incisional biopsy, and a large tissue sample should be taken to make an accurate diagnosis and grade and to allow any special studies that are needed. Care should be taken to obtain excellent hemostasis since hematoma resulting from biopsies of soft tissue sarcomas can spread the tumor along their paths. The incision should be placed longitudinally on the extremities. At other sites, the incision should be parallel to the long axis of the underlying principal muscle.

## Wide Excision

The tumor is removed along with the margin of normal surrounding tissues contiguous to the tumor. Every effort should be made to obtain clear margins. However, the neurovascular bundle is to be preserved, even if this requires leaving a gross tumor behind; this is possible in an organ-conserving approach because the tumor bed will receive a brachytherapy boost.

## Implantation of Catheters

High dose rate brachytherapy catheters should be placed parallel along the tumor bed, 1.0 to 1.5 cm apart. The margins of the tumor bed should be indicated by the application of radio-opaque surgical clips. The area to be implanted would include the tumor bed and a 2–5-cm margin. Orthogonal radiographs are obtained using dummy seeds. The target volume is drawn and an optimized treatment plan performed to allow a homogeneous dose within the target volume.

## Brachytherapy Dose

The optimal dose of brachytherapy to be used has not been established. Wayne State University in Detroit, Michigan, has used 200–400 cGy per fraction, given twice a day.[19] Patients receiving HDR brachytherapy alone received total doses ranging from 3,984 cGy over 12 fractions to 4,746 cGy over 14 fractions. Patients who received supplementary EBRT of 3,000–5,040 cGy also received HDR of 2,065 to 2,394 cGy over 7 fractions.

At McGill University, Montreal, Canada, 6–7 HDR treatments of 500 cGy each were delivered twice a day.[20] The patients who had received preoperative EBRT received only 4–5 HDR treatments of 500 cGy. The 500 cGy dose was applied to a continuous isodose curve surrounding the catheters by a 0.5-cm margin. No attempt was made to cover the scar or drain site with the prescription dose.

Although there is no consensus, the HDR Brachytherapy Working Group (HIBWOG) had proposed a trial of HDR brachytherapy of 3 Gy per fraction at 0.5 cm from the plane of implant to be delivered twice daily for 6 treatments (18 Gy total) for microscopic residual disease and 3 Gy twice daily × 7 (total 21 Gy) for gross residual disease. The brachytherapy would be started 5–7 days after surgery. This would be followed by postoperative EBRT.

### External Beam Radiation Therapy

Doses of 4,500–5,000 cGy in 25–28 treatments are generally used to boost brachytherapy doses. The target volume includes the tumor bed with margins sufficient to include all suspected or potential sites of occult tumor. If this results in irradiation of an excessively large amount of normal tissue, a margin of 10 cm measured from the tumor bed in the direction of the potential spread is suggested. If normal tissue consideration precludes the use of a 10-cm margin in some locations, a margin of 5 cm in the direction of potential spread is suggested as a minimum.

The scar area may be bolused for part of the treatment course in patients with proven or suspected areas of skin involvement. In most patients with deep-seated lesions, the skin incision need not be bolused. When extremities are irradiated, a peripheral strip of tissues must be spared to prevent lymphatic obstruction and distal edema. Ideally, one-third or more of the circumference of the extremities should be spared. If this is not feasible, the minimum width of the spared strip of tissue should be 2 cm for the forearm, 3 cm for the lower leg, and 4 cm for the thigh. Custom-made beam shaping blocks, compensating filters, wedges, immobilization devices, and the like are to be used to optimize the treatment.

# Results

There is very little experience in the use of HDR brachytherapy in soft tissue sarcomas; therefore, these results can be regarded as only preliminary and should be interpreted with caution. Of 13 patients treated, Wayne State University in Detroit, Michigan, reported wound complication with simple healing delay and hematoma, requiring premature removal of the implant and skin debridement in one patient. There were three local failures, and only one patient died of disease.[18]

At McGill University in Montreal, 19 patients have been treated with wide local resection and postoperative adjuvant HDR brachytherapy.[19] Two had preoperative EBRT. The first ten patients treated have a follow-up of at least 1 year. Postoperative EBRT was not an option in these patients because of the following conditions: proximity to radiosensitive tissue, that is, spinal cord and small bowel; previous radiation treatment for a different malignancy; recurrence after a wide local excision and EBRT; and recurrence after a wide local excision and [125]I brachytherapy. Of the 10 patients, only three have experienced local recurrence. Of these three, two were thought to have had radiation-induced sarcomas; and, in the third, recurrence developed in the tumor bed next to a grafted blood vessel that was not adequately treated with brachytherapy out of concern for possible morbidity to the graft. Of the 19 patients, three had wound complications. One had a dehiscence over the sacrum secondary to the patient lying continuously on this site after pelvic surgery. Two other patients had lymphedema and a wound infection. Both of these patients had continuous tumor growth during preoperative EBRT, and both were taken to surgery less than 1 week after a dose of 3,400 cGy was delivered to the area. None of these complications required surgery. Another patient with no evidence of recurrence developed a pathological fracture of the femur within the treated area.

## Discussion

The present trend in the management of soft tissue sarcoma is for organ-preserving surgery with adjuvant radiation therapy. The need for adjuvant therapy arises if the tumors are (a) high grade, (b) large, (c) recurrent, or (d) have close, microscopic, or grossly positive margins after resection. The radiation therapy can be in the form of EBRT,[6-10] LDR brachytherapy with or without EBRT,[11-18] intraoperative radiation therapy with EBRT,[21,22] or HDR brachytherapy.[19,20]

There is substantial experience (including a randomized trial) in the use of LDR brachytherapy in the management of soft tissue sarcoma after surgical resection. Remote afterloaded HDR brachytherapy has some theoretical advantages over manually afterloaded LDR (e.g., ability for optimization, elimination of radiation exposure hazard). However, of all these modalities, there is the least experience in the use of HDR brachytherapy in soft tissue sarcomas; therefore, caution must be exercised in its use, and further controlled clinical trials are required.

---

## REFERENCES

1. Lawrence W Jr, Donegan WL, Nachmuth N, et al. Adult soft tissue sarcomas: a pattern of care survey of the American College of Surgeons. Ann Surg 205:349-359, 1987.
2. Cantin J, McNeer GP, Chu FC, et al. The problem of local recurrence after treatment of soft tissue sarcoma. Ann Surg 168:47-53, 1968.
3. Shiu MH, Castro EB, Hajdu SI, et al. Surgical treatment of 297 soft tissue sarcomas of the lower extremity. Ann Surg 182:597, 1975.
4. Martin RG, Butler JJ, Albores-Saavedra J. Soft tissue tumors: surgical treatment and results. In: Tumors of Bone and Soft Tissue. Chicago, IL: Year Book Medical Publishers; 1965.
5. National Institutes of Health Consensus Development Panel of Limb-Sparing Treatment of Adult Soft Tissue Sarcomas and Osteosarcomas: introduction and conclusions. Cancer Treat Symp 3:1-5, 1985.
6. Windeyer SB, Dische S, Mansfield CM. The place of radiotherapy in the management of fibrosarcoma of the soft tissues. Clin Radiol 17:32-40, 1966.
7. Lindberg RD. Soft tissue sarcoma. In: Fletcher GH, ed. Textbook of Radiotherapy. Philadelphia, Pa.: Lea & Febiger; 1980, 922-942.
8. Tepper JE, Suit HD. Radiation therapy of soft tissue sarcomas. Cancer 55:2273-2277, 1985.
9. Suit HD, Mankin HJ, Schiller AL, et al. Results of treatment of sarcoma of soft tissue by radiation and surgery at Massachusetts General Hospital. Cancer Treat Symp 3:43-47, 1985.
10. Lindberg RD, Martin RG, Romsdahl MM, et al. Conservative surgery and postoperative radiotherapy in 300 adults with soft-tissue sarcomas. Cancer 47:2391-2397, 1981.

11. Shiu MH, Hilaris BS, Harrison LB, et al. Brachytherapy and function-saving resection of soft tissue sarcoma arising in the limb. Int J Radiat Oncol Biol Phys 21:1485-1492, 1991.
12. Habrand JL, Gerbaulet A, Pejovic MH, et al. Twenty years experience of interstitial iridium brachytherapy in the management of soft tissue sarcomas. Int J Radiat Oncol Biol Phys 20:405-411, 1991.
13. Zelefsky MJ, Nor D, Shiu MH, et al. Limb salvage in soft tissue sarcomas involving neurovascular structures using combined surgical resection and brachytherapy. Int J Radiat Oncol Biol Phys 19:913-918, 1990.
14. Gemer LS, Trowbridge DR, Neff J, et al. Local recurrence of soft tissue sarcoma following brachytherapy. Int J Radiat Oncol Biol Phys 20:587-592, 1991.
15. Nori D, Shupak K, Shiu MH, et al. Role of brachytherapy in recurrent extremity sarcoma in patients treated with prior surgery and irradiation. Int J Radiat Oncol Biol Phys 20:1229-1233, 1991.
16. Schray MF, Guunderson LL, Sim FH, et al. Integration of brachytherapy, resection, and external irradiation. Cancer 66:451-456, 1990.
17. Harrison LB, Franzee F, Gaynor J, et al. Results of a prospective randomized trial of adjuvant brachytherapy in the management of completely resected soft tissue sarcoma. Int J Radiat Oncol Biol Phys 24 (suppl.1):240, 1992 (abstract).
18. Schupak KD, Land JM, Weilepp AE, et al. The psychofunctional handicap associated with the use of brachytherapy in the treatment of lower extremity high grade soft tissue sarcomas. Int J Radiat Oncol Biol Phys 27 (suppl.):293, 1983 (abstract).
19. Alekhteyar KM, Porter AT, Ryan C, et al. Preliminary results of hyperfractionated high dose rate brachytherapy in soft-tissue sarcoma. Endocurie/Hypertherm Oncol 9:56, 1993 (abstract).
20. Donath D, Clark C, Kaufmann MD, et al. Postoperative adjuvant high dose rate brachytherapy in the treatment of poor-prognosis soft-tissue sarcoma. Endocurie/Hypertherm Oncol 9:48, 1993 (abstract).
21. Calvo FA, Ortiz de Urbina D, Beguiristain JL, et al. Soft tissue sarcomas of the extremities. In: Calvo FA, Santos M, Brady LW, eds. Intraoperative Radiotherapy. Berlin, Germany: Springer-Verlag; 1992, 91-97.
22. Calvo FA, Abuchaibe O, Serra JM, et al. Retroperitoneal and other central soft tissue sarcomas. In: Calvo FA, Santos M, Brady LW, eds. Intraoperative Radiotherapy. Berlin, Germany: Springer-Verlag; 1992, 85-90.

## Chapter 20

# High Dose Rate Remote Brachytherapy in the Treatment of Pediatric Tumors

*Subir Nag, Frederick B. Ruymann, and James Fontanesi*

## Introduction

External beam radiation therapy (EBRT), usually with generous tumor margins, is often used to treat patients with rhabdomyosarcoma (RMS). These treatments can often last 4–6 weeks, depending on the residual tumor status and planned total doses to be delivered. In the pediatric population, this can result in cosmetic deformity, altered dentition, altered organ function, and bone growth retardation.[1-3] Multimodality therapy including surgery, EBRT, and chemotherapy has improved survival in patients treated in the Intergroup Rhabdomyosarcoma Study (IRS) from 1972 to the present.[4-6] However, decreased survival has been reported in infants with RMS. A possible explanation for the poor local control in infants with RMS has been the reluctance to administer EBRT with its deleterious late effects on the growing child.[3] With the increased survival achievable in older children with multimodal therapy, it would be advisable to explore ways to reduce the dose to normal tissues and thereby preserve function (bone growth, sexual life, fertility, and endocrine function) in younger children.

With brachytherapy, it is possible to deliver a high dose of irradiation to a well-defined tumor volume with a low dose to the normal surrounding tissues and thus obtain a high tumor control with an acceptable rate of complications. These advantages of brachytherapy in comparison with EBRT are well known. Brachytherapy is routinely used in adults, but only a few authors have used this method of treatment in children.[7-29] Typically, manually afterloaded low dose rate (LDR) brachytherapy has been used.[7-27]

Experience with LDR brachytherapy in children has only recently been reported in significant numbers and with long enough follow-up to evaluate its efficacy and toxicity. The recent update of the St. Jude's Children's Research Hospital, Memphis, Tennessee, study documents its use in 46 children with a median follow-up of 39 months.[12] Forty-three of the 50 implanted regions have maintained continuous disease-free intervals of up to 115 months (median = 39 months). The failures have all occurred within 2 years

From: Nag, S. (ed.): *High Dose Rate Brachytherapy: A Textbook*, Futura Publishing Company, Inc., Armonk, NY, © 1994.

of implantation with only marginal success with salvage attempts (2 out of 7). The implants were evaluated for reason (1° treatment [primary], boost therapy in conjunction with EBRT or for metastatic and/or recurrent disease), dose rate, and total dose to determine the factors contributing to success and complications. No patient treated with primary implantation (11 sites) developed recurrence; 12 out of 15 patients treated with boost therapy remained in continuous local control, and 19 out of 24 recurrent and/or metastatic sites had documented local control. There was no statistical difference between treatment for gross versus microscopic residual disease or total dose or hourly dose rates in determining an influence on local control. However, there was an increased complication rate for those receiving a permanent iodine-125 implant. There was also a trend for the development of complications in the region of joints. Previous surgical intervention has been suggested in other series reviewing joint-related complications. There were no reports of infection or wound breakdown secondary to the placement of catheters.

Curran et al.[8] reported that seven of eight children who received interstitial radiation during initial therapy for soft-tissue sarcomas at the University of Pennsylvania, Fox Chase Cancer Center, in Philadelphia, Pennsylvania, demonstrated local control. Six of these children had no evidence of disease at a median follow-up of 5.8 years, but only one of the four patients treated for recurrent disease was alive. All of the patients developed self-limiting acute reactions, usually mucositis, but none required greater than a 2-week delay in the chemotherapy schedule. Functional and cosmetic effects from interstitial radiation were minimal at a median follow-up period of 6.5 years (range: 2 to 16 years).

Flamant et al.[9] treated 17 children with vulval and vaginal RMS with brachytherapy in addition to surgery and chemotherapy at the Institute Gustave-Roussy, Villejuif, France, between 1970 and 1978. One patient died of metastatic disease 1 year after diagnosis, and another patient died of infectious complications after chemotherapy. The remaining 15 patients are considered free of all disease. Four patients developed severe late effects (colorectal, vaginal, urethral, and ureteral stenosis); three patients had minimal vaginal stenosis requiring surgery for intercourse; another, in whom an ovarian transposition was not performed, developed partial ovarian insufficiency. The authors thought that advances in brachytherapy and improvements in dosimetry might reduce the occurrence of these complications.

Cherlow et al.[7] treated eleven pediatric patients with 40 Gy iridium-192 brachytherapy. Eight patients had no evidence of disease at 11–62 months (median = 38 months).

In an effort to reduce radiation exposure to the medical staff and parents, removable iodine-125, a low-energy radionuclide, has been used by Zelefsky et al.[27], and Marquez et al.[20] Nechuskin et al.[23] used LDR remote afterloading techniques of 30–35 Gy at 0.6–1.3 Gy/h over 20–25 hours in 4 children to eliminate radiation exposure to the parents. However, the treatments still required sedation or prolonged immobilization of small children.

# High Dose Rate Brachytherapy: Ohio State University (OSU)/Children's Hospital Experience—S. Nag, F. Ruymann, T. Olson, R.S. Pieters, and S. Teich

Although LDR brachytherapy can be used to obtain a high tumor control with an acceptable rate of complications, it is often difficult in younger children and infants primarily because they can require prolonged sedation and immobilization for the administration of LDR brachytherapy. In addition, the necessary close and frequent monitoring of these children increases the radiation exposure of nursing staff and parents. In an effort to reduce these problems, the use of high dose rate (HDR) brachytherapy has been undergoing evaluation at OSU and Children's Hospital, Columbus, Ohio, in pediatric patients.

High dose rate remote brachytherapy eliminates the radiation exposure hazard, and the treatment is delivered in minutes, obviating the need for prolonged sedation and immobilization while also allowing outpatient brachytherapy. High dose rate brachytherapy was, therefore, utilized as part of a multimodality treatment approach (eliminating EBRT) in seven young children at Children's Hospital and OSU.[28,29]

Seven children (six females, one male) with IRS group III RMS received a multimodality treatment regimen including organ-preserving surgery and aggressive chemotherapy according to the IRS III/IV, and HDR brachytherapy. The age at diagnosis ranged from 1 to 31 months. Age at the time of brachytherapy ranged from 6 to 36 months.

The primary tumors were in the base of the tongue (1), buccal mucosa (1), vagina (3), chest wall (1), and clitoris (1). All patients had received 2–6 cycles of multiagent chemotherapy for cytoreduction. Five patients had debulking surgery prior to brachytherapy, leaving only microscopic residual disease; two patients had biopsies only, leaving gross but small-volume (less than 2 cm) residual tumors. Amputation or bone resection was avoided, except in one patient who required a resection of her posterior chest wall including four ribs.

The brachytherapy techniques used were similar to those used in adults. Five patients had interstitial implantation of catheters in the operating room at the time of surgery. These catheters were left in the patient until the treatments were completed. The other two patients were treated by a custom-made intravaginal cylinder that was inserted into the vagina for each treatment.

The HDR treatment was performed utilizing a single-plane interstitial implant in three patients (Fig. 1), a three-plane volume implant in one patient (Fig. 2), a single line source for the intravaginal cylinder in two patients, and a combined intravaginal cylinder with an interstitial implant in one patient. The postchemotherapy residual tumor volume (with 0–0.5-cm margins) was implanted rather than the original tumor volume. The minimum peripheral dose was 36 Gy in 12 treatments (3 Gy for each treatment given twice a day, 6 hours apart) over 8 elapsed days. The New York System of dosimetry and dose optimization was used. Using the linear quadratic (LQ) model, the extrapolated response dose (ERD) was calculated to be equivalent to 50 Gy of continuous LDR

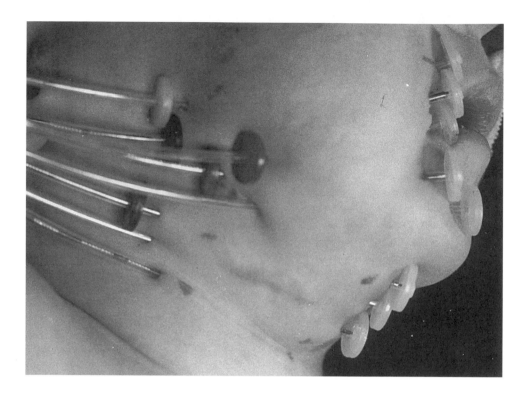

**Fig. 1.** A single-plane implant of the buccal mucosa and submandibular area, using eight catheters.

brachytherapy given over 5 days. Each treatment lasted 2 to 5 minutes and was given on an outpatient basis. Because slight movement of the patient during treatment was allowable, the brachytherapy was given using either mild sedation or temporary body restraint (e.g., papoose board or arm splint) (Fig. 3). General anesthesia was not required. The catheters were removed after all the treatments were completed. None of the patients received EBRT because a prime objective was preservation of organ and bone growth. The patient and treatment parameters are summarized in Table 1.

All seven children are alive and without evidence of tumor with a median follow-up time of 26 months (range: 12 to 32 months). One child had residual RMS on biopsy 11 months after brachytherapy. Surgical resection was performed, but only residual atypical cells were demonstrated in the final pathological specimens.

The treatments have been well tolerated with some acute skin toxicity and relatively good organ growth. The toxicities have been graded according to the Radiation Therapy Oncology Group (RTOG) Acute and Late Radiation Morbidity Scoring Criteria.[30]

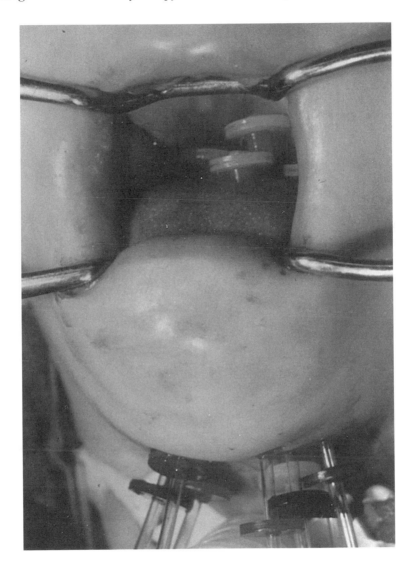

**Fig. 2.** Eight catheters implanted in the base of the tongue in a three-plane volume implant. The catheters project 0.5 cm superior to the dorsum of the tongue to avoid underdosing of the dorsum.

## Acute Reactions

Five patients experienced mucositis (one patient, grade 1; four patients, grade 2) within 2 to 4 weeks after brachytherapy. The reaction worsened in 3 patients who had received anthracycline-containing regimens, exhibiting a recall phenomenon.

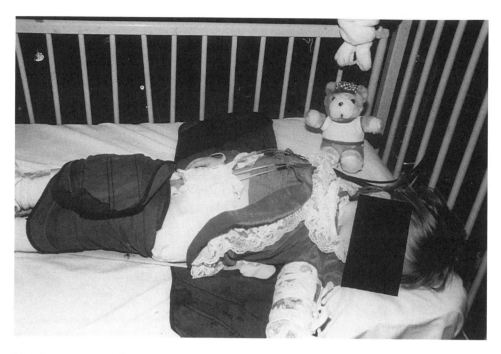

**Fig. 3.** A papoose board and arm splint is used for temporary body restraint during HDR treatment.

## Late Reactions

One patient developed Fanconi's Syndrome secondary to ifosfamide-based chemotherapy, and thus is small for her age due to renal rickets and associated metabolic acidosis. Radiation-related growth retardation has not been observed in this patient.

Two patients exhibited delayed dentition just adjacent to the implanted area. One patient had mild scoliosis/kyphosis as a result of a posterior chest wall and rib resection for the primary tumor. Two patients developed subcutaneous fibrosis (one grade 2 and one grade 3).

## Discussion

The standard treatment after surgery and chemotherapy in pediatric RMS is EBRT to the tumor with a generous (5-cm) margin for local control. This can require treatment over a 5-to-6-week period and the use of repeated deep sedation and can lead to unacceptable morbidity (especially organ- and bone-growth retardation) in infants and younger children.[1-3]

Limited volume irradiation over a short duration (a few days) by brachytherapy may be sufficient therapy for children treated with aggressive chemotherapy, as shown by the use of LDR brachytherapy.[7-27] This allows high

## Table 1
### Summary of Patient and Implant Parameters

| Pt No. | Sex | Age at Dx (Mo) | Age at IMP (Mo) | Site | Res. dis.[1] (M/G) | Histologic Subtype | No. of Cath | Implant Tech.[2] | Volume (cm) | F/U Mo |
|---|---|---|---|---|---|---|---|---|---|---|
| 1 | F | 3 | 6 | tongue | G | embryonal | 8 | 3-plane interst. volume | 2.5 × 2.5 × 3.0 | 32 |
| 2 | F | 14 | 16 | buccal mucosa | M | alveolar | 8 | single plane interst. | 4.0 × 7.0 × 1.0 | 28 |
| 3 | F | 31 | 36 | vagina | M | embryonal sarcoma botryoides | 1 | vag. cyl. | 4.0 × 1.5 × 1.5 | 27 |
| 4 | M | 1 | 6 | chest wall | M | undifferentiated sarcoma | 3 | single plane interst. | 6.0 × 2.5 × 1.0 | 26 |
| 5 | F | 27 | 33 | vagina | M | embryonal sarcoma botryoides | 1 | vag. cyl. | 5.5 × 2.1 × 2.1 | 23 |
| 6 | F | 12 | 14 | clitoris | M | embryonal | 4 | single plane interst. | 3.5 × 3.5 × 1.0 | 20 |
| 7 | F | 19 | 25 | vagina | G | embryonal sarcoma botryoides | 6 | vag. cyl. and single plane interst. | 4.0 × 3.0 × 1.0 | 12 |

[1]Residual disease at the time of implantation - microscopic (M) or gross (G).
[2]Implant technique - interstitial (interst.) or vaginal cylinder (vag. cyl.).
IMP: implant

doses of radiation to be limited accurately to the tumor bed only, sparing the surrounding normal tissues and thus minimizing the late sequelae. Manually afterloaded removable iridium-192 has been the most commonly applied isotope, but iodine-125, gold-198, cesium-137, and californium-252 have also been used with good results.[7-27]

The major disadvantage of the LDR technique is that younger children often must be sedated and immobilized during the entire period to prevent accidental removal of the implants. Radiation exposure to the medical personnel and the parents is another concern, although exposure can be reduced by placing a mobile lead shield at the bedside. The psychological effect of separating parents from their child can be significant and must be considered. The use of a low energy radionuclide like iodine-125 or LDR remote brachytherapy may reduce the hazards of radiation exposure, but prolonged sedation and immobilization are still required.[20,23,27]

The use of HDR in the OSU/Children's Hospital experience eliminated radiation exposure to the medical staff and the patients' families and allowed constant nursing care and interaction between the parents, nursing personnel, and the children. Each treatment took only a few minutes, and the treatment course was completed in 1 week without requiring prolonged sedation or immobilization. Treatment of narrow cavities did not present a problem.

The selection of a patient for HDR brachytherapy requires evaluation by a multidisciplinary team consisting of a pediatric surgeon, pediatric oncologist, and brachytherapist. The initial strategy for tumors that are unresectable by virtue of site or size is to achieve cytoreduction with active multiagent chemotherapy. The second phase of this standard approach is to use an effective local control strategy, such as surgery and radiotherapy, when the tumor has the least number of viable cells. An ideal candidate for HDR brachytherapy would be a child with a soft tissue sarcoma in whom organ preservation and function is a priority and in whom the tumor can be reduced by a surgical procedure to a microscopic residual tumor. This series demonstrates that organ-preserving surgery at selected sites in combination with HDR brachytherapy can be accomplished without fear of jeopardizing local control. In this regard, HDR brachytherapy has been used as an extension of the surgeon's scalpel without removing critical tissues. Because of technological advances, there are few sites that cannot be treated using HDR techniques.

The brachytherapist should be present at the initial resective surgery for optimal placement of the brachytherapy catheters into the tumor bed. This could be done at a subsequent surgery, but the result might be suboptimal. Patients with extensive residual tumors are not suitable candidates because marginal recurrence may result if small volumes are implanted, or treatment-related sequelae may result if large volumes are implanted. The seven patients in this study were carefully selected. The residual tumor volumes were microscopic or small. The volumes implanted were limited to the areas of suspected disease and not necessarily the entire prechemotherapy volume. A less favorable outcome might be expected if less rigid selection criteria were to be used.

The use of HDR also solved a logistical problem that may also be present at other institutions. The James Cancer Hospital, Columbus, Ohio, has brachytherapy facilities but does not have a pediatric surgical suite or a pediatric inpatient floor. Hence, surgical insertion of catheters or LDR brachytherapy cannot be performed in young children at the James Cancer Hospital. The Children's Hospital has surgical and inpatient facilities for young children but does not have radioactive licensing or brachytherapy facilities. Hence, surgical catheter insertion (if required) is performed at the Children's Hospital, and the HDR treatments are performed on an outpatient basis at the Cancer Hospital.

The use of EBRT in large volume fields can be myelosuppressive and thus limit subsequent administration of systemic multiagent chemotherapy. In this series, HDR brachytherapy did not impede the later use of maintenance therapy using alkylating agents. However, anthracycline-containing chemotherapy caused an increase in the radiation reaction in two of the children treated by HDR brachytherapy. Therefore, it is recommended that anthracycline-containing chemotherapy be eliminated from the immediate postbrachytherapy maintenance chemotherapy regimen of these patients. A similar recommendation might be applicable to other radiosensitizing agents such as actino-mycin D.

## Conclusions

The use of HDR brachytherapy has allowed the delivery of radiation to infants and younger children. Encouraging preliminary results have been observed in the initial seven patients treated at The Ohio State University. Normal organ and bone growth have been seen in this series with a short follow-up (10 to 30 months). Although the long-term sequelae of HDR brachytherapy in young children are not fully known, one may expect it to preserve organ function similar to the experience with LDR brachytherapy.[9] The use of HDR brachytherapy should be restricted to selected pediatric tumors in controlled clinical trials until long-term data are available.

## REFERENCES

1. Fromm M, Littman P, Raney RB, et al. Late effects after treatment of twenty children with soft-tissue sarcomas of the head and neck. Cancer 57:2070-2076, 1986.
2. Jaffe N, Toth BB, Hoan RE, et al. Dental and maxillofacial abnormalities in long-term survivors of childhood cancer: effects of treatment with chemotherapy and radiation to the head and neck. Pediatrics 73:816-823, 1984.
3. Pais RC, Ragab AH. Rhabdomyosarcomas in infancy. In: Maurer HM, Ruymann FB, Pochedly C, eds. Rhabdomyosarcoma and Related Tumors in Children and Adolescents. Boca Raton, FL: CRC Press; 1991, 373-384.
4. Maurer HM, Beltangady M, Gehan EA, et al. Intergroup rhabdomyosarcoma study-I: a final report. Cancer 61:209-220, 1988.
5. Maurer HM, Gehan E, Beltangady M, et al. The intergroup rhabdomyosarcoma study-II. Cancer 71:1904-1922, 1993.
6. Ragab A, Gehan E, Maurer H, et al. For the IRS Committee of CCSG, POG, & UKCCSG: intergroup rhabdomyosarcoma study (IRS) III: preliminary report of the major results. Proceedings of the American Society of Clinical Oncology; May 17-19, 1992; San Diego, CA, Pittsburgh, PA: W.B. Saunders; 1992, 1251.
7. Cherlow JM, Nisar Syed AM, Puthawala A, et al. Endocurietherapy in pediatric oncology. Am J Pediatr Hematol Oncol 2:155-159, 1990.
8. Curran WJ, Littman P, Raney RB. Interstitial radiation therapy in the treatment of childhood soft-tissue sarcomas. Int J Radiat Oncol Biol Phys 14:169-174, 1988.
9. Flamant F, Gerbaulet A, Nihoul-Fekete C, et al. Long-term sequelae of conservative treatment by surgery brachytherapy and chemotherapy for vulval and vaginal rhabdomyosarcoma in children. J Clin Oncol 8:1847-1853, 1990.
10. Flamant F, Chassagne D, Cosset JM, et al. Embryonal rhabdomyosarcoma of the vagina in the children. Eur J Cancer 15:527-532, 1979.
11. Fontanesi J, Kun L, Pao W, et al. Brachytherapy as primary or "boost" irradiation in 18 children with solid tumors. Endocurie/Hypertherm Oncol 7:195-200, 1991.
12. Fontanesi J, Rao B, Fleming I. Pediatric brachytherapy: update of SJCRH experience. Proceedings of 15th Annual Meeting of the American Endocurietherapy Society; 1992; Beaver Creek, Colo., 50.
13. Gerbaulet A. Pediatric neoplasms. In: Pierquin B, Wilson JF, Chassagne D, eds. Modern Brachytherapy. New York: Masson Publishing USA; 1987, 315-316.

14. Gerbaulet AP, Esche BA, Hail CM, et al. Conservative treatment for lower gynecological tract malignancies in children and adolescents: the Institut Gustave-Roussy experience. Int J Radiat Oncol Biol Phys 16:655-658, 1989.
15. Gerbaulet A, Panis X, Flamant F, et al. Iridium afterloading curietherapy in the treatment of pediatric malignancies. Cancer 56:1274-1279, 1985.
16. Gerbaulet A, Habrand JL, Haie C, et al. The role of brachytherapy in the conservative treatment of pediatric malignancies: experience of the Institut Gustave-Roussy. (Activity) Selectron Brachytherapy Journal 5:85-90, 1991.
17. Goffinet DR, Martinez A, Pooles D, et al. Pediatric brachytherapy. In: George FW III, ed. Modern Interstitial and Intracavitary Radiation Cancer Management. New York: Masson Publishing USA; 1981, 57-70.
18. Hilaris BS, Nori D, Anderson LL. Brachytherapy in pediatric oncology. In: Hilaris BS, Nori D, Anderson LL, eds. An Atlas of Brachytherapy. New York: Macmillan Publishing Co.; 1988, 294-302.
19. Knight PH, Doornbos JF, Rosen D, et al. The use of interstitial radiation therapy in the treatment of persistent, localized, and unresectable cancer in children. Cancer 57:951-954, 1986.
20. Marquez CM, Larson DA, Roberts LW, et al. Iodine-125 implant of a rhabdomyosarcoma of the prostate in a 20-month-old boy. Endocurie/Hypertherm Oncol 8:49-52, 1992.
21. Martinez A, Goffinet DR, Donaldson SS, et al. The use of interstitial therapy in pediatric malignancies. Front Radiat Ther Oncol 12:91-100, 1978.
22. Nag S, Rao B. Interstitial radiation implantation of pediatric solid tumors: preliminary results (abstract). Endocurie/Hypertherm Oncol 1:138, 1985.
23. Nechuskin M, Androsov N, Durnov L, et al. Initial experience in the USSR in the treatment of paediatric cancers using the microSelectron-LDR. Selectron Brachytherapy Journal (4):78-79, 1990.
24. Novaes PE. Interstitial therapy in the management of soft tissue sarcomas in childhood. Med Pediatr Oncol 13:221-224, 1985.
25. Pierquin B, Chassagne DJ, Chahbazian CM, et al. Embryonal sarcomas in children. In: Pierquin B, Chassagne DJ, Chahbazian CM, et al., eds. Brachytherapy. St. Louis, Mo.: Warren H. Green Inc.; 1978, 207-208.
26. Plowman PN, Doughty D, Harnett AN. The role of brachytherapy in the multidisciplinary therapy of localized cancers. Br J Radiol 62:218-222, 1989.
27. Zelefsky MJ, LaQuaglia MP, Harrison LB. Combination surgery and brachytherapy for pediatric soft tissue sarcomas. Proceedings of 15th Annual Meeting of the American Endocurietherapy Society; Beaver Creek, CO; 1992, 25.
28. Nag S, Ruymann F, Su CM, et al. The use of high dose rate remote brachytherapy in paediatric tumors. (Activity) Selectron Brachytherapy Journal 4:22-23, 1990.
29. Nag S, Grecula JC, Ruymann F. Aggressive chemotherapy, organ preserving surgery, and high dose rate remote brachytherapy in the treatment of rhabdomyosarcoma in infants and young children. Cancer 72:2769-2776, 1993.
30. Radiation Therapy Oncology Group. Radiation Therapy Oncology Group (RTOG) acute and late radiation morbidity scoring criteria. Philadelphia, Pa.: RTOG, 1991.

# Part III

# Special Topics

# Chapter 21

# High Dose Rate Brachytherapy Nursing

*Debra M. Brown, Janet Janes, and Cherylann Gregory*

## Introduction: An Overview of HDR Brachytherapy

Radiation therapy had its beginnings in the late 1800s with work of the Curies and Becquerel. Since then, major strides have been taken in the field of radiation therapy, including the concept and development of brachytherapy and, more specifically, high dose rate (HDR) remote afterloading brachytherapy. Remote afterloading of brachytherapy sources was first introduced about 30 years ago in Europe and Asia.[1] Henschke et al.[2] have been credited with first introducing HDR brachytherapy using remote afterloading techniques in the United States in the early 1960s.

Very little information is available on the role of nursing in the treatment of HDR brachytherapy patients. This chapter will introduce and discuss the role of the nurse in HDR remote afterloading brachytherapy, various applications of HDR remote afterloading, and the care of HDR brachytherapy patients.

## HDR Remote Afterloading Brachytherapy as a Treatment Modality

### Advantages

When compared to traditional low dose rate (LDR) brachytherapy, HDR remote afterloading brachytherapy has both advantages and disadvantages as a treatment modality for the patient and the family. Some of the advantages suggested with HDR remote afterloading include:

(1) treatments that can be given on an outpatient basis, which avoids hospitalization;

(2) shorter treatment times that are more tolerable for the patient;

(3) complete radiation protection for the staff;

(4) elimination of the need for general anesthesia or extended bed rest;

(5) greater accuracy of source and applicator position;

(6) ability to treat a large patient volume;

From: Nag, S. (ed.): *High Dose Rate Brachytherapy: A Textbook*, Futura Publishing Company, Inc., Armonk, NY, © 1994.

(7) availability for patients who may be poor surgical risks;

(8) containment of treatments within the radiation oncology department.

Treatments with HDR remote afterloading techniques can be relatively simple outpatient procedures. As such, they generally cause less fear, stress, and anxiety for the patient and family; however, this is not always true. Some patients prefer the security of being in the hospital, having full anesthesia, and having a nursing staff readily available.

### Disadvantages

Although there are many advantages to the use of HDR remote after-loading brachytherapy, there are also some disadvantages that should be considered.

(1) The patient usually receives several treatments and, therefore, must make multiple visits to the hospital.

(2) The patient can be exposed to radiation should the source get stuck in the ON position.

(3) Because of short treatment times, changes in the treatment plan are difficult to make before the end of treatment.[3]

(4) A nurse, physician, physicist, dosimetrist, and therapist are needed for each treatment, making HDR treatments more time consuming for department staff.[3]

It is also thought that HDR brachytherapy may be more toxic to normal tissue, when compared to LDR at the same total dose (A. A. Martinez, M.D., personal communication, 1993).

Generally, outpatient procedures are believed to be less expensive than in-patient procedures. However, the question of whether HDR techniques have a cost advantage over LDR techniques is highly controversial.[4] The total cost of the HDR remote afterloading procedures should be considered; the cost of equipment, source replacement, room shielding, and professional staff time should be factored into the cost of all HDR procedures.

Cost effectiveness, however, may not be the governing issue when considering this treatment technique. The significant benefits that HDR remote afterloading techniques offer to patients and staff may ultimately outweigh the comparative cost differences.

## Types of High Dose Rate Applicators and Treatments

### Intracavitary Treatment

HDR remote afterloading is being recognized as an effective treatment modality for cancers. The applicators and techniques used will vary greatly from one institution to another.

*Endometrial Applicators*

High dose rate techniques are used in the treatment of primary endometrial cancer and postoperative endometrial cancer, where the patient has already undergone a total abdominal hysterectomy. Implants can be done in combination with external beam radiation therapy (EBRT) or as the sole treatment modality in radiation therapy. The applicators used vary, and many are available commercially, for example, the vaginal applicator set, the shielded cylindrical applicator set, and the ring applicator set. Many institutions have also designed their own applicators to fit their specific needs.

*Cervical Applicators*

Several types of applicators can be used to deliver treatment to the cervix and vaginal apex or cuff with HDR remote afterloading systems. The ring applicator set and the standard applicator set are only two that are currently available. Other applicators have been made and used by their respective institutions.

*Vaginal Applicators*

There are several different applicators available to treat lesions within the vaginal canal. The vaginal applicator set is only one of the many that are available commercially.

*Endobronchial Applicators*

Endobronchial treatments are generally done with the assistance of a bronchoscope. Applicators that are placed into the bronchus are available, for example, bronchial applicator sets, as the scope is being removed. Placement of the catheter(s) should be checked before the start of each treatment, using fluoroscopy. These long, narrow catheters are secured in place for treatment and removed after each treatment is completed. The procedure is repeated for each treatment prescribed.

*Esophageal Applicators*

There are a number of esophageal applicators available to deliver the treatment dose to esophageal tumors, for example, the Rowland Oesophageal Applicator Set (Nucletron Corporation, Columbia, Maryland). Many institutions choose the technique and applicator according to their needs and comfort level. Esophageal applicators are placed in a variety of ways: by the patient swallowing a soft-tip, thin guide wire, after which the catheter is attached to the guide wire, or by passing the catheter through a fiberoptic scope to the tumor area, and, in some cases, by placing down the esophagus a nasogastric tube with the treatment catheter inside it. Regardless of the technique used, once the treatment dose is delivered, the applicator is removed. The applicator is placed each time for each prescribed treatment.

### Nasopharyngeal Applicators

Different types of applicators can be used with HDR remote afterloading systems to deliver treatment to the nasopharynx, for example, the nasopharyngeal applicator set (oral) or the nasopharyngeal applicator set (nasal). The applicator is passed through the nasal passage or oral cavity, which has been anesthetized, to the tumor area, and the treatment dose is delivered.

### Biliary Applicators

To deliver HDR brachytherapy treatments to the common bile duct or biliary system, a bile duct applicator can be used, for example, the Arnhem Bile Duct Applicator Set (Nucletron Corporation). In addition to commercially available sets, narrow bronchial catheters can be used. They are passed through an indwelling catheter that has been placed into the patient by a radiologist in the diagnostic radiology department. Different institutions have developed their own applicators and techniques.

## Interstitial Implants

For many years, interstitial implants have been a standard treatment for certain cancers in most radiation oncology centers. Most recently, the general trend in hospitals has been to do more and more outpatient procedures. Radiation oncology centers are not exempt from this trend. High dose rate remote afterloading technology allows many interstitial procedures to be done on an outpatient basis.

## Prostate Implants

In recent years, outpatient HDR remote afterloading interstitial prostate implants have been performed at a small number of institutions across the United States. This procedure involves the use of a perineal template that guides implanting needles into the prostate gland. The physician monitors the placement of the implants using ultrasound imaging. There are various templates available, for example, the MUPIT (Martinez Universal Peritoneal Interstitial Template) (Nucletron Corporation), which can be used with HDR remote afterloading techniques. The treatments can be done on an outpatient basis in combination with EBRT once a week for 3 consecutive weeks.

## Breast Implants

Traditionally, breast implants have been done as boost therapy using LDR brachytherapy techniques. Currently, some institutions have developed programs and techniques that use HDR remote afterloading as a primary and/or boost therapy to breast tumor areas. Special templates are placed on each side of the breast and are used as guides to implant needles into the breast. One- or two-plane implants are generally done, but templates have been designed to accommodate up to three-plane implants. Most templates and needles are reusable and are gas or steam sterilized. If plastic catheters are used, they are discarded.

## Superficial HDR Implants

Many institutions have used HDR remote afterloading to treat several types of superficial lesions. Applicators have been developed on the basis of need by individual institutions, and some have been manufactured commercially, for example, the surface mold applicator set. Many institutions have used various materials, for example, plastics and bolus materials, to design applicators that fit their need to deliver the best possible treatment to the patient. At William Beaumont Hospital in Royal Oak, Michigan, for example, a plastic mold of the patient's external auditory canal was constructed to treat a carcinoma of the external auditory canal. The mold was then drilled out to allow the placement of an HDR afterloading catheter.[5] The patient was given weekly treatments for 6 weeks. The mold was easily placed for each treatment, and the setup was reproducible.

## Other Types of Interstitial HDR Implants

Over the past few years, many institutions have begun using HDR remote afterloading in other tumor sites. A number of abstracts have suggested its use with and without hyperthermia in brain tumors, for carcinomas of the lower gynecologic tract, for certain head and neck cancers, and in anal canal cancers.[6] High dose rate remote afterloading schedules have been developed by a number of institutions in different parts of the world, and these exhibit a wide range of doses and numbers of applications.[3] The equipment and applicators used during each implant procedure are different at each institution. Some items are reusable, and others are disposable. Each institution has its own guidelines for cleaning, sterilizing, and processing the equipment and applicators.

# The Role of Nursing in High Dose Rate Brachytherapy

The role of the nurse in HDR brachytherapy is not well documented or defined in the literature. Nursing is central to the structuring of patient care and patient education programs. In part, the nurse's responsibility is to assure that the best quality of patient care and education is provided.

# Patient and Family Education

## Preprocedure Education

Patient education is essential for any HDR brachytherapy procedure to be effective. Preprocedure teaching by the nurse should be designed to be site specific since each radiation treatment is localized to a specific area. Effective site-specific teaching helps the patient know what to expect from beginning to end and helps to lessen any fears and anxieties the patient may be experiencing.

Before the treatment, the nurse plans to meet with the patient, family members, and/or other significant person(s). Usually, the nurse phones the patient at home and sets up an appointment. These arrangements can also be made during consultation or can be set up during the patient's course of EBRT. Since every HDR treatment plan is prescribed differently, it is essential for the nurse to know when the HDR treatments are planned: before, during, or after EBRT or as the primary treatment.

At this meeting, the complete procedure is discussed in detail, and any questions are answered. Most of the procedures are performed entirely in the radiation oncology department or in the brachytherapy suite. A few, however, are initially placed in the operating room. Specific written information should be given to the patient about the procedure. Some patients may find it helpful to see the implant equipment and treatment machine before treatment. The side effects that may occur are also discussed, as well as the management of any symptoms. Specific instructions regarding special diets, for example, NPO (nothing by mouth) after midnight, or specific bowel preps are individualized to each procedure. In some cases, special examinations or tests may be necessary (e.g., ultrasound, computed tomography scan, magnetic resonance imaging) before treatment planning can begin. Because some implants are done using spinal and local anesthesia with intravenous sedation, the patients should have advance testing done so that the necessary medical clearance is obtained for the patient to receive anesthesia or any necessary laboratory studies. The nurse intervenes in many ways to help the patients and their families cope with their knowledge deficiencies, anxieties, and fears.

## During the Procedure

The goal of patient and family teaching should be to alleviate the fear of the unknown. The patient needs to know that, while the treatment is in progress, monitoring will continue from outside the treatment room via camera and intercom systems. Treatment times will vary with each implant treatment but generally last between 5 and 10 minutes. The nurse plays a significant role in reinforcing information as the patient continues through treatment, and new information is added during the reinforcement process. Because we cannot assume that learning has occurred unless we continuously evaluate and assess the patient during treatment, the nurse always documents the teaching done and assesses the patient's level of learning.

### Postprocedure Information

Once the patient has completed the entire course of treatment, additional information, similar to discharge instructions, should be communicated to the patient. This information should be site specific and include:

(1) discussion of expected side effects;

(2) means of managing any occurring side effects, for example, medications, prescriptions, skin creams, or sitz baths;

(3) scheduling of follow-up appointments with their doctors;

(4) assurance that the patient or family member can call the nurse for any needed assistance or to answer questions.

All outpatient postprocedure HDR brachytherapy patients should be sent home with discharge instructions for proper care at home. The nurse reviews postprocedure instructions with the patient and their caregivers before leaving the radiation oncology department. A general example of a postprocedure information form is given in Fig.1.

The nurse becomes a liaison between the patient and other health care providers as the treatment course is completed. Setting up appropriate community services and/or resources can be invaluable to a patient's recovery at home.

| |
|---|
| Patient Name:                        Phone #: |
| Dr. Name:                            Phone #: |
| Procedure: |
| Medications: |
| Activity: |
| Side effects: |
| Additional Comments/Special Instructions: |
| Follow-up/treatment visit: |
| Phone number of Radiation Oncology Department   day:              night: |
| I have read, understood and received a copy of my post-procedure instructions:<br><br>_____   _____<br>Signature of patient or authorized representative   Date |

**Fig. 1.** An example of a postprocedure information form.

Patients have a real fear of becoming radioactive because of brachytherapy procedures. Discussing the safety aspects involved with HDR brachytherapy treatments may help to alleviate these fears.

A patient's progress can be followed through routine visits to the doctor and by telephone calls to the patient's home once treatment is completed. A telephone call within a week after the completion of treatment allows the nurse to reinforce follow-up and home care instructions and to assess any problems or answer questions the patient or family may have. Patients are generally scheduled for a follow-up appointment 2 to 6 weeks after treatment is completed. The patients are encouraged to resume normal activity as soon as possible and to call the nurse or doctor if any problems arise. All instructions given to the patients should be documented in the patient's chart.

## Patient Care and Implant Procedures

### Gynecologic Implants

*Endometrial Implants (Postoperative)*

The patients who receive intravaginal HDR brachytherapy may or may not have received EBRT. Once the procedure has been explained to them, they are scheduled for their HDR implants. Treatment planning that is done before the first treatment is generally done in the simulation room and may include the temporary insertion of markers into the bladder, vagina, and rectum. These markers are useful in determining the radiation dose to the surrounding organs and tissues.

On the days of the HDR brachytherapy procedure, the patient is escorted to the treatment room by the nurse and assisted into the treatment position. A nursing assessment is done before each treatment. No anesthesia or premedication is usually necessary. Once the assessment is completed and the patient is positioned appropriately, the physician places the vaginal applicator into the vaginal canal. The applicator is secured, and placement is verified using fluoroscopy. The patient is then connected to the HDR remote afterloading machine and left alone in the room for the prescribed treatment time. When the procedure is complete, the applicator is removed, and the patient may go home. The number of HDR treatments may vary, but patients are generally scheduled for one treatment weekly.

*Endometrial Implants (Primary)*

Women diagnosed with endometrial cancer may receive HDR brachytherapy as their primary treatment. The applicators vary and are generally inserted in the operating room. The treatment fractionation and the need for hospitalization will depend upon the applicator used, the dose prescribed, and the technique used.

The applicator placement is verified before treatment is started, and a nursing assessment of the patient is done. The patient is taken to the treatment room, connected to the HDR remote afterloading treatment machine, and left alone in the treatment room during the treatment, while being monitored closely from outside the room. The applicator is removed once the treatments are completed, and the patient may go home. The number of treatments varies from patient to patient and can be scheduled twice daily, once daily, or weekly.

### Cervical and Vaginal Implants

Patients who are to receive HDR brachytherapy for cervical or vaginal cancer also may or may not have received EBRT before HDR brachytherapy. Techniques and applicators, for example, the ring applicator, vary greatly from one institution to another. Depending on the applicator used, the patient may need to go to the operating room for placement of a cervical stent. The stent keeps the cervix dilated, allowing easier placement of the applicator. The nurse's responsibilities include the nursing assessment and teaching regarding the site and the treatment prescribed by the doctor.

The applicator placements are done in either the brachytherapy suite or the simulation room. After the patient is positioned and draped for the procedure, the physician places the applicator into the vaginal canal. For cervical cancers, the applicator is placed into the vaginal canal and through the cervix. The nurse assists the physician with the procedure as needed.

Placement is verified by fluoroscopy. If the placement of the applicator was performed in the simulation room, the patient is transported to the brachytherapy suite and connected to the HDR remote afterloading machine. The treatment dose is delivered as prescribed. Once the treatment is complete, the applicator is removed, and the patient is monitored for any problems, for example, changes in vital signs, cramping, and hemorrhage. When stable, the patient is assisted from the treatment room and may go home. Additional HDR brachytherapy treatments will be scheduled weekly until the prescribed dose is delivered.

## Endobronchial Implants

Patients who receive HDR endobronchial brachytherapy may or may not receive EBRT. High dose rate endobronchial brachytherapy treatments can be delivered during the course of EBRT, after EBRT, or as the primary treatment for palliation. The endobronchial treatments are performed as an out-patient procedure with the assistance of the endoscopy unit and a pulmonologist. Responsibility for patient and family teaching is shared by the brachytherapy and endoscopy nurses. Information about the actual bronchoscopy procedure is given to the patient by the endoscopy nurse or pulmonologist, and the brachytherapy nurse addresses the delivery of the radiation treatments.

For each treatment, the patient registers with the hospital and reports to the endoscopy department. The patient is assessed by the nurse, prepared for intravenous access, and premedicated as ordered by the pulmonologist. The patient is brought to the radiation oncology department by the endoscopy nurse. The pulmonologist and radiation oncologist collaborate in the performance of the procedure. The patient's throat is anesthetized with viscous lidocaine (Xylocaine™), and the pulmonologist performs the bronchoscopy, introducing the flexible scope into the patient's bronchus. The area to be treated is visualized, and photographs of the treatment area can be obtained. The radiation oncologist then places the bronchial catheter/applicator to deliver the treatment. The treatment catheter is secured, and its placement is verified under fluoroscopy. The radiation oncology nurse assists the endoscopy nurse in monitoring the patient's progress and tolerance of the procedure throughout the procedure, keeping track of vital signs, oxygen saturation, ECG display, and the need for suction. Because the flexible scope is placed down the patient's throat, oral communication is not possible; therefore, the nurse must establish effective hand signals so that the patient can communicate during the procedure.

When the procedure is completed, the patient returns to the endoscopy unit for observation, and the endoscopy nurse delivers the usual postbronchoscopy care. The patient is usually discharged within a couple of hours after the procedure. The patient is followed closely by the radiation oncology nurse and physician after treatments are completed. Routine follow-up with the pulmonologist is also recommended.

## Esophageal Implants

The treatment of esophageal cancer using HDR remote afterloading techniques will vary in each institution. The applicators may vary as much as the techniques. Regardless of the applicator used, the patient will have a treatment catheter or applicator placed into the esophagus, either through the nasal passage or the mouth. The procedure is done in the radiation oncology department, the brachytherapy suite, or the simulation room. The nurse assesses the patient before the start of each treatment or procedure and assists during the procedure as necessary.

The procedure can also be performed with the assistance of the endoscopy department, which uses a flexible gastroscope to place the applicator. The patient is scoped in the endoscopy department by the gastroenterologist, and the applicator is placed in position. The patient is then brought to the radiation oncology department for treatment. An endoscopy nurse accompanies the patient and closely monitors the patient during the procedure.

In either case, the physician will need to anesthetize the throat and/or the nasal passage with an numbing spray or solution, for example, viscous lidocaine (Xylocaine™). A guide wire and sterile esophageal applicator or catheter are used. After the applicator has been placed, the position of the applicator is usually confirmed by fluoroscopy, and the treatment can be given.

Postprocedure care will differ depending on the nature of the procedure (i.e., with or without gastroscope) and the administration of any premedication.

The patients are treated as outpatients, regardless of the recovery time. If the procedure was performed using the gastroscope and guide wire for placement of the esophageal applicator, the patient's recovery may be longer. During the period before discharge, the nurse monitors the patient frequently. Usually, weekly treatments are scheduled until the prescribed total dose is given.

### Nasopharyngeal Implants

Patients who receive HDR brachytherapy treatments to the nasopharynx generally receive a course of EBRT. On the day of the HDR treatment, the patient comes directly to the radiation oncology department. The nurse reviews the procedure with the patient and assesses the patient for any problems or concerns. The patient is accompanied by the nurse to the brachytherapy suite or treatment room for placement of the applicator and treatment. The patient is requested to remove any dentures or partial dental work and then is treated either in a supine position or sitting in a chair. The nurse assists the physician and the patient during the procedure. The patient's throat and oral cavity are anesthetized with a numbing spray, for example, Cetacaine™ and lidocaine (Xylocaine™) jelly, and the nasopharyngeal applicator is passed into the nasopharyngeal area. On some applicators, a balloon is inflated with sterile water to help keep the applicator in place during the treatment.

When the treatment is completed, a postprocedure assessment is performed, and the nurse gives the patient specific postprocedure instructions, for example, refrain from taking anything by mouth for 2 to 3 hours or until the numbness has worn off. The patient can then go home. Treatments are generally scheduled weekly, depending on the course of treatment established.

### Biliary Implants

Patients with carcinoma of the common bile duct are treated with HDR brachytherapy in combination with EBRT. Before the HDR brachytherapy procedure, the patient undergoes placement of a number 12 catheter into the common bile duct. This is done under fluoroscopy by the diagnostic radiology department. A treatment applicator is placed into the catheter to deliver treatment to the obstructed area.

The patient is escorted to the brachytherapy suite, assisted to the treatment table, and placed in the supine position. The nurse assists the physician during the procedure by preparing the patient and equipment. The dressings over the catheters are removed, and the catheters are cleaned and disinfected, including the cap, with a sterile povidone-iodine (Betadine™) solution. The cap is removed, and the biliary treatment applicator inserted into the indwelling catheter. The exact treatment depth and plan have been calculated before treatment. When the treatment is complete, the applicator is removed, the biliary catheter is cleansed again with povidone-iodine (Betadine™), the cap is replaced, and a dressing is applied.

Since the catheters are kept in place and irrigation of the catheter and dressing changes will be done at home, the nurse needs to teach these procedures to the patient or family member. The patient may also be placed on antibiotic therapy for 5 days after insertion of the treatment catheter. The nurse closely monitors the patient after the procedure, until the patient is ready to go home. The number of fractions or treatments will vary, depending on the dose prescribed by the physician and the institution's protocols or guidelines.

## Prostate Implants

Preassessment is done by a certified registered nurse anesthetist (CRNA) and an anesthesiologist on the day of the implant procedure. An intravenous solution is started, and the patient is given spinal anesthesia. The patient is connected to a monitoring system through which vital signs, oxygen saturation, and cardiac status are continuously monitored. An indwelling catheter is placed into the bladder, and the bladder is distended with a sterile fluid and clamped. Antiembolism stockings are also used to promote circulation in the lower extremities. The patient is then placed in the lithotomy position with the legs in stirrups. Next, the scrotum is taped up toward the abdomen, fully exposing the perineum; the area is prepped with a povidone-iodine (Betadine™) solution, and the patient is draped. The template is affixed to the table with the rectal ultrasound probe in place. The prostate gland is visualized, and the needles are placed. The needle placement is verified by the ultrasound probe scanning the prostate; a c-arm x-ray film is taken, and a cystoscopic examination is done by a urologist.

Once the needle placement is completed, the patient is connected to the HDR remote afterloading machine, and the treatment is delivered as prescribed. The patient is monitored continuously from outside the treatment room via camera and intercom systems. The implant is removed quickly, all needles being removed at once. The patient is taken out of the lithotomy position, moved onto a stretcher, and taken to the postanesthesia care unit (PACU). The patient is discharged to a short stay unit or observation area from PACU. Once the hospital's discharge criteria have been met, the patient is encouraged to drink fluids, put on oral antibiotic therapy, and sent home. At home, the patient may experience fatigue, soreness in the perineal area that evening and the next day, and slightly pink-tinged urine. Some current protocols suggest that three outpatient HDR prostate treatments are needed, once a week or in combination with EBRT.[7]

## Breast Implants

Breast implants are done as either primary or boost therapy. In either case, the patient is taken to the operating room or to the brachytherapy suite where the implant is done. Once the patient is seen by the CRNA and anesthesiologist, vital signs are assessed, and anesthesia is given. The breast templates are held in place by the doctor, and the needles or plastic catheters are placed interstitially. Radiographs are taken to verify the placement. The films are done in the brachytherapy suite with a c-arm x-ray machine, or the patient is taken to the simulator. The patient is then connected to the HDR remote afterloading machine, and the treatment dose is delivered as prescribed. The patient is monitored via intercom and camera systems during each treatment.

Because the actual procedure and, accordingly, the dose fractionation may vary from one institution to another, patients may either be discharged the same day or may require a hospital stay. The implant is removed after the last fraction is given. The patient should be premedicated before removal of the implant. A sterile dressing is applied over the implanted site, and the patient is discharged home, with a companion. The patient should keep the dressing on for 24 hours and then may shower, using a mild soap if needed. The patient is to observe the area for any signs of infection.

## Research

Historically, the nurse's involvement in clinical research was task oriented and limited to providing nursing care to patients participating in clinical trials.[8] Nurses need to become more aware and involved in current research protocols. In many different institutions and universities, research in HDR remote afterloading brachytherapy is currently underway. These clinical investigations are exploring new and better ways to treat cancer patients.

Currently, there are many research protocol groups established. The Community Clinical Oncology Program (CCOP) and the Southwest Oncology Group (SWOG) provide opportunities for physicians to participate in cancer treatment research. More nurses need to be involved in these types of research groups. Being more aware and having a greater understanding of cancer research, the nurse gains the knowledge needed to develop new nursing research protocols.

Patient-oriented protocols are needed to assess the effects of toxicities and to monitor emotional status, patient tolerance, and performance status related to the HDR remote afterloading brachytherapy procedures. Nurses are engaged in patient care, patient education, ongoing monitoring, and interventions. Their knowledge and expertise are needed in using research data to effectively enhance patient care in the future.

## Staff Education

The increased nursing responsibilities that have developed with the increasing use of HDR remote afterloading have necessitated additional nursing education. It is necessary to have nursing in-service training within the radiation oncology department at least twice a year for radiation oncology staff nurses. Also, a teaching outline and program should be developed to be used when newly hired nurses join the radiation oncology department. In this way, nurses can have current knowledge of new procedures and developments relating to HDR brachytherapy.

Not only is nursing education within the radiation oncology department important, but this education should extend to the rest of the hospital nursing staff. Once a year all nursing personnel within the hospital should receive in-service training regarding HDR brachytherapy. This training will help the nurse to deliver the optimum nursing care. The nursing education in HDR brachytherapy can be accomplished through the use of lectures, written material, diagrams, and visits to the radiation oncology department, especially the brachytherapy suite. Maintaining continued contact between the individual nursing units and the radiation oncology department and being available to answer staff questions ensures smoother patient care and provides reassurance for the nursing staff.[9] Also, being a part of the nursing unit's general orientation program for new employees would be beneficial for the new staff.

Continuing education is essential for those nurses already working in the radiation oncology specialty. Memberships in nursing societies such as the Oncology Nursing Society, which includes subscriptions to their newsletter and the Oncology Nursing Forum journal, can contribute to the nurse's continuing education. Through the publications of such organizations, the nurse can keep up to date on the latest developments in oncology. Through seminars and various lecture series that are offered at different times of the year all over the country, the oncology nurse can keep abreast of current trends. In the field of brachytherapy, especially HDR brachytherapy, one cannot overemphasize the need for continuing education.

## Future Directions of Nursing in Brachytherapy

Brachytherapy has evolved rapidly over the last decade. With newer technologies such as HDR remote afterloading, the nurse's involvement with research, patient education, and patient care has grown and will continue to change and expand tremendously. We have already seen the shift to many more outpatient procedures, a shift that has resulted in a change in the focus of patient teaching and care. General care guidelines are no longer applicable in an outpatient setting. New guidelines and standards of care need to be determined.

The need for qualified expert nurses in radiation oncology is evident now more than ever. The clinical nurse specialist (CNS) has become more prominent in many nursing units. Unfortunately, it can be quite costly to employ a staff of master prepared nurses. The certification of radiation oncology nurses, like the certification needed to administer chemotherapy, would assure the nursing profession of well-qualified nurses within the oncology field and would provide affordable experience and expertise within radiation oncology centers. These nurses would be recognized worldwide as experts in their specialty.

The new advances and technologies in brachytherapy have made it necessary for nurses to become more specialized. The knowledge and experience of a brachytherapy nurse clinician is an integral part of any brachytherapy program and is needed to effectively enhance patient care in the future of HDR remote afterloading programs and procedures. Continuing education programs, within an institution and/or at local or national conferences, should be required of all nurses caring for brachytherapy patients.

*Acknowledgment*

The authors wish to thank Ms. Jan Rupert, Nurse Manager, Division of Radiation Oncology, The Ohio State University, for her review and valuable comments.

---

# REFERENCES

1. Fu KK, Phillips TL. High-dose-rate versus low-dose-rate intracavitary brachytherapy for carcinoma of the cervix. Int J Radiat Oncol Biol Phys 19(3):791-796, 1990.
2. Henschke UK, Hilaris B, Mahan DG. Remote afterloading with intracavitary applicators. Radiology 83:344-345, 1964.
3. Stitt JA. High-dose-rate intracavitary brachytherapy gynecologic malignancies. Oncology 6(1):59-70, 1992.
4. Orton CG. Remote afterloading for cervix cancer: the physicist's point of view. Activity/Selectron Brachytherapy Journal, Gynaecological High Dose Rate Brachytherapy 5(suppl. 2):53-55, 1991.
5. Martinez AA, Edmundson GE, Borrego JC, et al. High dose rate treatment of ear canal carcinoma: a case report. Activity/Selectron Brachytherapy Journal 5(1):2-6, 1991.
6. Mould RF. International brachytherapy: programme and abstracts. Presented at the Seventh International Brachytherapy Working Conference. Veenendaal, The Netherlands; 1992; Nucletron International B.V.;74-80; 109-111; 356-381; 421-426; 485-487.
7. Martinez AA, Gonzalez J, et al. A phase II non-randomized study of combined external beam radiation and [192]Ir high dose rate brachytherapy for locally advanced adenocarcinoma of the prostate. William Beaumont Hospital Protocol: HIC Project No. 92-07. Departments of Radiation Oncology, Urology, and Anesthesia, 1991.
8. Hubbard SM. Principles of clinical research. In: Johnson B, Gross J, eds. Handbook of Oncology Nursing. New York, NY: John Wiley & Sons; 1985; 67-69.
9. Dow KH. Principles of brachytherapy. In: Dow KH, Hilderley LJ, eds. Nursing Care in Radiation Oncology. Philadelphia, PA: WB Saunders; 1992, 24.

## Chapter 22

# Intraoperative High Dose Rate Remote Brachytherapy

*Subir Nag, Peter Lukas, David S. Thomas, and Louis Harrison*

## Introduction

The term intraoperative radiation therapy (IORT) refers to the delivery of a single, large dose of radiation to a surgically exposed tumor or tumor bed while some or all of the dose-limiting, radiosensitive normal tissues are displaced or shielded. IORT has generally been delivered by electron beam in the 6 to 18 MeV range from a linear accelerator. This treatment may be performed either in a shielded operating room in centers using a dedicated linear accelerator or in a radiation therapy suite to which the anesthetized patient is moved for treatment.

Intraoperative radiation therapy can also be delivered by brachytherapy using afterloading catheters or permanent radioactive seeds. In most centers, the catheters are inserted in the operating room, and the radiation is delivered subsequently. Hence, it is not strictly intraoperative brachytherapy, but rather perioperative brachytherapy. Intraoperative brachytherapy in the strict sense of the word, that is, with the entire treatment delivered under anesthesia, is performed in very few centers.[1-3]

The technique, as used at The Ohio State University (OSU), Columbus, the Institut und Poliklinik für Strahlentherapie und Radiologische Onkologieder Technischen Universität München, Munich, Germany, Georgetown University, Washington, D.C., and Memorial Sloan-Kettering Cancer Center, New York, and the preliminary results at these centers will be described in this chapter.

## Methods

### OSU Technique—Subir Nag

*Operating Room*

Intraoperative high dose rate (IOHDR) brachytherapy is performed at this institution in a concrete shielded room in the operating suite of the hospital.

From: Nag, S. (ed.): *High Dose Rate Brachytherapy: A Textbook*, Futura Publishing Company, Inc., Armonk, NY, © 1994.

The control panel for IOHDR brachytherapy is located in an adjacent room, which also has scrub facilities and is considered a substerile area. The room has five video cameras to allow monitoring of the patient by the anesthesiologist and brachytherapist and to provide a permanent record of the procedure on videotape. A clone monitor duplicates the readout of the actual anesthesia monitor, thus allowing constant monitoring of the patient during the entire treatment time when all personnel are required to leave the operating room. Since a HDR brachytherapy machine is available in the radiation oncology department, a dedicated one is not required for the operating room; therefore, only a terminal was installed there. The HDR machine is small and mobile and can be easily transported between the radiation therapy department (where it is normally used) to the operating room and connected to the appropriate HDR terminal. A mobile cart has been constructed for transportation of the control panels, cables, and so forth. The radioactive license was modified to allow transportation of the HDR machine between the department and the operating suite.

*Applicators*

Since the patient is under anesthesia, the entire treatment must be performed accurately, but rapidly. This has been accomplished by the development of IOHDR brachytherapy applicators. Initially, these were made of 1-cm thick, gelatinous Super-flab (Nuclear Associates, Carle Place, New York), with parallel catheters embedded 1 cm apart. Although these applicators were flexible and could be contoured to the body surface, they could not be easily sterilized. Therefore, they could not be used unless they were placed in a presterilized plastic sleeve. To overcome this problem, a number of surface applicators of a material made of delron (a rigid, sterilizable plastic) with parallel catheters embedded 1 cm apart were made in different sizes to encompass different treatment volumes. However, their rigidity limits their use to flat areas of the body.

Applicators made of Silastic block (Dow Corning Operation Medical Products, Midland, Michigan) are slightly flexible. These applicators were made in various sizes with similarly embedded catheters; however, the embedded catheters made the applicators rather long and cumbersome for sterilization. Hence, we now have the Silastic block with predrilled parallel holes 1 cm apart into which presterilized flexiguide catheters are inserted in the operating room. The Silastic block can be cut in the operating room if fine adjustment is required. Although these applicators are not rigid, they have only limited flexibility.

Foam-based applicators were developed for use in areas where the Silastic applicators could not be used. The 1-cm-thick foam is more flexible and can be contoured to the tumor bed by packing the foam applicators with gauze to establish contact with a curved surface. The foam material is also easily cut and tailored to the tumor surface in the operating room. The advantage of the foam applicator, flexibility, can also be a relative disadvantage. If the applicator is compressed, the catheter may not maintain its 1-cm separation. This risk can be minimized by passing the catheter through a rigid template to help maintain the 1-cm spacing.

Localization radiographs are obtained using dummy sources. In conventional HDR brachytherapy, the dosimetry is performed after obtaining orthogonal radiographs, digitizing the data, and then performing the treatment planning. Since the patient is under anesthesia, the time required for this process must be minimized. To accomplish this, we have precalculated dosimetry tables for various-size applicators, thus saving the time required for dose calculation and allowing the treatment to be performed without delay. The localization radiographs are used for verification.

*IOHDR Brachytherapy Treatments*

A close collaboration is required between surgeons, radiation oncologists, and radiation physicists and nursing, anesthesia, and the hospital scheduling personnel. The patient must be evaluated by the brachytherapist and informed consent obtained. It is preferable that the patient be scheduled in the shielded operating suite. Although a patient can be moved from an adjacent operating room to the shielded room for treatment, this should preferably be avoided.

The brachytherapist should be called to the operating room just before the tumor resection to see the relationship of the tumor to the surrounding tissues. The brachytherapist and the surgeons jointly decide on the volume of tissue that can and should be removed and which tissues should be preserved. In general, we prefer the maximum debulking that is feasible without substantial destruction of functional tissue.

The tumor bed is measured, and an appropriate applicator (Silastic, rigid delron, or foam-based) is placed on the tumor bed. Localization radiographs with dummy sources are obtained for verification. After the applicator has been secured on the tumor bed (with stay sutures or by packing with gauze, if necessary), care is taken to reduce the dose to surrounding normal radiosensitive structures by displacement using gauze or retractors or by shielding with sterilized lead foils.

In the meantime, the microSelectron HDR machine is transported by the physicist and brachytherapy technologist and cleaned with an antiseptic before entering the operating room. The operating room personnel leave the room briefly to allow quality assurance checks mandated by the Nuclear Regulatory Commission to be performed on the HDR machine and the door interlock system. Then the preplanned treatment program is retrieved from the computer and transferred on a disk to the treatment-control panel. The transfer cables from the IOHDR brachytherapy applicator are then connected to the microSelectron HDR machine. All personnel again leave the room, and the treatment is performed within a few minutes with the anesthetized patient being closely monitored.

## Munich Technique—Peter Lukas

In Munich, we began intraoperative radiotherapy in patients with recurrent tumors of the rectum in 1986, using polyglactin 910 (Vicryl™) mats for flexible catheter implants, a method described by Meerwaldt et al. in 1989.[4] Experience showed a high complication rate (fistulae or radiation necrosis) due to hot spots near the surface of these flexible catheters. In order to achieve a homogeneous dose distribution, we developed a moulage technique[2,5-7] using commercially available, 1.0–1.5-cm thick, gelatinous Super-flab ranging in area from 5 × to 16 × 16 cm with embedded, flexible, parallel catheters 1 cm apart. This system is extremely flexible and contours perfectly to any underlying flat or curved surface. The dose distribution on the surface is homogeneous (Fig.1). The decrease of dose with depth depends on the thickness of the moulage. To optimize dose distribution at the edges of the moulage, we developed several computer programs (P. Kneschaurek, personal communication, 1993) to be used on a personal computer system in the operation theater. Doses in the range of 12 to 15 Gy on the surface are delivered intraoperatively.

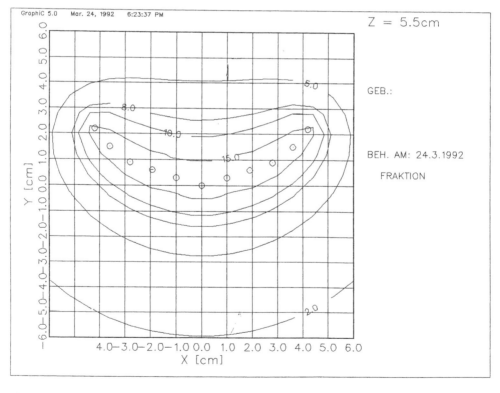

**Fig. 1.** Dose distribution of a flab of 1-cm thickness. The dose distribution is homogeneous on the surface of the flab, delivering 15 Gy on the convex surface of the flab, 10 Gy at 7-mm depth and 8 Gy at 12-mm depth.

As a radiation source we use iridium-192 in a GammaMed IIi, 12-channel afterloading system. Two different operating rooms in our hospital were specially equipped for the application of HDR intraoperative therapy. One of these is situated in the operating suite of the department of surgery, the other in the operating suite of the department of gynecology. Those operating rooms are shielded for radiation as prescribed by Bavarian laws.

One of the problems that had to be solved was sterilization of our moulages (so-called flabs). The following procedure was tested and found to be sufficient.

(1) The flabs were brushed in warm water immediately after surgery and IORT.

(2) The flabs were carefully air dried for several hours and placed in disinfectant (70% alcohol) for 2 to 4 hours.

(3) The flabs were then carefully air dried again for several hours.

(4) The flabs were packed into doubled sterilization packs and gas sterilized using 15% ethylene oxide and 85% carbonic acid at 1.7 bar and 45°C for 3 hours.

(5) After this procedure, the flabs were aerated for more than 15 hours (24 hours is preferable).

We found steps (2) and (3) to be essential; that is, the flabs must be perfectly dry before packing. Tests showed that flabs treated in the manner described above turned out to be absolutely sterile. To further assure sterility, the flabs can be packed into sterile plastic sleeves (bags) during the procedure.

## Patients

From August 5, 1988, until January 11, 1993, we treated 112 patients intraoperatively with our flab method. Indications were colorectal cancer (61), soft tissue sarcoma (20), recurrence of gynecologic tumors (11), tumors of the liver or the biliary system (10), bronchial tumors (3), metastasis (3), and other tumors (4).

Tumor biology and staging required establishing different treatment protocols for four main groups of patients.

*(1) Rectal Cancer:* There are two protocols for patients with rectal cancer. (a) If tumors are staged T3, patients undergo surgery and receive IORT of 15 Gy either prophylactically to the presacral region or to those parts of the tumor bed where resection borders are suspected to be marginal. After surgery, IOHDR brachytherapy, and a 3-to-4-week recovery interval, a course of external beam radiotherapy (EBRT) combined with radiosensitizing 5 Fluorouracil (5-FU) chemotherapy is administered. Radiotherapy is delivered in single doses of 1.8 Gy per day up to a 50.4 Gy total dose. Chemotherapy (5-FU) is given at 375 mg/m$^2$ per day on days 1–3 and 22–24 through a central venous catheter. The aims of the treatment protocol for T3 rectal carcinoma are avoidance of

local recurrence and prolongation of survival times. (b) The objective for tumors staged T4 is to make the tumor resectable. Therefore, these patients receive a combined modality treatment preoperatively: hyperfractionated radiotherapy with single doses of 1.1 Gy twice daily (at a 6-hour interval) to a total dose of 39.6 Gy and 5-FU of 400 mg/m$^2$ every 24 h continuously by a Port-A-Cath system (Pharmacia Deltec, Inc., St. Paul, Minnesota) on every treatment day. After a 3-week interval, which includes restaging examinations, the patients undergo surgery. IOHDR brachytherapy of 15 Gy is applied to the critical area of suspected tumor infiltration.

*(2) Soft Tissue Sarcoma* : Patients with soft tissue sarcoma undergo radical surgery (compartment resection) and receive IOHDR brachytherapy of 15 Gy. After a 3-week interval, hyperfractionated, accelerated radiotherapy in 1.3 to 1.6 Gy single fractions is given twice daily to a total dose of 51 to 54 Gy. There is an interval of at least 6 hours between the two daily fractions.

*(3) Recurrent Gynecologic Tumors* : These were mainly patients with tumors of the uterine cervix with recurrence at the pelvic wall or in the para-aortal or paracaval region. After radical resection that leaves the tumor less than 3 mm thick, the tumor bed is electrocoagulated and then treated with IOHDR brachytherapy of 15 Gy. Then, after a wound-healing period of 2 to 3 weeks, percutaneous radiotherapy with single doses of 1.8 Gy to a total dose of 50.4 Gy is added to the pretreated region marked by surgical clips.

*(4) Upper Abdominal Tumors* : This group includes tumors of the pancreas, bile duct, or biliary system, and primary hepatocellular carcinoma. Seven patients with orthotopic liver transplantation (OLT) and 3 patients with Whipple's operation were treated intraoperatively with single doses of 12 to 15 Gy, followed by percutaneous radiotherapy combined with radiosensitizing 5-FU 3 to 6 weeks later. As described by Moertel et al.,[8] this combined modality treatment was applied in two courses with 1.1 Gy twice a day to a total dose of 19.8 Gy in each course with a treatment break of 2 weeks between the courses. Alternatively, daily normal fractionated radiation therapy with single doses of 1.8 Gy to a total dose of 39.6 Gy may be given. 5-Fluorouracil was given continuously via a Port-A-Cath system, 300 mg/m$^2$ per day on days 1 to 5 of each course. The target volume is the region of the residual lymphatic drainage (N1-region). Irradiation during OLT is done after resection of the host liver and before replacement with the donor liver.

## The Georgetown Technique—David S. Thomas

At Georgetown University Hospital two shielded rooms were built for IORT. The first was a standard operating room converted in 1985 specifically for intraoperative HDR brachytherapy by lining the walls with lead shingles.[1] The second was an operative suite built in the radiation oncology department to house a linear accelerator with intraoperative electron beam capability. Each room was equipped with two cameras and audio and anesthetic monitors for remote observation in the adjacent substerile room or corridor. The transportable HDR device could thus be employed in either room. The HDR operational console and a personal computer with a treatment-planning program were also transportable between the treatment locations.

Therapeutic intent in most cases has been radical with the predominant treatment site in the liver as detailed in Chapter 14. Nonhepatic tumors, however, have also been treated with success. Selection criteria include unresectable or residual tumors, single or limited sites of abdominal or pelvic involvement, and significant likelihood of prolonged survival should local-regional control be achieved (i.e., absence of metastatic disease).

Whenever feasible, surgical resection precedes HDR irradiation. Areas of involved margin, incomplete excision, or unresectable disease undergo free-hand implantation with beveled, closed-end, hollow 1.7-mm diameter needle applications. Either planar or volumetric implants are employed, with the usual spacing between needles of 1.0 to 1.5 cm. Care is taken to encompass the tumor periphery and to maintain the parallel orientation of the needles with gauze packing for stability. Additional gauze packing displaces uninvolved critical structures such as the bowel from the treatment volume. The needles are then attached to translucent cables that are connected to the afterloader. Sterility of the needles and cables is maintained up to the insertion of the cable hub to the afterloader. Then, with all personnel absent from the treatment room and with the patient monitored remotely, a single fraction of HDR irradiation is delivered. While preplanning is done, the operative findings generally differ from computed tomography (CT) and magnetic resonance imaging scans, and thus intraoperative treatment planning is necessary. Developed at Georgetown, this software runs on a transportable personal computer. The usual spacing between dwell positions is 0.8 to 1.0 cm. Needles are then withdrawn, and pressure or cautery are sufficient to control bleeding.

Stage III ovarian cancer patients with diaphragmatic implants have been treated with a specially designed applicator.[9] This lucite diaphragmatic applicator was constructed with flexible joints and thus permits insertion of straight needles or curved needles up to an arc of 90°. When the needles are inserted, the applicator assumes a rigid configuration (Fig.2). Because this configuration is predetermined by the shape of the needle, accurate dosimetry is performed before operation.

The dose range has been 10 to 30 Gy. The primary factors involved in determining the dose are the normal tissue tolerance of the treated and adjacent structures and the combined use of external beam irradiation. The higher dose is employed in treating hepatic lesions when external beam irradiation is not employed. Doses between 10 to 20 Gy have been employed for extrahepatic sites, particularly if external beam irradiation was also used. While extrapolation from intraoperative electron beam data may be possible, no definitive rec-

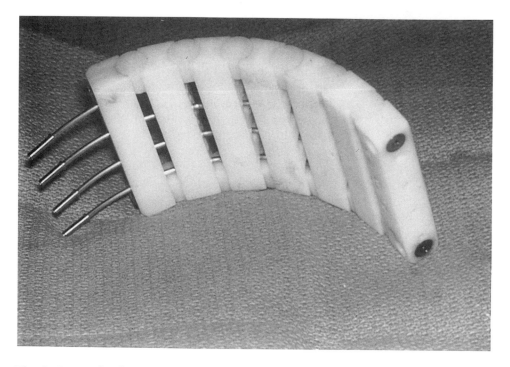

**Fig. 2.** Lucite diaphragmatic applicator with flexible joints for the treatment of curved surfaces.

ommendation can be made on the optimal safe and effective dose for the various abdominal and pelvic sites. Further investigation is needed to determine safety and efficacy.

## Memorial Sloan-Kettering Technique—Louis Harrison

Intraoperative HDR brachytherapy is performed in a specially shielded operating room in the department of radiation oncology in the brachytherapy suite. This room is concrete shielded for the delivery of radiation therapy. The room is equipped with a HDR remote afterloader radiation machine (GammaMed).

After the surgeon completes the procedure pertinent to the specific case, the radiation oncologist performs the intraoperative brachytherapy procedure. Once the decision is made to proceed with treatment, special retractors are used to move all or as much as possible of the normal tissue out of the way, and the tumor bed is exposed. The Harrison-Anderson-Mick (HAM) applicator, (Mick Radio-Nuclear Instruments, Inc., Bronx, New York) a flexible and transparent applicator made of 1-cm thick Super-flab with source-guide channels 5 mm from the surface, is sutured onto the tumor bed. The HAM applicator comes in a variety of sizes to suit any anatomical situation; it is sterilized and disposable. The catheters protruding from the applicator are attached to specially designed tubing that attaches to the HDR remote afterloader. Then, intraoperative, fluoroscopic radiographs are taken of the tumor bed with the applicator in place and dummy sources within the lumen of the catheters. The information provided by these x-rays helps the oncologist to determine the preferred dose distribution. A medical physicist is present throughout the procedure to assist the physician in planning the dose distribution and the appropriate arrangement of radioactive sources required to achieve that dose distribution. In a relatively short time, usually between 5–40 minutes, the entire dose of intraoperative irradiation will be delivered.

Depending upon the anatomical area involved, the complexity of the applicator-implantation procedure, the process of determining the dosimetry, and the time required to move the normal tissue structures from the radiation field, the radiation oncologist's intraoperative time could range from 1–3 hours.

# Results

## OSU Experience

The above technique has been used to treat tumor beds in 32 patients in the first year (March 1992–March 1993). The experience with 13 patients in the first 4 months after installation was recently analyzed.[10] All patients had gross disease removed and were treated for a microscopic residual tumor at sites inaccessible to the IORT machine. The sites of treatment included the superior orbit (1), pelvis (4), retroperitoneum (1), base of skull (4), liver hilum (1), and supraclavicular fossa (2). Six patients had previously received 45–55 Gy fractionated EBRT and were treated for recurrence; seven patients had not received prior EBRT.

The minimum peripheral dose used at 0.5 cm depth within tissue was 10 Gy in 7 patients. The plan was to use 45 Gy supplementary EBRT. However, three patients did not receive the intended EBRT. One patient received 30 Gy EBRT since he was in the pediatric age group and was receiving aggressive chemotherapy. The five patients who were not to receive the EBRT boost received 15 Gy IOHDR brachytherapy, and one patient with gross residual tumor received 20Gy.

A foam-based applicator was used in five patients, foam/template in one, a delron applicator in three, and a Silastic applicator in one patient. One patient did not have an applicator and was treated with interstitially placed catheters. Treatment areas have ranged from $3 \times 2$ cm to $6 \times 11$ cm. Treatment times have ranged from 4–24 minutes (median: 9 minutes) and source activity from 4.5 Ci to 9.7 Ci (there was a change of source during this period).

Dose reduction to normal tissues has been achieved by physical displacement of 2–10 cm by tissue retraction or packing with gauze in three patients. A 2-cm displacement of tissue typically results in 80% dose reduction to normal tissues (bowel, bladder, skin flap). Tissue displacement of 3 or 4 cm typically results in an 87% or 93% dose reduction, respectively.

In nine patients where tissues could not be physically displaced, 1–5 mm sterilized lead foil was inserted to reduce the normal tissue dose by about 20–80%. Physical displacement is, therefore, generally used whenever possible to provide a greater dose reduction.

The treatments were well tolerated acutely with no hemorrhage or mortality. Two patients died with distant disease during the 1–6 month follow-up period. Morbidity included ptosis (1), postop ileus (1), diarrhea (1), bowel perforation (1), leg pain and edema (1).

## Munich Experience

### Rectal Carcinoma

Out of the group of 61 patients with colorectal carcinomas, 30 patients with more than 6 months follow-up were evaluated. The median observation time was 18.8 months. Sixteen patients had primary rectal carcinoma, ten had clinically staged T4, and six had clinically staged T3. Of 14 patients with recurrent rectal carcinoma, 7 were clinically staged T4 as invading the surrounding organs, and 7 were not further classified.

*Downstaging* : The histological findings of the 10 patients with primary T4 rectal carcinoma were: pT4:O, pT3:9, and pTx:1. Eight patients had macroscopically and microscopically tumor-free margins ($R_o$) (no residual disease). Of the 14 patients with recurrent tumors, 6 had tumor-free margins.

*Recurrences* : Recurrence was observed in 1 of the 16 primary rectal tumors (6.25%) and in 3 of the 14 recurrent tumors (21.4%).

*Survival* : Survival rates of patients with primary rectal carcinoma (n=16) and patients with recurrent tumors computed according to Kaplan-Meier are given in Figs. 3 and 4, respectively.

*Complications* : The postoperative complication rate, including minor and major complications, for these radiotherapy patients was 47%, similar to the complication rate of 48% for patients treated with surgery (without the addition of intraoperative radiotherapy).

### Soft Tissue Sarcoma

Out of the group of 20 patients with primary or recurrent soft tissue sarcoma, 14 patients were evaluated, with a median follow-up of 14.5 months. At follow-up, 12 patients were free of tumor and alive. Two patients suffered from tumor recurrence. In both patients, distant metastases were known at the time

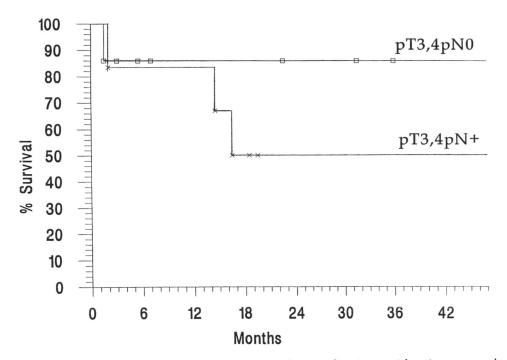

**Fig. 3.** Rectal carcinoma. Kaplan-Meier survival rates of patients with primary rectal carcinoma depending on lymph node status.

of surgery, and recurrence occurred in both before the beginning of percutaneous radiotherapy. Both patients died. Minor complications (secondary wound healing) occurred in two patients.

### Recurrent Gynecologic Tumors

Data on 11 patients with recurrent gynecologic tumors are being evaluated for survival and recurrence. There was no "in-field" recurrence during the first 6 months after treatment. No major complications have been observed.

### Tumors of the Upper Abdomen

Of ten patients with cancer of the biliary system or primary hepatocellular cancer, seven patients who underwent OLT have been evaluated. Three patients underwent the complete course of the treatment, three patients had IOHDR brachytherapy only, and one patient completed only one course of percutaneous therapy (because of a vanishing bile duct syndrome in the transplanted liver outside the radiation field).

The mean survival in the treated group of cancer patients was 304 days in comparison to 493 days in the nononcologic patient group. In no case was the cause of death tumor related (acute and chronic rejection and infection). At re-

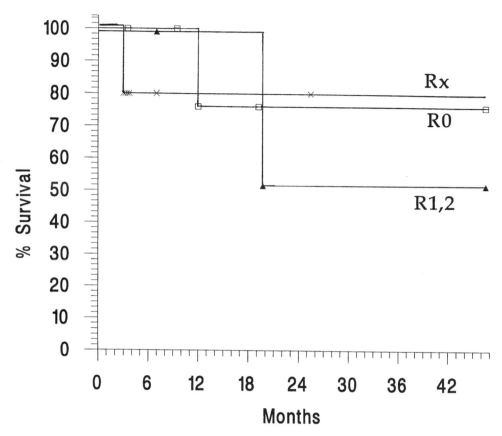

**Fig. 4.** Recurrent rectal carcinoma. Kaplan-Meier survival rates of patients with recurrent rectal carcinoma, depending on resection borders. It is remarkable that patients with positive margins survive as well as patients with negative margins. This may have been influenced by IOHDR brachytherapy.

peat laparoscopy or autopsy, no local tumor recurrence in the N1-region was evident in six of seven patients.

A C14 aminopyrine breath test[11] was used to evaluate the influence of percutaneous treatment on the transplanted liver (see Fig. 5). No influence of percutaneous radiotherapy on liver function could be seen. There were no cases of rejection caused by radiation. There were no major complications related to IOHDR brachytherapy.

## Georgetown Experience

Three patients, ages 56, 67, and 82, with pancreatic carcinoma underwent interstitial irradiation of the pancreatic primary. The largest dimension of tu-

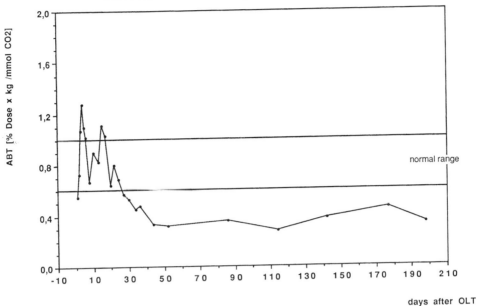

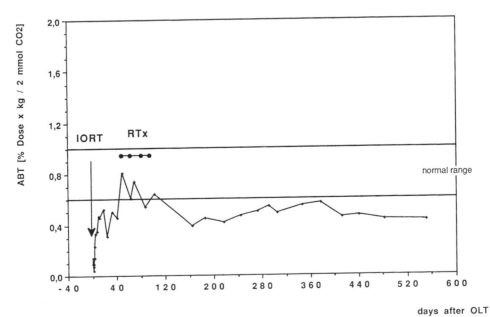

**Fig. 5.** C14 Aminopyrine breath test in patients after OLT with (top) and without (bottom) radiotherapy.

mor in each patient was 6, 3.5, and 6 cm, and the interstitial dose was 12, 20, and 20 Gy, respectively. The younger two patients also received EBRT to a dose of 41.4 and 39.6 Gy in 1.8 Gy fractions. In the first patient, the primary disease site clearly remained controlled until death at 11 months from hepatic disease progression. In the second patient, progressive disease possibly occurred in the pancreas at 9 months (the CT scan findings were equivocal), but death at 11 months was due to hepatic progression. The third, more elderly, patient experienced postoperative gastric atony and early recurrence at the gastric suture line as well as in the pancreas. Owing to poor performance status, no external irradiation was administered, and the patient died at 3.5 months. No acute or late complication attributable to the interstitial irradiation was detected. Specifically of concern are the possibilities of duodenal hemorrhage from the close proximity of the radiation field to the medial duodenal wall and of pancreatic fistula formation. Attention must always be paid to these potential complications when the needles are placed and the dose selected.

Five other cases are illustrative of interstitial HDR irradiation. A 52-year-old man with common bile duct carcinoma received 15 Gy interstitial irradiation to a 2-cm diameter primary lesion. Reestablishment of common bile duct patency was documented before 40 Gy EBRT. Progressive hepatic disease caused death at 6 months, and an autopsy revealed diminished tumor primary. A 62-year-old man with an 8-cm cholangiocarcinoma involving primarily the left hepatic lobe was treated with 10 Gy interstitial irradiation and 41.4 Gy EBRT. At 8 months, death occurred from other hepatic progressive disease, but the irradiated site remain controlled. A 60-year-old man with hepatic and right adrenal gland metastases from colorectal carcinoma underwent interstitial irradiation to all known sites of disease. A single 20-Gy dose was delivered to the 5-cm right adrenal gland metastasis. Dosimetry and intraoperative measurements indicated that the spinal cord and mid-to-inferior kidney received an acceptable dose. Although progressive hepatic metastases subsequently developed, no toxicity was encountered, and tumor control was established in the adrenal gland for the remaining 14.5 months of life. A 65-year-old woman with recurrent vaginal carcinoma received 45-Gy preoperative EBRT. At operation, biopsy-proven residual disease involved the upper vagina and measured 3.7 cm in maximum dimension. A dose of 10-Gy interstitial irradiation was given. The patient remains alive and well with no evidence of disease at over 5 ¾ years. A 71-year-old man with recurrent colonic carcinoma involving the anterior abdominal wall at the level of the bladder underwent gross resection by blunt dissection alone. The lucite applicator allowed for HDR treatment of the inner aspect of the abdominal wall. The dose delivered was 15 Gy at a tissue depth of 0.5 cm. Although pulmonary lesions subsequently developed, no further recurrence was seen at the site of HDR treatment with the last follow-up at over 20 months.

At Georgetown University, intraoperative HDR irradiation has safely been delivered with a unique interstitial technique and with an innovative applicator for intra-abdominal and intrapelvic use. Final dose recommendations cannot be made at this time. More patients must be treated and followed for a longer time before optimal therapies are established.

## Memorial Sloan-Kettering Experience

The operating room used for HDR intraoperative radiation is in the department of radiation oncology. Since this operating suite opened in November of 1992, seven cases have undergone treatment. Six of these were either advanced or recurrent rectal tumors; one was a recurrent retroperitoneal sarcoma. All of the rectal cases were completely resected and received adjuvant intraoperative radiation. The retroperitoneal sarcoma was unresectable; this patient received a permanent $^{125}$I implant in addition to HDR intraoperative radiation to the entire tumor bed. A dose of 1,500 cGy was delivered intraoperatively to patients who had prior radiation therapy. Patients who were to undergo further EBRT or who had preoperative EBRT received an intraoperative dose of 1,000–1,200 cGy. These doses were delivered 5 mm from the HAM applicator or 1 cm from the source plane.

To date, there have been no acute complications or prolonged hospital stays. It is too early to comment on long-term results or morbidity. At this center, we will be using this treatment for colorectal tumors, retroperitoneal sarcomas, recurrent extremity sarcomas, some pediatric malignancies, some thoracic tumors, and selected liver tumors and metastases. Protocols for other sites are also under discussion.

# Discussion

Maximal surgical debulking with IOHDR brachytherapy presents several advantages over surgery, EBRT, perioperative brachytherapy, or electron beam IORT.

## Advantages Over Surgery as the Only Treatment Modality

IOHDR brachytherapy allows less radical surgery to be performed, thus preserving normal structure and function, which is especially important if the tumor is close to bones, blood vessels, and other vital organs. Surgery in combination with IOHDR brachytherapy, however, may enhance the efficacy of IOHDR brachytherapy in that the debulking surgery removes the hypoxic, radioresistant tumor, leaving only a microscopic residual for IOHDR brachytherapy to treat.

## Advantages Over EBRT as the Only Treatment Modality

IOHDR brachytherapy reduces the dose of EBRT required, thus lowering the total dose delivered to the surrounding normal tissues while a high dose of radiation is delivered to the tumor bed. It allows radiosensitive normal structures to be displaced or shielded by lead, further lowering the dose received by the normal tissues. The target volume is accurately defined visually, minimizing the risk of a geographical miss.

For all practical purposes, the intraoperative radiation dose must be delivered in a single fraction (see "Disadvantages" section). Hence, whenever feasible, IOHDR brachytherapy is given as a boost to be followed by a moderate dose (45–50 Gy) of EBRT.

## Advantages Over Perioperative Brachytherapy

Compared to perioperative brachytherapy, IOHDR brachytherapy has advantages in normal tissue protection, mechanical procedure, and total dose delivered. IOHDR brachytherapy allows displacement of tissues by packing or retraction or protection of tissues with lead shielding, thus reducing the dose to the radiosensitive adjacent normal structures. The catheters do not need to be individually sutured to the tumor bed if IOHDR brachytherapy surface applicators are used. Hence, the process is rapid and allows the treatment to be delivered to sites into which catheters cannot be sutured. The catheters are not left behind in the patient, hence reducing the risk of infection, as well as minimizing the risk of catheter displacement or extrusion during the short period of time required for treatment to be completed.

The linear-quadratic (L-Q) bioeffect dose model[12] with $\alpha/\beta$ for tumor set at 10 Gy shows that a 10-Gy single dose of IOHDR brachytherapy is equivalent to a low dose rate (LDR) brachytherapy dose (at 0.5 Gy/h) of 18.7 Gy, and 15 Gy is similarly equivalent to 35 Gy at LDR. These values have been calculated assuming a half-time for repair of tumor cells of 0.5 h. With a half-time for repair of 1.5 h, these LDR doses are 16.6 Gy and 31 Gy, respectively.[3]

Although there are some apparent disadvantages of IOHDR brachytherapy when compared to perioperative HDR brachytherapy, these can be mitigated by combined therapies, dose-planning preparation, and developments in technology and technique.

(a) There is the inherent radiobiological disadvantage of using a large single fraction (see "Disadvantages" section). If substantial tissue displacement or shielding of normal tissues are not obtained, IOHDR brachytherapy could be combined with perioperative fractionated HDR brachytherapy or radiosensitizers.

(b) Since the patient is under anesthesia, elaborate treatment planning cannot be performed. However, this disadvantage has been solved by the use of preplanned dosimetry for each IOHDR brachytherapy applicator, thus allowing treatments to be performed without delay.

(c) Since the treatments are given intraoperatively, a shielded operating room is required. If a shielded operating room is not available, the anesthetized patient must be transported to the radiation oncology suite, a time consuming and potentially hazardous procedure. This necessity limits the widespread use of this technique. However, the development of a low-energy radionuclide like iodine-125 for IOHDR brachytherapy will obviate the need for a shielded operating room. Another possibility is the construction of a large, mobile lead shield that could be placed over the treatment site to reduce radiation exposure.

## Advantages Over IORT

Delivery of IORT by conventional electron beam requires accessibility of the cone to the tumor or tumor bed. Hence, it is not possible to treat a steeply sloping surface (inferior pelvic side wall) or narrow cavities (e.g., paranasal sinuses). The electron beam cannot bend around curves and, therefore, cannot be used to treat locations like the posterior wall of pubis symphysis, dome of the liver, or similar areas that are often the sites of residual disease after resection. IOHDR brachytherapy can overcome these limitations by the use of the flexible applicators to access these sites.

Since the brachytherapy dose follows the inverse square law, there is better sparing of normal tissues beyond the tumor when compared to electron beam treatments (Table 1). Although the dosimetry is less homogenous than that of an electron beam, portions of the tumor receive higher doses than the prescribed dose (at 0.5 cm depth), without delivering higher doses to the surrounding normal tissues. This could improve the therapeutic ratio. The dosimetry of Super-flab or foam-based IOHDR brachytherapy applicators, unlike that of the electron beam, can conform to curved surfaces.

IOHDR brachytherapy is far more cost effective than IORT. The remote afterloader costs less than a linear accelerator. Furthermore, since the HDR machine is mobile, dedicated equipment is not required. The HDR equipment from the radiation oncology department can be transported to the shielded operating room, increasing its utilization. By contrast, use of a linear accelerator is limited to the room in which it is installed.

### Table 1

**Percentage Depth Dose for Electron Beam IORT Versus IOHDR Brachytherapy with Dose Prescribed at 0.5 cm for IOHDR Brachytherapy and at $D_{max}$ for IORT**

| Depth (cm) | HDR Brachytherapy | IORT |
|---|---|---|
| 0 | 200% | 75% |
| 0.5 | 100% | 85% |
| 1.0 | 60% | 95% |
| 1.5 | 40% | 100% |
| 2.0 | 30% | 90% |
| 2.5 | 20% | 50% |
| 3.0 | 15% | 20% |

**Disadvantages**

The major disadvantage of IOHDR brachytherapy (also shared by IORT) is the radiobiology of a large single dose. A general principle of radiation therapy is that the radiation dose is fractionated to allow repair of sublethal damage of the normal tissues, to permit reoxygenation of the hypoxic radioresistant cells, and to allow radioresistant cells in the S phase to progress to the more radiosensitive mitotic phase of the cell cycle. However, this disadvantage is minimized if the IORT/IOHDR brachytherapy is given as a boost to the immediate tumor bed to supplement moderate doses (45 Gy) of EBRT to a greater volume. In those patients who cannot receive further EBRT, perioperative fractionated HDR brachytherapy may be added by surgically placed catheters.

The radiobiological disadvantage of a single large dose fraction of IOHDR brachytherapy can also be overcome by the dose reduction to normal tissues achieved by shielding and physical displacement. The effect on the dose to the normal tissues of even a small physical displacement can be dramatic. For example, a displacement of 1, 2, 3, and 4 cm can reduce the dose to normal tissue by about 60%, 80%, 87% and 93%, respectively.[3] Therefore, if the dose at the applicator is 15 Gy and the normal tissue is displaced by 2 cm, the dose to the normal tissue will be only 3 Gy, which is acceptable even if given as a single fraction. Although normal tissues should be displaced as far as possible, a 2–3 cm displacement is generally sufficient, depending on the size of the implant and the radiosensitivity of the concerned normal tissue.

One millimeter of lead foil reduces the dose by about 20%. However, the dose reduction achieved by the combined effects of shielding and distance can be substantial. For example, 3 mm and 6 mm of lead will reduce the dose to normal tissues by 63% and 85%, respectively, when both the shielding and distance effects are taken into account.

L-Q model calculations[12] using an $\alpha/\beta$ of 3 Gy for late-reacting normal tissue cells show that the dose reduction for isoeffect needs to be only 20% if a half-time for repair of tumor cells of 0.5 h is assumed or 25% for a 1.5-h half-time.[3]

Another possible method of overcoming hypoxia is the use of radiosensitizers like SR 2508. The Radiation Therapy Oncology Group (RTOG) is currently studying the effects of combining the radiosensitizer SR 2508 with IORT. Similar trials could be undertaken to combine a radiosensitizer with IOHDR brachytherapy to more effectively treat the hypoxic tissues.

## Conclusion

IOHDR brachytherapy is a simple technique to deliver a single, large fraction radiation dose to the tumor or a surgically resected tumor bed. The reduction of dose to the normal tissues achieved by physical displacement and shielding overcomes the radiobiological disadvantage of the lack of fractionation. The development of intraoperative applicators and preplanned dosimetry has simplified administration and standardization of the treatments. It is far more economical than electron beam IORT. However, unless a low-energy radionuclide source is developed, the need for a shielded operating room will limit the widespread use of the technique.

This preliminary report deals principally with the development of the facilities and techniques. Obviously, further experience must be gained, and continued follow-up will be required to address the efficacy and morbidity results. A multi-institution trial is warranted to determine whether the theoretical advantages of IOHDR brachytherapy will lead to increased tumor control and lower morbidity

## REFERENCES

1. Dritschilo A, Harter KW, Thomas D, et al. Intraoperative radiation therapy of hepatic metastases: technical aspects and report of a pilot study. Int J Radiat Oncol Biol Phys 14:1007-1011, 1988.
2. Lukas P, Kneschaurek P, Ries G, et al. A new modality for intraoperative radiotherapy using a high dose rate afterloading unit. In: Proceedings of Sixth International High Dose Rate Remote Afterloading Conference; May 2-4, 1991; Budapest, Hungary, 62-66.
3. Nag S, Orton C. Development of intraoperative high dose rate brachytherapy for treatment of resected tumor beds in anesthetized patients. Endocurie/Hypertherm Oncol 9:187-193, 1993.
4. Meerwaldt JH, Wiggers T, Westenberg H, et al. Intraoperative brachytherapy: application of vicryl mats for flexible catheter implants. In: Mould RF, ed. Brachytherapy 2. Leersum, The Netherlands: Nucletron International B.V.; 1989, 592-597.
5. Lukas P, Kneschaurek P, Ries G, et al. A new modality for intraoperative radiotherapy of rectal carcinoma. In: E.O.R.T.C. Symposium on Advances in Gastrointestinal Tract Cancer Research and Treatment, Résumés. Strasbourgh, France, 1989.
6. Lukas P, Kneschaurek P, Kaciniel E, et al. Eine neue Technik zur intraoperativen Strahlentherapie des Rektumkarzinoms. Zbl Radiol 14:228-229, 1990.
7. Lukas P, Stepan R, Ries G, et al. A new modality for intraoperative radiation therapy with a high-dose-rate-afterloading unit. Radiology 181:251, 1991.
8. Moertel CT, Childs DS, Reitmeier RJ, et al. Combined 5-Fluoruracil and supervoltage radiation therapy of locally unresectable gastrointestinal cancer. Lancet 2:865, 1969.
9. Pirkowski M, Holloway R, Delgado G, et al. Radiotherapy of malignant subdiaphragmatic implants in advanced ovarian carcinoma: a new technique. Int J Rad Onc Biol Phys 22:1105-1108, 1992.
10. Nag S, Martin EW, Schuller DE, et al. High dose rate remote brachytherapy as an ecomomic alternative to electron beam for intraoperative radiation therapy. Endocurie/Hypertherm Oncol 9:56, 1993.
11. Adolf J, Martin WG, Müller DF, et al. Influ β der akuten zellulären Absto βung auf die Leberfunktion nach orthotoper Lebertransplantation: quantitative Funktionsuntersuchungen mit dem 14C-Aminopyrin-Atemtest. Dtsch Med Wochenschr 117:1823-1828, 1992.
12. Dale RG. The application of the linear-quadratic dose-effect equation to fractionated and protracted radiotherapy. Br J Radiol 58:515-528, 1985.

# Chapter 23

# The Future of High Dose Rate Brachytherapy

*Subir Nag, Alvaro A. Martinez, Arthur T. Porter, and Basil S. Hilaris*

## Introduction

During the last decade, there have been tremendous technological improvements and an increase in the use of high dose rate (HDR) brachytherapy. High dose rate treatments have the advantages of total elimination of radiation exposure, short treatment times, and out-patient optimized treatment. These advantages will make HDR equipment a standard component of the resources available in most radiation oncology departments. We predict major developments in the following areas of HDR brachytherapy: optimized treatment planning; computed tomography (CT)-based three-dimensional planning; ultrasound-based real-time optimization; radiologically guided brachytherapy; molds, templates, and intraoperative applicators; a combination of surgery and brachytherapy; integration of HDR brachytherapy and external beam radiation therapy (EBRT); HDR brachytherapy and hyperthermia; HDR brachytherapy and radiosensitizers; low-energy radionuclides; the integrated brachytherapy unit (IBU); and cooperative clinical trials.

## Optimized Treatment Planning

In HDR brachytherapy, a single high-intensity stepping source of iridium-192 is used to treat the target volume. The dose to a point is changed by varying the dwell time of the source in that position. Hence, it is possible to precisely shape the dose distribution within the target volume by changing the dwell times in each position. The oscillation of the source would lead to a more homogeneous implant, decreasing "hot spots" within the tumor volume and lowering the dose to surrounding normal tissues. We hope it will lead to lower morbidity without sacrificing tumor control rates. The ability to optimize the dose distribution within the treatment volume by the use of the stepping source may ultimately lead to a better therapeutic ratio. Chapter 6 on treatment planning and optimization in this book provides further details on optimization.

From: Nag, S. (ed.): *High Dose Rate Brachytherapy: A Textbook*, Futura Publishing Company, Inc., Armonk, NY, © 1994.

# Computed Tomography (CT)-Based Three-Dimensional Treatment Planning[1]

For accurate preplanning of needle position, three-dimensional (3-D) information is required. This can be provided by using a close-cut CT scan of the anatomical area. The information will be directly fed into the treatment-planning computer. The target volume in each cut can be outlined, hence obtaining a 3-D view of the target volume and surrounding radiosensitive normal tissues. Computerized dosimetry is then performed, and a 3-D surface isodose contour is obtained. When the 3-D isodose curves are superimposed onto the patient's anatomy, one can determine whether the entire target volume is adequately encompassed and whether critical normal tissues are being overdosed. The isodoses can be rotated on any axis on the computer for critical evaluation. This may further be combined with an optimization program for further benefit.[1]

Although an implant can be preplanned three-dimensionally, tissue motion and/or displacement as the needles are inserted remains a problem; therefore, the final needle positioning may not be exactly the same as the preplan. Alternatively, by taking the patient to the CT scanner, preplanning can be performed after the needles have been positioned. In this case, however, the artifacts caused by the needles can sometimes make it difficult to properly visualize the tumor boundaries. These difficulties must be overcome before 3-D CT-based dosimetry is routinely implemented.

# Ultrasound-Based Real-Time Optimization[2]

An ultrasound-based real-time optimization program has been developed at William Beaumont Hospital, Royal Oak, Michigan,[2] for use in transperineal HDR prostate implantations. The details are in Chapter 6 on treatment planning and optimization. A personal computer, used in the operating room, is connected to the Nucletron planning system. Each time a needle position is entered, the coordinates of the new dwell positions and an optimized isodose distribution is calculated and displayed in a few seconds. This is a significant improvement in that it allows the brachytherapist to visualize a 3-D isodose distribution within the tumor volume and to perform optimum placement of radioactive sources.

# Radiologically Guided Brachytherapy

The traditional methods of brachytherapy have used inspection and palpation to define the tumor volume for implantation. With advances in radiological technology, CT scans, fluoroscopy, and ultrasound are used to guide the needles into the tumor volume. An example is a transperineal implantation of the prostate. Chapter 16 on the prostate provides further details. Similar methods are used to implant needles in the chest wall, abdominal wall, and so forth.

An intravascular route for brachytherapy administration is also possible.[3] The interventional radiologist or cardiologist performs the angiogram and advances the catheter to the site of the tumor. Once the position of the catheter within the tumor area is confirmed, the required area can be irradiated.

## Molds, Templates, and Intraoperative Applicators

Molds and templates serve to maintain a preset separation of the catheters. Intraoperative applicators have catheters implanted parallel, thus minimizing any delay related to geometrical reconstruction of the implant and allowing the use of preplanned dosimetry.[4] Catheters implanted in dental molds can be used to deliver brachytherapy to head and neck tumors.[5] The molds allow fractionated HDR brachytherapy on an outpatient basis. Provided the fitting of the mold does not change, repeat dosimetry is unnecessary because of the fixed geometry mold. The prosthesis can also be used to increase the distance between the tumor and the normal uninvolved structures, thus reducing the dose to normal tissues. The mold is placed over the tumor site daily for HDR brachytherapy. This concept can be adapted to other areas of the body for tumors in the vaginal areas, skin nodules, or superficial tumors.[6,7]

## Combination of Surgery and Brachytherapy

Brachytherapy has the advantage of delivering a high radiation dose to a defined volume. However, tumor size is the limiting factor for controlling the disease. The larger the lesion, the lower the tumor control is. Hence, for large tumors, it is advisable to reduce the tumor burden to microscopic levels by surgery whenever possible, without sacrificing vital structures. The residual microscopic tumor volume can be successfully irradiated by implanting afterloading catheters for fractionated HDR brachytherapy subsequently,[8] or by intraoperative radiation therapy with the patient still under anesthesia.[4] Chapter 22 on intraoperative brachytherapy gives further details. This technique has much promise since, in addition, normal tissues can be displaced and/or partially shielded during the radiation, and no residual radioactivity is left in the patient.

## Integration of HDR and EBRT

Brachytherapy has two disadvantages: (1) it can only treat relatively small tumors; (2) it does not treat lymphatic areas at risk. A method of overcoming these disadvantages is to combine EBRT to moderate dose levels to the tumor volume and nodal areas. Then brachytherapy can be used as a boost to the primary tumor. In contrast to low dose rate (LDR) brachytherapy, HDR brachytherapy can be used concurrently with EBRT. A concurrent EBRT/HDR program is used to treat carcinoma of the cervix.[9] A common regimen would be to deliver EBRT 4 days a week and HDR brachytherapy once weekly over a 6-week period. Concurrent programs have been used for some cancers, such as lung, esophagus, and prostate.

## Combination of HDR Brachytherapy and Hyperthermia

Although hyperthermia can be cytotoxic on its own, there is some synergism between hyperthermia and radiation therapy, probably because hypoxic and poorly nourished cells, which are radioresistant, are more sensitive to hyperthermia. In addition, cells in the radioresistant S phase are sensitive to hyperthermia; however, effective delivery of heat to deeper structures is difficult. Catheters implanted for interstitial HDR brachytherapy can be used to deliver interstitial hyperthermia.[10] This is the most efficient way of delivering hyperthermia to deeper structures. Hence, a combination of interstitial hyperthermia with HDR brachytherapy should be beneficial. A controlled trial is required to confirm this.

## Combination of HDR Brachytherapy and Radiosensitizers

One of the disadvantages of intraoperative HDR brachytherapy is that the dose is not fractionated. Since the dose is given as a single fraction, cells that are hypoxic and radioresistant may be spared from radiation. Radiosensitizers should make these cells more vulnerable to radiation. The value of combining intraoperative radiation therapy (IORT) with radiosensitizers is currently being investigated by the Radiation Therapy Oncology Group (RTOG) for recurrent rectal cancers. This approach requires further attention.

## Low-Energy Radionuclides

A disadvantage of HDR brachytherapy is that it requires a shielded room. The use of HDR brachytherapy would be even more popular if a shielded room were not required. For example, intraoperative brachytherapy could be performed in a nonshielded operating room, and fractionated HDR brachytherapy could be performed in smaller hospitals that do not have teletherapy equipment. The ideal radionuclide for HDR brachytherapy would be one with a low energy emission (such that shielding would not be required), a long half-life (so that frequent source exchanges would not be required), and high specific activity. Palladium-103 and Iodine-125 have low energy but, because of their short half-lives, frequent source exchanges would be required. Further, they do not have a high specific activity. Hence, it will be not possible to obtain a very high dose rate.

Samarium-145 is attractive because it has a low energy emission and a long half-life. In addition, if combined with iodo-deoxyuridine (IUdR) it can induce photon activation, leading to an enhanced cytotoxic effect.[11] However, samarium has a low specific activity and is not yet commercially available.

The low energy of americium-241 (60 keV) reduces radiation shielding requirements, and its long half-life (432 years) eliminates the problem of source exchanges.[12] However, like samarium, it has the disadvantage of low specific activity and, therefore, cannot produce sufficiently HDR radiation. Although ytterbium-169 has a high specific activity, its short half-life (32 days) necessitates frequent source exchanges.[13] The energy of its emission (93 keV) is intermediate between iodine-125 and iridium-192.

## Integrated Brachytherapy Unit

High dose rate remote brachytherapy machines have become popular only recently. Therefore, they are usually installed in existing teletherapy (linear accelerator or cobalt) rooms. These rooms usually do not have fluoroscopy or diagnostic x-ray capabilities and are not equipped as an operating room. Ideally, a dedicated HDR brachytherapy room should be properly shielded and constructed to the specifications of an operating room. The table should be such as to allow fluoroscopy capability and the ability to obtain orthogonal diagnostic radiographs. The information should be directly transferred to the treatment planning computer. The development of such an IBU has been recently published.[14] This should improve the accuracy of the brachytherapy treatment and patient scheduling and allow intraoperative radiation therapy.

## Cooperative Clinical Trials

One of the main obstacles to the development of brachytherapy is the lack of clinical trials in brachytherapy.[15] Most of the trials in brachytherapy are retrospective Phase II studies evaluating the technique. However, Phase III trials are lacking. With the present environment and new health care reforms, we will be under increasing pressure to demonstrate the efficacy of a procedure to obtain reimbursement.

As HDR brachytherapy grew, the need for national guidelines became evident. To meet this need, the HDR Brachytherapy Working Group (HIBWOG) was formed under the leadership of Dr. Subir Nag in January 1990.[16] This group had set up some guidelines for HDR brachytherapy. The HIBWOG merged with the Clinical Research Committee of the American Endocurietherapy Society (AES) in September 1992, and currently this committee has reported the consensus guidelines for HDR brachytherapy in carcinoma of the cervix, endometrium, and lung.[17] Another group, the International High Dose Rate Cooperative Group, is also currently working on guidelines in HDR brachytherapy under the leadership of Dr. Anas El-Mahdi.[18] The Radiation Therapy Oncology Group has one active HDR brachytherapy protocol: evaluation of the efficacy of LDR and HDR intraluminal brachytherapy in the treatment of the carcinoma of the esophagus. If brachytherapy is to become a recognized modality, further efforts have to be expended in setting up cooperative clinical trials on a national and international basis. Some collaboration between the AES and its European counterpart, the European Society of Therapeutic Radiologists and Oncologists (ESTRO) will be a positive step.

## Conclusion

High dose rate brachytherapy will have a prominent position in cancer management, with HDR machines becoming standard equipment in most radiation oncology departments in the next decade. There will be new and exciting developments in the field. We are sure many of the techniques that have been touched on briefly in this chapter will be in commonplace use in a few years, and the next edition of this book will have the updated results.

---

## REFERENCES

1. Hilaris BS, Tenner M, High M, et al. Three-dimensional brachytherapy treatment planning. In: International Brachytherapy: Programme & Abstracts. Presented at the Seventh International Brachytherapy Working Conference; Sept. 6-8, 1992; Baltimore, MD, Veenendaal, The Netherlands: Nucletron International B.V.; 1992, 117-118.
2. Edmundson RT. Ultrasound in treatment planning: a prototype real-time planning system. In: International Brachytherapy: Programme & Abstracts. Presented at the Seventh International Brachytherapy Working Conference; Sept. 6-8, 1992; Baltimore, MD, Veenendaal, The Netherlands: Nucletron International B.V.; 1992, 119-121.
3. John M, Flam M, Holinbeck L, et al. Intravascular radiotherapy for pulmonary artery sarcoma. In: International Brachytherapy: Programme and Abstracts. Presented at the Seventh International Brachytherapy Working Conference; Sept. 6-8, 1992; Baltimore, MD, Veenendaal, The Netherlands: Nucletron International B.V.; 1992, 541-544.
4. Nag S, Orton C. Development of intraoperative high dose rate brachytherapy for treatment of resected tumor beds in anesthetized patients. Endocurie/Hypertherm Oncol 9:187-193, 1993.
5. Jolly DE, Nag S. Technique for construction of dental molds for high-dose-rate remote brachytherapy. Special Care in Dentistry 12:219-224, 1992.
6. Nag S, Grecula J, Ruymann FB. Aggressive chemotherapy, organ preserving surgery, and high dose rate remote brachytherapy in the treatment of rhabdosarcoma in infants and young children. Cancer 72:2769-2776, 1993.
7. Pisch J, Alfieri AA, Harvey J, et al. Use of vicryl/dexon mesh for afterloading HDR and LDR catheter placement in planar implants. In: International Brachytherapy: Programme and Abstracts. Presented at the Seventh International Brachytherapy Working Conference; Sept. 6-8, 1992, Baltimore, MD, Veenendaal, The Netherlands: Nucletron International B.V.; 1992, 545-547.
8. Nori D, Williams H. Intraoperative brachytherapy: rationale and future directions. In: International Brachytherapy: Programme and Abstracts. Presented at the Seventh International Brachytherapy Working Conference; Sept. 6-8, 1992; Baltimore, MD, Veenendaal, The Netherlands: Nucletron International B.V.; 1992, 132-137.

9. Stitt JA. High-dose-rate intracavitary brachytherapy for gynecologic malignancies. Oncology 6:59-81, 1992.

10. Hilaris BS, Moorthy C, Tchelebi A, et al. Pilot study on combined hyperthermia and HDR interstitial brachytherapy in the management of superficial malignancies. In: International Brachytherapy: Programme and Abstracts. Presented at the Seventh International Brachytherapy Working Conference; Sept. 6-8, 1992; Baltimore, MD, Veenendaal, The Netherlands: Nucletron International B.V.; 1992, 389-393.

11. Fairchild RG, Kalef-Ezra J, Packer S, et al. Samarium-145: a new brachytherapy source. Phys Med Biol 32:847, 1987.

12. Nath R, Bongiorni P, Rockwell S. Enhancement of IUdR radiosensitization by low energy photons. Int J Radiat Oncol Biol Phys 13:1071, 1987.

13. Battista JJ, Mason DLD. New Radionuclides for brachytherapy. In: International Brachytherapy: Programme and Abstracts. Presented at the Seventh International Brachytherapy Working Conference; Sept. 6-8, 1992; Baltimore, MD, Veenendaal, The Netherlands: Nucletron International B.V.; 1992, 125-127.

14. van't Hooft E. The concept of an integrated brachytherapy unit. In: International Brachytherapy: Programme and Abstracts. Presented at the Seventh International Brachytherapy Working Conference; Sept. 6-8, 1992; Baltimore, MD, Veenendaal, The Netherlands: Nucletron International B.V.; 1992, 138-141.

15. Porter AT. Clinical trials in brachytherapy. In: International Brachytherapy: Programme and Abstracts. Presented at the Seventh International Brachytherapy Working Conference; Sept. 6-8, 1992; Baltimore, MD, Veenendaal, The Netherlands: Nucletron International B.V.; 1992, 142-144.

16. Nag S, Abitbol A, Clark D, et al. High dose rate brachytherapy working group (HIBWOG) of North America. In: International Brachytherapy: Programme and Abstracts. Presented at the Seventh International Brachytherapy Working Conference; Sept. 6-8, 1992; Baltimore, MD, Veenendaal, The Netherlands: Nucletron International B.V.; 1992, 525-526.

17. Nag S, Abitbol A, Anderson LL, et al. Consensus guidelines for high dose rate remote brachytherapy (HDR) in cervical, endometrial, and endobronchial tumors. Int J Radiat Oncol Biol Phys 27:1241-1244, 1993.

18. El-Mahdi A. International high dose rate cooperative group. Presented at the Seventh International Brachytherapy Conference and GammaMed User Meeting; May 6-9, 1992; Luzern, Switzerland, Abstract No. 64.

# Index

Absolute dose, 80–81
Absorbed dose rate, 65–67
Absorption, 64
Accelerator room, 29–30
Accessories, 28, 30–31
Accredited Dosimetry Calibration Laboratory, 70
Actinomycin D, 407
Afterloading. *See* Remote afterloading
Air-kerma rate, 42, 73–74, 91–93
Air-kerma strength, 60–61, 62–63, 64–65, 66
ALARA principle. *See* As Low As Reasonably Achievable principle
Americium-241, 451
Aminopyrine breath test, 438, 439
Anal cancer, 349
Analgesia, 365
Anaplastic astrocytoma, 215, 223, 230
Anaplastic oligodendroglioma, 215, 223, 226
Anderson natural volume dose histogram, 118–122
Anesthesia, 241, 242, 305
Anthracycline-containing chemotherapy, 406
Antitussives, 314–315
Applicators
  Arnhem, 414
  biliary, 414
  bronchial, 54
  cervical, 413
  in cervical carcinoma, 375–376, 377
  cylinder, 52
  Delron, 428, 429
  endobronchial, 304–305, 413
  endometrial, 53, 54, 413
  esophageal, 54, 413–414
  in esophageal cancer, 283
  Finzi, 283
  Fletcher-Suit, 53, 377
  foam-based, 428–429
  future of, 449
  Guisez, 283
  Harrison-Anderson-Mick, 434–435
  Hartigan, 283
  insertion of, 148, 200–201
  intraoperative, 449
  in intraoperative brachytherapy, 428–429
  intrauterine, 52, 53
  localization measurements for, 196, 198, 199
  lucite diaphragmatic, 433, 434
  nasopharyngeal, 414
  for Omnitron 2000, 56
  in ovarian cancer, 433, 434
  perineal, 54, 55
  preparation of, 199–200
  quality assurance and, 165–172, 190, 191, 193
  rectal, 52
  in remote afterloading, 50–56
  ring, 53, 54, 375–376, 377
  silastic block, 428, 429
  transvaginal, 375
  vaginal, 413
Argon laser, 298

Arnhem Bile Duct Applicator Set, 414
As Low As Reasonably Achievable principle, 153
Astrocytoma, anaplastic, 215, 223, 230
Atelectasis, 301, 308
Audioradiography method for quality assurance, 163, 164
Audio-visual communications, 153, 187, 190
Autoradiography method of positional accuracy, 163

Barium swallow, 283–284
Base of skull
  dose calculation in, 243
  in endocavitary brachytherapy, 240, 243, 244, 245
Base of tongue
  cancers of, 245–248
  implant in, 252–253. *See also* Interstitial tongue implants
Battery for backup power system, 36
Beam radiation, external. *See* External beam radiation therapy
BED. *See* Biologically effective dose
Bile duct carcinoma, 331–338
Biliary applicators, 414
Biliary implants, 421–422
Biologically effective dose, 13
  pulsed brachytherapy and, 22–23
Biopsy
  endobronchial, 296
  in soft tissue sarcomas, 394–395
Bladder dose monitoring, 377, 378
Bleomycin, 297
Boost therapy, 324–326
BOT. *See* Base of tongue
Brachytherapy
  afterloading, 225–226
  endocavitary, 238–245
  high dose rate. *See* High dose rate brachytherapy
  integrated, 451
  intracavitary, 347, 349–350, 391
  palliative, 282–284
  perioperative, 442–443
  pulsed, 22–23
  radiologically guided, 448–449
  surgery and, 449
Brachytherapy esophageal tube, 286
Brachytherapy physicist
  operating room responsibilities of, 201
  patient setup and treatment rules of, 205
  pretreatment planning and, 203–205
  quality assurance and, 192–194
Brachytherapy physics, 41–43
Brachytron, 5
Brain Tumor Study Group, 215
Breast cancer, 321–329
  boost therapy in, 324–326
  conserving therapy in, 321–324
  interstitial implants in, 326–329
  recurrence in, 322–324
Breast implants, 415, 422–423
Breath test, 438, 439
Brenner and Hall formula, 251

Bronchial applicator, 54
Bronchial carcinoma, 297–298
Bronchial obstruction, 308
Bronchitis, radiation, 314–315
Bronchodilators, alkalinized, 314
Bronchoscopic cryotherapy, 297–298
Bruel and Kjaer ultrasound machine, 363

Calibration, 59–78
    clinical problems in, 67–69
    concepts and quantities in, 60–67
    defined, 70
    distance for, 68, 69
    institutional, 60
    interim, 70–74
    re-entrant well ionization chambers for, 74–76
    source. See Source calibration
Californium-252, 405
C14-aminopyrine breath test, 438, 439
Cancer
    anal, 349
    bile duct, 331–338
    breast, 321–329. See also Breast cancer
    bronchial, 297–298
    cervical, 373–383. See also Cervical carcinoma
    colorectal. See Rectal cancer
    endometrial, 385–392. See also Endometrial carcinoma
    of esophagus, 275–294. See also Esophageal carcinoma
    of head and neck, 237–273. See also Head and neck cancer
    hepatocellular, 432
    inoperable corpus, 140–142
    lung, 295–319. See also Lung cancer
    mouth, 258, 259, 263–266
    nasopharyngeal, 259–263, 266–272
    ovarian, 433
    pancreatic, 438–441
    primary hepatocellular, 432
    prostate, 355–371. See also Prostate cancer
    rectal, 347–353. See also Rectal cancer
    rectosigmoid, 349
Capital costs
    of dedicated high dose rate brachytherapy program, 29, 30, 32
    of integrated high dose rate brachytherapy program, 34–35
Carbon monoxide afterloading technique, 389–390
Carcinoma. See Cancer
Catheters
    in base of tongue, 252, 253
    in bile duct cancer, 333, 334, 335
    in dosimetry systems, 85
    in endobronchial brachytherapy, 303–306
    in endocavitary brachytherapy, 240, 246
    flexiguide, 254
    in pediatric tumors, 401–402, 403
    in soft tissue sarcomas, 395
    in transhepatic cholangiocatheter technique, 332
Cathetron, 7
Cell survival
    dose-rate effect and, 11, 12
    fraction curves for, 17, 18
    linear-quadratic model of, 11, 12, 13–15
    pulsed brachytherapy and, 22–23
Cellular repair rates, 15, 16, 19–22
Cerra ion chamber method for dosimetry measurements, 181–183
Cervical applicators, 413
Cervical carcinoma, 138–140, 373–383
    Madison system in, 377–381
    resource utilization in, 381–382
    University of Miami protocol in, 374–377
Cervical implants, 419
Cervitron, 8
Cesium
    calibrations for, 69, 71
    in endobronchial brachytherapy, 302
    in esophageal cancer, 277–278, 284
    in head and neck cancer, 259, 260, 261

    in pediatric tumors, 405
    physical properties of, 43–44
    reference exposure rate for, 63
Cetacaine, 421
Chamber, 51, 68, 69, 71–72
Charged-particle equilibrium, 71
Check phantom, 173, 186
Chemotherapy
    in bronchial carcinoma, 297–298
    in esophageal cancer, 276, 292
    in obstructive jaundice, 333
    in pediatric tumors, 404, 406
    in rectal cancer, 431
Cholangiocatheter, transhepatic, 331, 332–333
Cholangiopancreatography, 333
Clinical trials, cooperative, 451–452
Cobalt-60
    calibrations for, 69, 71–72
    in endobronchial brachytherapy, 301
    in esophageal cancer, 285–286
    physical properties of, 43–44
    reference exposure rate for, 63
[57]Co-Bleomycin, 297
Collimator, 186, 187
Colorectal cancer. See Rectal cancer
Colorectal metastases, 339, 340–342
    hepatic, 342–344
Colpostat, 169, 170, 389
Computer treatment planning systems, 184, 185
Consensus standard, 70
Console of afterloader, 36, 153
Contained activity, 66
Continuing education, 424
Control console, 7, 36, 153
Cord dose calculation, 243
Corpus carcinoma, 140–142
Correction factors versus source-to-chamber distance, 69
Costs
    of dedicated high dose rate brachytherapy program, 29, 30, 32
    of high dose rate brachytherapy, 8
    of integrated high dose rate brachytherapy program, 34–35
    of low dose rate brachytherapy, 381–382
Cough, 308
CPE. See Charged-particle equilibrium
Cryosurgery, 296–298, 339
Cs. See Cesium
Curative endobronchial brachytherapy, 307–312
Curie, 41–42
Curietron 192 Oris, 8, 47–49
Cylinder applicators, 52
Cystoscopy, 365

Delron applicators, 428, 429
Detectors, 206
Diaphragmatic applicator, 433, 434
Differential volume-dose histogram, 115–118
Diode dosimetry, 183
Distance, source-to-chamber, 67, 68, 69
Door interlock, 153, 156–157, 187, 190, 193
Dose
    absolute, 80–81
    for Cobalt 60 tubes, 286
    monitoring of, 377, 378
    per fraction, 9
    reference, 89–90
    relative, 81
    in soft tissue sarcomas, 395
    transit, 174–180
    in University of Miami protocol for cervical carcinoma, 376–377
Dose calculation, 91–103
    air-kerma strength and, 65–67
    dwell position and, 91–93
    in stepping-source unit, 93–103. See also Dose during transit for stepping-source unit
Dose component, 98–101
Dose-delivery accuracy, 151–152
Dose distribution, 90–91

visual evaluation of, 113–114
Dose during transit for stepping-source unit, 93–103
  clinical example of, 101–103
  considerations for, 93–94
  determination of, 94–96
  distribution of, 101
  dosimetric considerations in, 94
  dwell points for, 96–97
  fractions in, 98
  general solution for, 98–101
  patient planning for, 103
  prescribed, 98
  source activity in, 98
  source speed for, 96
Dose homogeneity, 85–89
Dose nonuniformity ratio, 136
Dose optimization nasopharynx fractioned high dose
    rate, 240, 243
Dose rate
  effect of, 11, 12
  high, 46
  intermediate, 17, 312
  therapeutic ratio for, 19
Dose specification
  in inoperable endometrial carcinoma, 391 392
  in Madison system, 377–381
  prescription and, 83–91. *See also* Stepping Source
    Dosimetry System
Dosimetrist, 194
Dosimetry
  computers in, 126
  in head and neck cancer, 243–245, 263
  Manchester, 81–82
  Paris, 83–91, 327
  quality assurance and, 151
  selection and verification of, 181–183
  Stepping Source, 83–91. *See also* Stepping Source
    Dosimetry System
Dummy ribbon in positional accuracy verification,
    169–171
Dummy source. *See* Simulators
Dwell points, 96–97
Dwell position, 91–93
Dwell-time accuracy, 173, 198
Dyspnea, 308

EBRT. *See* External beam radiation therapy
Education
  family and patient, 416–418
  staff, 423–424
Electrical emergencies, 38
Electrocoagulation, 296
Electron beam intraoperative radiation therapy, 443
Electrons, 323, 325, 326
Emergency equipment, 37, 38
  in quality assurance, 186, 188, 190
  response and error-detection, 153–157
Emergency procedures in radiation safety, 38–39
Emergency source container, 51
Emergency system, 45
Encapsulation, 42, 64–65
Endobronchial applicators, 304–305, 413
Endobronchial brachytherapy, 301–315
  clinical results in, 306–312
  complications of, 312–315
  curative, 307–312
  obstruction score definitions in, 308
  outcome data for high dose rate, 307, 310
  symptom index in, 308
  technical considerations in, 303–306
  techniques in, 301–302
Endobronchial brachytherapy data sheet, 309
Endobronchial disease, 295–301
Endobronchial implants, 419–420
Endobronchial occlusion, 295
Endobronchial prosthesis, 300–301
Endobronchial tumors, 297
Endocavitary brachytherapy, 238–245
Endometrial applicators, 53, 54, 413
Endometrial carcinoma, 385–392
  adjuvant treatment in, 385–390

inoperable, 391–392
  recurrent vaginal disease and, 390–391
Endometrial implants, 418–419
Endoscopy in biliary carcinoma, 331, 333–334
Equivalent mass of radium, 64–65
ERD. *See* Extrapolated response dose
Esophageal applicators, 54, 413–414
Esophageal carcinoma, 275–294
  China experience with, 284–290
  Exeter experience with, 282–284
  history of, 275–276
  new therapeutic trends in, 276–277
  protocols for, 290–292
  Vancouver experience with, 277–282
Esophageal fistula, 315
Esophageal implants, 420–421
Esophageal tube with balloon dilator, 286
Esophagectomy, 276
Esophagitis, 287
Exposure
  constants for, 64–65
  radiation, 3
  reference, 63
  in uncontrolled areas, 152–153
External beam radiation therapy, 449–450
  in bile duct carcinoma, 331–334, 335
  in cervical carcinoma, 373, 374, 378, 379
  in endobronchial disease, 301
  in esophageal cancer, 288–289, 288–290, 292
  in head and neck cancer, 254–256, 257, 258–259
  in inoperable endometrial carcinoma, 391
  integration of high dose rate brachytherapy and,
    449–450
  intraoperative brachytherapy versus, 441–442
  in mouth cancer, 263–264
  in nasopharyngeal carcinoma, 239, 266–272
  in non-small cell lung cancer, 310
  in Ohio State experience, 435
  in pediatric tumors, 399–400
  in prostate carcinoma, 355, 356, 362, 363, 365,
    369–370
  in rectal cancer, 348, 350–352, 431
  in soft tissue sarcoma, 394, 395, 396–397
External photon beam irradiation, 339
Extrapolated response dose, 13

Family education, 416–418
Farmer-type ionization chamber, 68, 69
Fentanyl, 381, 389
Finzi applicator, 283
Fire emergencies, 38
Fistulae, 315
Flab in rectal tumors, 430–431
Fletcher-Suit applicator, 377
Fletcher-Suit-Delcios-style gynecology applicator, 53
Fletcher-Suit shielded colpostat, 169, 170
Flexible cystoscopy, 365
Flexiguide catheters, 254
Flexiguide needles, 363, 364, 365
Fluoroscopy, 306, 389
5-Fluorouracil
  in obstructive jaundice, 333
  in rectal cancer, 349, 431
  in upper abdominal tumors, 432
Flutamide, 356
Foam-based applicators, 428–429
Fractional decay rate per unit time, 41
Fractional repair, 15, 16
Fractionated high dose rate brachytherapy
  for head and neck tumors, 245–253
  of nasopharynx, 238–245
Fractionation schema, 81
Fraction size, 9
French Van Andel catheter, 333
FU. *See* 5-Fluorouracil

GammaMed I, 302
  in esophageal cancer, 283
  fatal hemoptysis and, 314
GammaMed 12i, 47, 48, 49–50
  applicators for, 54

development of, 6
quality assurance for, 149, 154
source localization procedure for, 171–172
GammaMed II
in endobronchial brachytherapy, 303
in prostate carcinoma, 359
GammaMed IIi
dosimetry measurements and, 181–183
quality assurance and, 154, 160, 165, 181–183
in rectal tumors, 431
Geiger-Müller detector, 206
Geometric optimization, 91, 108–113
Glioblastoma multiforme, 215, 223, 226
Gliomas, malignant, 215–235. See also Malignant
gliomas
Glycopyrrolate, 305
Gold
in endobronchial brachytherapy, 302
in esophageal cancer, 283
in pediatric tumors, 405
Grid points through implant volume, 114–115
Guisez applicator, 283
Gynecologic applications
optimization in, 138–142
rectal retractor and, 53
resource utilization for, 381–382
Gynecologic implants, 418–419
Gynecologic tumors, 432

Half-life of radionuclide, 41
HAM applicator. See Harrison-Anderson-Mick appli-
cator
Harrison-Anderson-Mick applicator, 434–435
Hartigan applicator, 283
HDR. See High dose rate brachytherapy
Head and neck cancer, 237–273
China experience with, 266–272
fractionated endocavitary brachytherapy in,
238–245
high dose rate-interstitial brachytherapy in,
245–253
New York experience with, 254–256, 257, 258
Rotterdam experience with, 238
survival in, 253
Vancouver experience with, 258–266
Hematoporphyrin derivatives, 300
Hemoptysis, 308
fatal, 312–314
Hepatic metastases, 339–345
Hepatic tumors, 339–346
Hepatocellular carcinoma, 432
Hepatoma, 344–345
High dose rate boost, 325–326
High dose rate brachytherapy
for breast cancer, 321–329. See also Breast cancer
for cervical carcinoma, 373–383. See also Cervical
carcinoma
contraindications for, 254
endobronchial, 307, 310
endocavitary, 238–245
for endometrial carcinoma, 385–392. See also Endometrial carcinoma
equipment for, 29–30, 36
for esophageal carcinoma, 275–294. See also
Esophageal carcinoma
evolution of, 3–10
external beam radiation therapy in. See External
beam radiation therapy
fatal hemoptysis and, 312–314
fractionated, 238–253. See also Fractionated high
dose rate brachytherapy
future of, 447–453
for head and neck cancer, 237–273. See also Head
and neck cancer
hyperthermia and, 449–450
intraoperative, 427–445. See also Intraoperative
high dose rate brachytherapy
in linear quadratic model, 14
for lung cancer, 295–319. See also Lung cancer

operating room for, 30–34
for pediatric tumors, 399–408. See also Pediatric
tumors
program for, 27–40. See also Program for high
dose rate brachytherapy
for prostate carcinoma, 355–371. See also Prostate
cancer
pulsed, 248–253
quality assurance for, 147–212. See also Quality
assurance
for rectal cancer, 347–353
for soft tissue sarcomas, 393–398
treatment planning for, 79–145. See also Treatment
planning
unit for, 34–35
High dose rate brachytherapy nursing, 411–425
applicators and, 412–415
education of, 423–424
future directions of, 424–425
in patient and family education, 416–418
in patient care and implant procedures, 418–423
in research, 423
role of, 415
treatment modality in, 411–412
High dose rate computer calculations, 206–209
High dose rate interstitial irradiation. See Interstitial
irradiation therapy
High dose rate remote afterloading. See Remote
afterloading
High dose repair, 15–17
Hot room, 5–6
Hyperdose sleeve, 243, 248
Hyperthermia, 292, 336, 449–450

IBT. See Intracavitary brachytherapy
IBU. See Integrated brachy therapy unit
I-125 implant, 323–324
IIRT. See Interstitial irradiation therapy
Implantation
in endobronchial brachytherapy, 302
in hepatic tumors, 339
in lung cancer, 300–301
in soft tissue sarcomas, 395
Implants
base of tongue, 252–253. See also Interstitial
tongue implants
biliary, 421–422
breast, 415, 422–423
in breast cancer, 323–324
cervical, 419
distribution of grid points through, 114–115
endobronchial, 419–420
endometrial, 418–419
esophageal, 420–421
gynecologic, 418–419
interstitial, 414, 415
localization and stimulation of, 201–202
nasopharyngeal, 421
patient care and, 418–423
in pediatric tumors, 401–402, 403, 405
prostate, 414, 422
rectangular single-plane, 209
single-plane, 209, 401, 402–403
superficial, 415
vaginal, 419
Indexer of movement, 155–156
Institutional calibration, 60
Integrated brachytherapy unit, 34–35, 451
Intercom system, 153
Interim calibration technique, 70–74
Interlocking door, 153, 156–157, 187, 190, 193
Intermediate dose rate, 17
fatal hemoptysis and, 312
Interstitial brachytherapy for head and neck tumors
fractionated high dose rate, 245–253
pulsed dose rate, 248–253
Interstitial hypothermia, 221, 223
Interstitial implants, 414, 415
of base of tongue. See Interstitial tongue implants

in breast cancer, 324–329
in hepatic tumors, 339
prostate, 414
treatment planning for, 201
tubing for, 54
Interstitial irradiation therapy
for head and neck tumors, 245–253
for hepatic tumors, 339–346
high dose rate, 254–256, 257, 258
for pancreatic carcinoma, 438–440
for pediatric tumors, 400
Interstitial needles, 54
Interstitial tongue implants, 126–138
description of, 126–128
evaluation of, 137
optimization for, 128–136
Intracavitary brachytherapy
in inoperable endometrial carcinoma, 391
in rectal cancer, 347, 349–350, 352
Intracavitary irradiation
in esophageal cancer, 281
in nasopharyngeal carcinoma, 271–272
Intracavitary therapy, 412–414
localization and simulation for, 201–202
prescription parameter in, 64
Intraductal component, 321–324
Intraluminal applications, 142–143
Intraoperative applicators, 449
Intraoperative high dose rate brachytherapy, 427–445
external beam radiation therapy for, 441–442
Georgetown technique for, 432–434
Memorial Sloan-Kettering technique for, 434–435
Munich technique for, 430–432
Ohio State University method of, 427–429, 435
perioperative, 442–443
radiation therapy for, 427, 443
results of, 435–441
surgery for, 441
Intraoperative radiation therapy, 427, 443
brachytherapy versus, 443
disadvantages of, 444
for gynecologic tumors, 432
for hepatic tumors, 339
Memorial Sloan-Kettering experience with, 441
in rectal cancer, 431, 432
Intrauterine applicators, 52, 53
Iodine, 450
in endobronchial brachytherapy, 302
in hepatic tumors, 339
in malignant glioma, 216, 224
in pediatric tumors, 400, 405
IOHDR brachytherapy. *See* Intraoperative high dose rate brachytherapy
Ion chamber measurements, 173, 174, 181–183
Ionization, 68, 69
source velocity from, 176–180
IORT. *See* Intraoperative radiation therapy
[$^{192}$]Ir. *See* Iridium-192
Iridium-192
afterloading and, 4
in bile duct cancer, 335, 336
in breast cancer, 323, 324, 326
calibrations for, 69, 72–74, 75, 181–183
in endobronchial brachytherapy, 302
in endometrial carcinoma, 387
in esophageal cancer, 277–278, 279
fatal hemoptysis and, 314
in head and neck cancer, 259
in malignant glioma, 216, 224–229
in nasopharyngeal carcinoma, 267–269
oscillating source of, 8
in pediatric tumors, 400, 405
physical properties of, 43–44
in prostate carcinoma, 355–357, 359–362, 365, 369–370
in rectal tumors, 431
Iridium wires in endocavitary brachytherapy, 243, 249
Irradiation
ablative, 339

in breast cancer, 321
in esophageal cancer, 278–281
external beam. *See* External beam radiation therapy
external photon beam, 339
in hepatic tumors, 339–346
interstitial. *See* Interstitial irradiation therapy
intracavitary, 271–272
intraoperative. *See* Intraoperative radiation therapy
photon beam, 339
Isocentric method in endobronchial brachytherapy, 304
Isodose planning system, 46, 130–131
Isotopes, radioactive, 277

Joule-Thompson effect, 297

Kaplan-Meier survival curves
for brain tumor, 223
for head and neck tumors, 253, 257
for nasopharyngeal tumors, 246
for rectal carcinoma, 436, 437, 438
Kondo-Randolph effect, 69, 72
Kubo and Chin mathematical formulas, 207

Laser therapy, 298–299, 302
LDR. *See* Low dose rate brachytherapy
Leakage currents in dosimetry system, 68–69
Linear quadratic model, 13–23
of cell survival, 11, 12, 13–15
conventional treatments in, 14
high dose rate versus low dose rate treatment in, 17–22
incomplete repair in, 14–15
interstitial brachytherapy in, 251
pulsed brachytherapy in, 22–23
Localization procedure, 79–80, 201
Low dose rate boost, 326
Low dose rate brachytherapy
for breast cancer, 324
endobronchial, 307, 309
fatal hemoptysis and, 312–314
in linear quadratic model, 14, 17–22
for pediatric tumors, 399–400
Low dose remote afterloading, 8
Low dose repair, 15–17
Low-energy radionuclides, 450–451
Lucite diaphragmatic applicator, 433, 434
Lung cancer, 295–319
endobronchial brachytherapy in, 301–315. *See also* Endobronchial brachytherapy
management of, 295–301

Madison system of dose specification, 377–381
Malignant gliomas, 215–235
multiple catheter technique in, 216–224. *See also* Multiple catheter technique
single and multiple catheter technique in, 224–231. *See also* Single and multiple catheter technique
Manchester dosimetry system, 81–82, 179
Manchester Rectal Applicator, 55
Martinez Universal Peritoneal Interstitial Template, 414
Mediastinal fistula, 315
Medium dose rate, 17
Metastases, hepatic, 339–345
Microprocessor, dedicated, 45–46
MicroSelectron high dose rate, 47, 48, 49
applicators for, 54
in bile duct cancer, 334
dosimetry measurements and, 183
in endobronchial brachytherapy, 303, 304
in endocavitary brachytherapy, 240, 246
in intraoperative brachytherapy, 429
in nasopharyngeal carcinoma, 266–271
quality assurance for, 149–150, 154, 157–163
in rectal cancer, 352
source localization procedure for, 167–169, 172
transit dose in, 175–176

Mitomycin C, 349
Molds, 449
Monitoring
  in catheter placement, 305
  in cervical carcinoma, 376–377
  dose, 377, 378
  in intraoperative brachytherapy, 428
  radiation, 37, 187, 190
Monte Carlo photon-transport simulation, 183
Mortality. See Survival
Moulage in rectal tumors, 430–431
Mouth cancer, 258, 259, 263–266
Movement indexer, 155–156
Mucosa, 247
  sloughing of, 315
Multiple catheter technique, 216–224
  brachytherapy treatment and, 220, 221
  explanation, discharge, and follow-up in, 221
  hyperthermia treatment and, 221
  implantation in, 216–219, 220
  patient characteristics and, 221–222
  survival in, 222
  treatment summary of, 222
  tumor response and, 222–224
MUPIT. See Martinez Universal Peritoneal Interstitial
  Template

Na. See Nasopharyngeal-point
Nasopharyngeal applicators, 414
Nasopharyngeal cancer, 259–263
  China experience with, 266–272
  endocavitary brachytherapy of, 238–245
Nasopharyngeal dose calculation, 243
Nasopharyngeal implants, 421
Nasopharyngeal-point, 240, 243, 244, 245
Nasopharyngeal tumors, 246
Nd:YAG laser. See Neodymium:yttrium-aluminum-
  garnet laser
Neck cancer. See Head and neck cancer
Needles
  flexiguide, 363, 364, 365
  interstitial, 54
  trochar point, 363
Neodymium:yttrium-aluminum-garnet laser,
  298–299, 302
Non-small cell lung cancer, 297, 310–312
Nose, 243
NPS. See Nucletron Planning System
Nucletron micro-Selectron/HDR. See MicroSelectron
  high dose rate
Nucletron Planning System, 304, 327, 365
Nursing. See High dose rate brachytherapy nursing

Obstruction
  bronchial, 308
  endobronchial, 295
  tracheal, 308
Obstructive jaundice, 333
Oligodendroglioma, anaplastic, 215, 223, 226
Omnicath, 56
Omnitron 2000, 50
  applicators for, 56
  in endobronchial brachytherapy, 303
  quality assurance for, 150, 154, 160, 165
  source localization procedure for, 171–172
Operating room
  dedicated, 30–34
  in intraoperative brachytherapy, 427–428
  physics team and, 201
Optic chiasm, 243
Optimization, 104–113
  evaluation of, 113–125. See also Optimized plan
  general, 104–108
  geometric, 91, 108–113
  in gynecologic applications, 138–142
  of interstitial implants of base of tongue, 126–138.
    See also Interstitial tongue implants
  in intraluminal applications, 142–143
  in malignant glioma, 220, 221

manual dose verification methods for, 206–209
  ultrasound-based, 448
Optimized plan, 113–125
  Anderson natural volume-dose histogram in,
    118–122
  differential volume-dose histogram in, 115–118
  distribution of grid points in, 114–115
  in future of brachytherapy, 447
  visual evaluation of dose distributions in, 113–114
  volume gradient ratio in, 122–125
Output specification, 62
Ovarian cancer, 433

Palate, 243
Palladium-103, 450
Palliative brachytherapy, 282–284
Pancreatic carcinoma, 438–441
Paris Dosimetry System, 83–84, 327
  differences between Stepping Source Dosimetry
    System and, 85–91
Paterson-Parker calculations of transit time, 179
Patient care and implant procedures, 418–423
Patient-controlled analgesia, 365
Patient education, 416–418
Patient planning, 108
Patient safety, 191
Patient setup and treatment, 205–206
PDR. See Pulsed dose rate brachytherapy
PDS. See Paris Dosimetry System
Pediatric tumors, 399–408
  external beam radiation therapy in, 399–400
  Ohio State University Children's Hospital experi-
    ence with, 401–404
  patient and implant parameters in, 405
Perineal applicators, 54
Perioperative brachytherapy, 442–443
Personnel requirements, 192
Personnel safety, 191
Photodynamic therapy, 299–300
Photofrin-II, 300
Photon beam irradiation, 339
Photons, 323
Physical dose distribution, 9
Physicist, brachytherapy
  operating room responsibilities of, 201
  patient setup and treatment rules of, 205
  pretreatment planning and, 203–205
  quality assurance and, 192–194
Pituitary gland, 243
Plastic interstitial needles, 54
Pneumonia, 308
Pneumonitis, 301
Point source model, 65–67
Polyglactin 910 mats, 430
Polynomial optimization, 106–108
Porter Perineal Applicator, 55
Positional accuracy, 158–172
  clinical, 165–172
  intrinsic, 159–165
  quality assurance and, 150–151, 186–191
  re-entrant chamber modified to verify, 186, 189
Positional uncertainty, 68, 69
Postprocedure information, 417–418
Posttreatment quality assurance, 206
Power failures, 36, 38, 187, 190
Preprocedure education, 416
Pretreatment physicist review, 203–205
Primary hepatocellular carcinoma, 432
Program for high dose rate brachytherapy, 27–40
  criteria for, 27–28
  implementation of, 28–35
  safety policies and procedures in, 35–39
Programmable source-train machines, 157
Prostate cancer, 355–371
  American Joint Committee staging system of, 362
  Kiel experience with, 356–361
  Royal Oak experience with, 367–369
  Seattle experience with, 361–367
  University of Keil treatment of, 369–370

William Beaumont Hospital treatment of, 369–370
Prostate implants, 414, 422
Prosthesis, endobronchial, 300–301
Protection, radiation, 30
PulmoCath, 56
Pulsed brachytherapy, 22–23, 248–253
Pulsed dose rate brachytherapy, 248–253

Quality assurance, 147–212
    in applicator insertion process, 148
    checklists for, 196, 197, 200
    in computer treatment planning systems, 184, 185
    for dose delivery accuracy, 180–184
    in high dose rate computer calculations, 206–209
    machine, 148–149
    periodic, 184–191
    in personnel requirements, 192–194
    for positional accuracy, 158–172. *See also* Positional accuracy
    posttreatment, 206
    procedure-specific, 149
    program endpoints for, 149–152
    in remote afterloading, 152
    in safety of patient and public, 152–157
    for temporal accuracy, 172–180. *See also* Temporal accuracy
    in treatment planning and delivery, 148, 195–198
    treatment specific, 199–206
    treatment team organization and, 149

Radiation bronchitis, 314–315
Radiation emergencies, 38
Radiation exposure, 3
Radiation monitor, 37, 187, 190
Radiation oncologist, 192, 205
Radiation protection, 30
Radiation safety, 152–153
    policies and procedures for, 35–39
Radiation scatter, 73–74
Radiation stenosis, 314–315
Radiation survey meter, 37
Radiation therapy. *See* Irradiation
Radioactive decay of radionuclide, 41
Radioactive isotopes, 277
Radiobiology, 9, 11–25. *See also* Linear quadratic model
Radiographs, orthogonal, 304
Radiolabeled Bleomycin, 297
Radiologically guided brachytherapy, 448–449
Radionuclides
    activity of, 41–43
    half-life of, 41
    low-energy, 450–451
    physical properties of, 43–44
    radioactive decay of, 41
Radiopaque internal stiffening cable, 306
Radiosensitizers, 444, 450
Radiotherapy, 322–323
Radium
    equivalent mass of, 64–65
    in head and neck cancer, 259, 261
    reference air-kerma rate and, 63–64
RD. *See* Reference dose
Rectal applicator, 52
Rectal cancer, 347–353
    intraluminal brachytherapy in, 349
    Munich technique in, 431–432
    survival rates of, 436, 437, 438
Rectal dose monitoring, 377, 378
Rectal tumors, 430–432
Rectangular single-plane implants, 209
Rectosigmoid cancer, 349
Recurrence
    of breast cancer, 322–324
    of endometrial carcinoma, 386, 387
    of esophageal carcinoma, 289–290
    of gynecologic tumors, 432
    of vaginal disease, 390–391
Re-entrant chambers

for calibration, 74–76
    positional accuracy and, 186, 189
Reference air-kerma rate, 63–64
Reference dose, 89–90
Reference exposure rate, 63
Reference points, 151
Relative dose, 81
Remote afterloading, 4–8
    advantages and disadvantages of, 8
    in bile duct carcinoma, 331–338
    in biliary cancer, 336
    development of, 4
    in endometrial carcinoma, 387, 388, 389–390
    equipment for. *See* Remote afterloading equipment
    low dose, 8
    principle of, 3
    radiobiological controversies in, 9
    in rectal cancer, 348
    in soft tissue sarcoma, 394
    technique of, 225–226
    as treatment modality, 411–412
Remote afterloading equipment, 5, 41–57
    applicators and accessories in, 50–56
    brachytherapy physics in, 41–43
    control panel of, 7
    in endobronchial brachytherapy, 303
    features of, 43–50
    with high-activity oscillating iridium-192 source, 8
    quality assurance for, 148–149
    testing and commissioning of, 152
    treatment room for, 6
Remote afterloading interstitial prostate implants, 414
Remote control unit, 45
Repair, fractional, 14–15, 16
Retina, 243
Rhabdomyosarcoma, 399, 400. *See also* Pediatric tumors
Ring applicators, 53, 54, 375–376, 377
RMS. *See* Rhabdomyosarcoma
Room-scatter radiation, 73–74
Rotterdam Nasopharynx Applicator, 240, 241, 242, 246
Rouviere node, 243, 244
Rowland Oesophageal Applicator Set, 413
R/Silisonde, 240
R/Xylometazoline hydrochloride, 241, 242

Safety
    of patient and public, 150, 152–157
    of personnel, 191
    radiation, 35–39, 152–153
Salpingo-oophorectomy, 385
Samarium-145, 450–451
Sarcomas, soft tissue, 393–398, 432
Scatter
    air-kerma rate and, 73–74
    air-kerma strength and, 64
    corrections for, 68, 69
Seattle fractionation scheme, 365
Selectron machine, 283
Semiorthogonal method in endobronchial brachytherapy, 304
Shielding, 30
Silastic block applicators, 428, 429
Silisonde, 240
Simulation source localization procedure, 150–151
Simulators, 30–31, 45, 50
    safety features of, 36
Single and multiple catheter technique, 224–231
    afterloading brachytherapy treatment and, 225–226
    complications of, 226–231
    implantation in, 225
    results of, 226
Single catheter treatments, 207
Single-plane implants, 209, 401, 402–403
Single-stepping source machines, 154–157
Skull

dose calculation in, 243
in endocavitary brachytherapy, 240, 243, 244, 245
Soft tissue sarcoma, 393–398, 432
Software tests, 184, 185
Source
    distance from, 67
    encapsulated, 42
    exposure rates in areas adjacent to, 152–153
    penetrability of, 42
Source activity, 98
Source calibration
    in daily quality assurance, 186, 187
    in quality assurance, 180–181
    quality assurance and, 192, 193
Source capsule, 44
Source collimator, 186, 187
Source container, 51
Source-drive cables, 44
Source-drive mechanism, 44
Source encapsulation, 64–65
Source exchange, 37–38
Source-guide tubes, 44
Source localization
    applicator-dependent parameters affecting,
        165–172
    simulation procedure for, 150–151, 190, 191, 193
Source movement, 45
Source output standards, 62
Source position verification device, 51
Source speed, 96
Source strength
    calibration quantities of, 61–65
    quality assurance and, 186, 187, 190
    specification quantities for, 59–60, 61
    terms for, 59
Source-to-chamber distance, 68, 69
Source velocity, 176–180
Square single-plane implants, 209
Staff education, 423–424
Stenosis, radiation, 314–315
Stent implantation, 300–301
Stepping Source Dosimetry System, 83–91
    comparison of, 85–91
    dose during transit for, 93–103. See also Dose dur-
        ing transit for stepping-source unit
    geometric optimization in, 91
    Paris Dosimetry System and, 83–85
Steroids
    in prostate cancer, 365
    in radiation bronchitis and stenosis, 314
Super-flab in rectal tumors, 430–431
Survival
    in endometrial carcinoma, 386, 387
    in nasopharyngeal tumors, 246
    in rectal cancer, 348–349
    in rectal carcinoma, 436, 437, 438

Target volume
    dose homogeneity over, 85–89
    in dosimetry systems, 85
    quality assurance and, 151
    treated volume and, 85
Task assignment for high dose rate brachytherapy,
    195
Television system
    in positional accuracy, 163–165
    quality assurance and, 153, 161
Templates, 363, 449
Temporal accuracy, 172–180
    evaluation of transit dose in, 174–180
    quality assurance in, 151
    timer accuracy and linearity in, 172–174
Test jig, 186
Theraplan VO5 planning system, 341
Thermoluminescent dosimetry, 176, 183
Three-dimensional treatment planning, 448
Time interval and dose, 9
Timer accuracy
    linearity and, 172–180

in quality assurance, 186, 188, 194
Timer linearity, 173
TLD. See Thermoluminescent dosimetry
Tongue
    cancers of, 245–248
    interstitial implants of. See Interstitial tongue
        implants
Traceability, 70
Tracheal obstruction, 308
Tracheoesophageal fistula, 315
Tracheomediastinal fistula, 315
Transduodenal endoscopic technique, 335
Transfer standard, 70
Transfer tubes, 44
    quality assurance and, 165–172, 190, 191, 193
Transformation constant, 41
Transhepatic cholangiocatheter, 331, 332–333
Transit dose, 174–180
Transit exposure, 68
Transplantation, orthotopic liver, 432
Transrectal ultrasound, 355, 356, 357
Transvaginal applicator, 375
Treated volume, 85
Treatment delivery process, 148
Treatment distance, 67
Treatment length calculations, 196, 198, 199
Treatment planning, 79–145
    computer, 184
    dose calculation in, 91–103. See also Dose
        calculation
    dose specification and prescription in, 80–91. See
        also Stepping Source Dosimetry System
    execution in, 125–126
    gynecologic applications in, 138–142
    intraluminal applications in, 142–143
    localization in, 79–80
    optimization in, 104–125. See also Optimization
    quality assurance in, 148, 194, 195–198
    three-dimensional, 448
    for tongue cancer, 126–138. See also Interstitial
        tongue implants
Treatment specific quality assurance, 199–206
Treatment team organization, 149
TRUS. See Transrectal ultrasound
Tumors. See also Cancer
    abdominal, 432
    endobronchial, 297
    gynecologic, 432
    head and neck, 253. See also Head and neck cancer
    hepatic, 339–346
    nasopharyngeal, survival of, 246
    pediatric, 399–408. See also Pediatric tumors
    rectal, 430–432

Unit of activity of radionuclide, 41–42
Upper abdominal tumors, 432
Uterovaginal applications, 377

Vaginal applicators, 413
Vaginal cylinder applicator, 52
Vaginal disease, 390–391
Vaginal implants, 419
Van Andel catheter, 333
Versed, 381
VGR. See Volume gradient ratio
Vicryl mats, 430
Volume dose histogram
    Anderson natural, 118–122
    for base of tongue, 134–136
    differential, 115–118
Volume-dose table for base of tongue, 131–134
Volume gradient ratio, 122–125

Wayne State University formula for treatment time,
    209
Well-ionization chamber, 51
Williamson dosimetry measurements, 183

X-rays, 240, 244, 245. See also Irradiation
Xylometazoline hydrochloride, 241, 242